A Clinician's Guide to Urological Disorders

A Clinician's Guide to Urological Disorders

Editor: Ember Sawyer

AMERICAN
MEDICAL PUBLISHERS
www.americanmedicalpublishers.com

AMERICAN
MEDICAL PUBLISHERS
www.americanmedicalpublishers.com

Cataloging-in-Publication Data

A clinician's guide to urological disorders / edited by Ember Sawyer.
p. cm.
Includes bibliographical references and index.
ISBN 978-1-63927-848-0
1. Urinary organs--Diseases. 2. Urinary organs--Diseases--Treatment. 3. Urinary organs--Diseases--Diagnosis.
4. Urology. I. Sawyer, Ember.
RC900 .C55 2023
616.6--dc23

American Medical Publishers,
41 Flatbush Avenue,
1st Floor, New York,
NY 11217, USA

ISBN 978-1-63927-848-0 (Hardback)

Contents

Preface

Urological disorder refers to any condition that affects the urinary tract and its functioning. The urinary tract consists of kidneys, ureters and bladder. Some common urologic disorders are urinary incontinence, urinary tract infections, kidney stones and prostate cancer. Urinary incontinence involves the loss of bladder control. In this condition, a patient experiences uncontrolled leakage of urine. Diabetes, pregnancy or childbirth, overactive bladder, enlarged prostate, and weak bladder muscles are some common causes of urinary incontinence. Kidney and ureteral stones is another urological condition that develops stones in the kidney. These stones can result in the blockage of the tubes which carry urine and cause a substantial amount of pain. Extracorporeal shock wave lithotripsy (ESWL) is a common technique used to remove large stones. A urinary tract infection (UTI) is an infection caused by bacteria that infect the lining of the urinary tract. It may result in hematuria or bloody urine. Treatment of UTI depends on the analysis of urine. Antibiotic therapy is a common treatment used for UTI infections. This book includes some of the vital pieces of work being conducted across the world, on various topics related to urological disorders. It will provide comprehensive knowledge to the readers.

After months of intensive research and writing, this book is the end result of all who devoted their time and efforts in the initiation and progress of this book. It will surely be a source of reference in enhancing the required knowledge of the new developments in the area. During the course of developing this book, certain measures such as accuracy, authenticity and research focused analytical studies were given preference in order to produce a comprehensive book in the area of study.

This book would not have been possible without the efforts of the authors and the publisher. I extend my sincere thanks to them. Secondly, I express my gratitude to my family and well-wishers. And most importantly, I thank my students for constantly expressing their willingness and curiosity in enhancing their knowledge in the field, which encourages me to take up further research projects for the advancement of the area.

Editor

1

Botulinum toxin A for the Treatment of Overactive Bladder

Po-Fan Hsieh [1], Hung-Chieh Chiu [1], Kuan-Chieh Chen [2], Chao-Hsiang Chang [1,3] and Eric Chieh-Lung Chou [1,3,*]

1 Department of Urology, China Medical University Hospital, Taichung 40447, Taiwan; phdoublem@yahoo.com.tw (P.-F.H.); b101091082@tmu.edu.tw (H.-C.C.); urology8395@yahoo.com.tw (C.-H.C.)
2 Department of Surgery, China Medical University Hospital, Taichung 40447, Taiwan; kuanchieh_c@hotmail.com
3 School of Medicine, China Medical University, Taichung 40402, Taiwan
* Correspondence: ericchou66@yahoo.com.tw

Academic Editor: Hann-Chorng Kuo

Abstract: The standard treatment for overactive bladder starts with patient education and behavior therapies, followed by antimuscarinic agents. For patients with urgency urinary incontinence refractory to antimuscarinic therapy, currently both American Urological Association (AUA) and European Association of Urology (EAU) guidelines suggested that intravesical injection of botulinum toxin A should be offered. The mechanism of botulinum toxin A includes inhibition of vesicular release of neurotransmitters and the axonal expression of capsaicin and purinergic receptors in the suburothelium, as well as attenuation of central sensitization. Multiple randomized, placebo-controlled trials demonstrated that botulinum toxin A to be an effective treatment for patients with refractory idiopathic or neurogenic detrusor overactivity. The urinary incontinence episodes, maximum cystometric capacity, and maximum detrusor pressure were improved greater by botulinum toxin A compared to placebo. The adverse effects of botulinum toxin A, such as urinary retention and urinary tract infection, were primarily localized to the lower urinary tract. Therefore, botulinum toxin A offers an effective treatment option for patients with refractory overactive bladder.

Keywords: botulinum toxin A; overactive bladder; detrusor overactivity

---

1. Introduction

Overactive bladder (OAB) is a clinical diagnosis defined by the International Continence Society as "urgency, with or without urge incontinence, usually with frequency and nocturia" [1]. The overall prevalence of OAB was 12%–17% in the general population and it poses a great impact on daily activities and quality of life (QOL) [2–5]. In contrast to the clinical diagnosis of OAB, detrusor overactivity (DO) is a urodynamic observation characterized by involuntary detrusor contraction during the filling phase which may be spontaneous or provoked [1]. There is a substantial overlapping between OAB and DO, and DO is generally regarded as a major underlying physiology of OAB [6]. The standard treatment for OAB starts with patient education and behavior therapies. Among pharmacologic treatments, antimuscarinic agents are widely used but associated with adverse effects such as dry mouth, constipation, and blurred vision [7,8]. Due to the bothering side effects, the long-term adherence was consequently very low for antimuscarinic agents (12.0% to 39.4% at 12 months and 0% to 16% at 36 months) [9]. Beta3-adrenoceptor agonist is an alternative to antimuscarinic agents. The efficacy was similar among beta3-adrenoceptor agonists and antimuscaniric agents, but beta3-adrenoceptor agonists produce less rates of dry mouth and constipation [7].

Botulinum toxin was first isolated from *Clostridium botulinum* by van Ermengem [10]. There were seven serotypes of botulinum toxin, and botulinum toxin A (BoNT/A) was used most frequently in the urologic field. The efficacy of BoNT/A in treating OAB has been supported by literatures [11–13]. Currently both AUA and EAU guidelines suggested that intravesical injection of BoNT/A should be offered to patients with urgency urinary incontinence (UUI) refractory to antimuscarinic and beta3-adrenoceptor agonist therapy, and the FDA approved dose was 100 U of BoNT/A for idiopathic detrusor overactivity (IDO) and 200 U for neurogenic detrusor overactivity (NDO) [7,14]. In this article we will review the mechanism of BoNT/A in the treatment of OAB and evaluate randomized, placebo-controlled trials for the applicability of BoNT/A in IDO and NDO.

2. Mechanism of Action

BoNT/A is composed of a 100 kDa heavy chain polypeptide and a 50 kDa light chain polypeptide, as is joined via a disulfide bund [15]. The initially-proposed mechanism of BoNT/A was that by attachment of the heavy chain to the protein receptor SV2 on axon terminals, the toxin could enter the neuron by endocytosis [16]. Then the light chain cleaves synaptosomal-associated protein (25 kDa) (SNAP-25), a protein from the soluble *N*-ethylmaleimide-sensitive factor attachment receptor (SNARE) family. As a result, the fusion of neurosecretory vesicles and release of acetylcholine(Ach) from presynaptic nerve terminals are blocked [17]. With inhibition of Ach release, the effect on suburothelial afferent and detrusor parasympathetic nerve endings was abolished, which was similar to the action of anticholinergic agents [8,18]. However, emerging studies indicated that BoNT/A also exerts complex inhibitory effects on other neurotransmitters, neuropeptides, and receptors mediating neurotransmission [19]. In a rat model, BoNT/A injection was shown to reduce capsaicin or ATP-induced contraction frequencies and amplitudes [20]. Patients with DO had increased expression of the capsaicin receptor TRPV1 and purinergic receptor P2X3 in the suburothelial nerve fibers, and intradetrusor injection of BoNT/A resulted in decreased levels of these sensory receptors [21–23]. The change in P2X3 immunoreactivity was correlated with improved sensation of urgency in patients with intractable neurogenic or idiopathic DO [23]. Besides, women with DO had increased densities of suburothelial substance P (SP) and calcitonin gene related peptide (CGRP) immunoreactive fibers [24]. BoNT/A injection could reduce the release of CGRP with improvement in the intervals between bladder contractions in a rat model [25]. Inhibition of SP by BoNT/A would reduce the activation of TRPV1 and P2X3 receptors in suburothelium and detrusor muscle via decreased activation of NK1 receptors as was shown in a guinea pig model [26]. In addition, intravesical BoNT/A leaded to neurotrophic growth factors (NGF) deprivation up to 3 months, which was correlated with clinical response in patients with DO [27,28]. Last but not least, a recent study showed that there was a significant accumulation of the radiolabelled BoNT/A in the lumbosacral dorsal root ganglia following intradetrusor injection in rats [29]. In other words, BoNT/A works through not only localized peripheral mechanism but also a CNS effect through retrograde axonal transport.

In summary, it was proposed that the action of BoNT/A on human overactive bladders followed a sequential mechanism [19]. First, the immediate effect of BoNT/A is inhibition of vesicular release of Ach, ATP, and SP and the axonal expression of TRPV1 and P2X3, leading to peripheral denervation [18,30,31]. Second, after SNAP-25 was cleaved by BoNT/A, this exocytosis inhibitor could persist for a long time (up to 40 days in a mouse model) [17]. Third, through retrograde transport into CNS BoNT/A would result in attenuation of central sensitization, leading to further peripheral desensitization.

3. Application of Botulinum Toxin A

3.1. *Idiopathic Detruosr Overacitity*

Radziszewski *et al.* conducted the first trial of BoNT/A for patients with IDO. All seven patients became continent after treatment with 300 U of BoNT/A [32]. In November 2015, we searched randomized, placebo-controlled trials of BoNT/A on Pubmed using the keywords "Botulinum toxin A" and "detrusor overactivity". Relevant literature in the reference lists were also reviewed. Finally, eleven randomized, placebo-controlled trials of BoNT/A for IDO to date were identified and summarized in Table 1 [33–43]. The definition of refractory IDO/OAB varied among studies. Most studies enrolled patients with OAB symptoms inadequately responded to anticholinergic therapy or those who had intolerable side effects [33,35,37–43]. Failed behavioral modification in addition to anticholinergic therapy was used as inclusion criteria in two studies [34,36].

Sahai *et al.* reported the first randomized, double-blind, placebo-controlled trial to compare the efficacy of BoNT/A *versus* placebo in treating patients with refractory IDO of either sex [33]. BoNT/A of 200 U (10 U/mL) was injected at 20 sites with trigone sparing. Significant increases in maximum cystometric capacity (MCC) from 182 mL to 313 mL were observed at 4 weeks. BoNT/A also reduced episodes of frequency (mean change from 15.44 to 7.93 times per day), urgency (mean change from 11.69 to 9.21 times per day) as well as UUI (mean change from 4.98 to 1.9 times per day) at 4 weeks, and a significantly better improvement in QOL as compared with placebo was noted. The beneficial effects persisted for at least 24 weeks. Brubaker *et al.* also compared 200 U intradetrusor BoNT/A injection at 15 to 20 sites *versus* placebo in women with refractory idiopathic UUI [34]. Based on the Patient Global Impression of Improvement, they found a greater clinical response rate and a greater reduction in mean incontinence episodes in those who received BoNT/A compared to those who received placebo. The median duration of responses was 373 days, significantly longer than 62 days for placebo. Later Tincello *et al.* conducted a larger study to evaluate the efficacy of BoNT/A 200 U for the treatment of refractory IDO [35]. In this study, 122 women received BoNT/A injection at 20 sites and 118 women received placebo. In the treatment group, patients experienced greater reduction of median voiding frequency, urgency episodes, and leakage episodes compared with placebo (difference 1.34, 2.50, and 4.33 respectively). Continence was more common after BoNT/A injection. Flynn *et al.* used 200 U and 300 U BoNT/A of higher concentration (66–100 U/mL in 10–12 sites) *versus* placebo to treat 22 female patients with refractory OAB [36]. The combined results of the two different doses showed that there were significant improvements in daily incontinence episodes (mean change from 7.9 to 3.4 times), pads changed per day (mean change from 4.4 to 2.2) and QOL questionnaires in the treatment group.

On the other hand, some trials were designed to evaluate the benefit of BoNT/A 100 U in the treatment of refractory IDO. In a small-scaled study (10 BoNT/A *versus* 11 placebo), Dowson *et al.* reported that BoNT/A could significantly increase the mean MCC by 105 mL, but the storage symptoms and QOL remained statistically unchanged following BoNT/A 100 U injection [37]. However, Chapple *et al.* conducted a study of BoNT/A 100 U *versus* placebo in 558 patients of either sex and showed different results [43]. BoNT/A 100 U not only decreased urinary incontinence (UI) episodes (mean change from 5.5 to 2.55 times per day for BoNT/A *versus* mean change from 5.7 to 4.67 times per day for placebo) at 12 weeks but also improved the treatment benefit scale, other OAB symptoms (episodes of UUI, micturition, urgency, and nocturia) and health-related quality of life (HRQOL). Nitti *et al.* also tested BoNT/A 100 U *versus* placebo in 557 patients of either sex with idiopathic OAB and confirmed the benefit of BoNT/A in decreasing daily frequency of UI episodes vs placebo (mean change from 5.5 to 2.85 times per day for BoNT/A *versus* mean change from 5.1 to 4.23 times per day for placebo) [38]. All other OAB symptoms including frequency, urgency, and nocturia episodes as well as HRQOL were also improved greater by BoNT/A 100 U compared with placebo.

Table 1. Randomized controlled trials of botulinum toxin A for idiopathic detrusor overactivity.

Authors/Year	No. Patients	Injection Method	UI Episode (%Change)	Frequency (%Change)	MCC (%Change)	Pdetmax (%Change)	Urinary Retention Requiring CIC (%)	Duration of Benefit
Sahai *et al.*/2006 [33]								
Placebo	18	Intravesical injection (trigone sparing)	−18	−7	−15	−4	None	NA
Botox 200 U	16		−70	−49	+72	−59	37.5%	>24 weeks
Brubaker *et al.*/2008 [34]								
Placebo	15	Intravesical injection (trigone sparing)	−5	NA	NA	NA	None	62 days
Botox 200 U	28		−75	NA	NA	NA	43%	373 days
Flynn *et al.*/2009 [36]								
Placebo	7	Intravesical injection (trigone sparing)	9.3	−6.8	NA	NA	None	NA
Botox 200 U or 300 U	15		−57.5	−12.2	NA	NA	7	>6 weeks
Dmochowski *et al.*/2010 [39]								
Placebo	44		−17.4	NA	NA	NA	0	NA
Botox 50 U	56		−20.7	NA	NA	NA	5.4	18 weeks
Botox 100 U	55	Intravesical injection (trigone sparing)	−18.4	NA	NA	NA	10.9	24 weeks
Botox 150 U	50		−23	NA	NA	NA	20	36 weeks
Botox 200 U	52		−19.6	NA	NA	NA	21.2	36 weeks
Botox 300 U	55		−19.4	NA	NA	NA	16.4	36 weeks
Dowson *et al.*/2010 [37]								
Placebo	13	Intravesical injection (trigone sparing)	45	0	0	NA	0	12 weeks
Botox 100 U	10		−8.3	−4.5	+40.9	NA	30	12 weeks
Rovner *et al.*/2011 [40]								
Placebo	44		−51.7	−15.6	+4.7	−10.7	0	NA
Botox 50 U	57		−69.9	−23.9	+8	0	3.6	12 weeks
Botox 100 U	54	Intravesical injection (trigone sparing)	−64.6	−26.4	+15.1	+24	9.1	12 weeks
Botox 150 U	49		−89.6	−14.4	+19.3	+3.4	12.7	36 weeks
Botox 200 U	53		−80	−24.8	+17.2	+5.5	18.2	36 weeks
Botox 300 U	56		−77.6	−27.1	+21.8	+23.1	16.4	36 weeks
Fowler *et al.*/2012 [41]								
Placebo	44		−53.5	NA	NA	NA	0	NA
Botox 50 U	57		−68.3	NA	NA	NA	14.6	12 weeks
Botox 100 U	54	Intravesical injection (trigone sparing)	−66.2	NA	NA	NA	-	24–36 weeks
Botox 150 U	49		−81.3	NA	NA	NA	-	24–36 weeks
Botox 200 U	53		−73	NA	NA	NA	-	24–36 weeks
Botox 300 U	56		−72.3	NA	NA	NA	-	24–36 weeks

Table 1. *Cont.*

Authors/Year	No. Patients	Injection Method	UI Episode (%Change)	Frequency (%Change)	MCC (%Change)	Pdetmax (%Change)	Urinary Retention Requiring CIC (%)	Duration of Benefit
Denys *et al.*/2012 [42]								
Placebo	31	Intravesical injection (trigone sparing)	29% had UUI reduction > 50%		+10.5	−49.3	3.2	NA
Botox 50 U	23		37% had UUI reduction > 50%	NA	+8	−51.2	13	6 months
Botox 100 U	23		65% had UUI reduction > 50%	NA	+8	−36.5	4.3	6 months
Botox 150 U	30		56% had UUI reduction > 50%	NA	+9.5	-49.5	13.3	6 months
Tincello *et al.*/2012 [35]								
Placebo	118	Intravesical injection (trigone sparing)	−3.2	−9.6	NA	NA	4	NA
Botox 200 U	122		−73.1	−19.1	NA	NA	16	6 months
Chapple *et al.*/2013 [43]								
Placebo	271	Intravesical injection (trigone sparing)	−13.9	-6	NA	NA	0.7	NA
Botox 100 U	277		−53.2	−19.7	NA	NA	6.9	12 weeks
Nitti *et al.*/2013 [38]								
Placebo	277	Intravesical injection (trigone sparing)	-17.1	4.1	NA	NA	0.4	NA
Botox 100 U	280		-48.2	−16.9	NA	NA	5.4	12 weeks

To assess the dose response relationship of intradetrusor BoNT/A, Dmochowski *et al.* conducted a trial using BoNT/A of doses ranging from 50 U to 300 U administered as 20 intradetrusor injections for male and female patients with idiopathic OAB and UUI [39]. They found durable efficacy for all BoNT/A dose groups of 100 U or greater. However, doses greater than 150 U contributed minimal additional or clinically relevant improvement in symptoms and HRQOL. On the other hand, use of clean intermittent catheterization (CIC) was dose dependent. Therefore, 100 U of BoNT/A may be the appropriate dose balancing the benefits and safety profiles. Rovner *et al.* tested the same dose range and also found that dose of 100 U or more led to significant improvements in OAB symptoms [40]. Dose-response relationship was observed in the changes of mean MCC and the volume at first involuntary detrusor contraction. Fowler *et al.* confirmed that BoNT/A at doses of 100 U or more produced significantly greater improvements than placebo in HRQOL by week 2, and the effect could sustain for up to 36 weeks [41]. Denys *et al.* performed a trial to evaluate the efficacy and tolerability of low doses of BoNT/A (50 U, 100 U and 150 U) compared to placebo in patients with idiopathic OAB [42]. They reported more than 50% improvement *versus* baseline in urgency and UUI at month 3 in 65% and 56% patients receiving 100 U and 150 U BoNT/A injections. Complete continence was achieved in 55% and 50% patients after 100 U and 150 U BoNT/A, respectively. These benefits persisted up to 6 months.

Recently, a meta-analysis including eight publications to evaluate the safety and efficacy of BoNT/A in treating idiopathic OAB was published [12]. It was reported that BoNT/A significantly decreased the mean number of UI per day (−2.77 *versus* −1.01, the standard mean difference [*SMD*] = −1.68) and the mean number of micturitions per day (−1.61 *versus* −0.87, *SMD* = −1.82); increased MCC (91.39 *versus* 32.32, *SMD* = 63.82) and volume voided (44.29 *versus* 7.36, *SMD* = 33.05) compared with placebo. Besides, 29.20% of patient treated with BoNT/A became incontinence-free *versus* 7.95% of patients with placebo (odds ratio [*OR*] = 4.89). In addition, the injection method of all the above studies was intradetrusor injection with trigone sparing in order to reduce the potential complication of vesicoureteral reflux. However, two RCTs by Kuo *et al.* and Maneckshа *et al.* revealed that bladder base/trigone injection of BoNT/A was as safe and effective as bladder body injections with or without trigone involvement [44,45].

3.2. Neurogenic Detruosr Overacitity

In 2000, Schurch *et al.* reported a preliminary study of BoNT/A in treating NDO patients. In their initial experience, BoNT/A of 200 U to 300 U significantly increased MCC and decreased detrusor voiding pressure, and complete continence was restored in 17 of 19 cases by 6 weeks [46]. On searching with "Botulinum toxin A" and "detrusor overactivity" on Pubmed in November 2015 and reviewing relevant articles in the reference lists, we identified that at present there are four randomized, placebo-controlled trials which examined the efficacy of BoNT/A for NDO (Table 2) [47–50].

Schurch *et al.* conducted the first randomized trial to determine the efficacy of two doses of BoNT/A (200 U and 300 U administered as 30 intradetrusor injections) in patients with urinary incontinence caused by NDO [47]. Both BoNT/A treatment groups had significantly decreased UI episodes (mean change −58% and −54% for 200 U and 300 U respectively), increased MCC (mean change 174.2 mL and 92.9 mL for 200 U and 300 U respectively), and improved QOL. There was no clinically relevant difference between the two doses of BoNT/A. The other two clinical trial by Cruz *et al.* and Ginsberg *et al.* also tested 200 U and 300 U BoNT/A in patients with NDO [48,49]. Significantly greater improvements in UI episodes, QOL, and urodynamic parameters including MCC and maximum detrusor pressure during the first involuntary detrusor contraction compared with placebo were noted in both doses of BoNT/A in both studies. Again, both 200 U and 300 U of BoNT/A yielded similar efficacy and duration of benefits.

Consistent with above findings, Herschorn *et al.* performed a trial using BoNT/A 300 U with intradetrusor injection at 30 sites for NDO patients [50]. After injection of BoNT/A, there was a lower frequency of UI episodes, greater improvements in urodynamic and QOL parameters compared with placebo. Interestingly, the clinical benefits lasted for up to 9 months.

Table 2. Randomized controlled trials of botulinum toxin A for neurogenic detrusor overactivity.

Authors/Year	No. of Patients	Patients Type	Injection Method	Continence (%)/ UI Episode (%Change)	MCC (%Change)	Pdetmax (%Change)	Urinary Retention Requiring CIC (%)	Duration of Benefit
Schurch *et al.*/2005 [46]		53 SCI, 6 MS	Intravesical injection (trigone sparing)					
Placebo	21			24/−10	+18	−13	-	NA
Botox 200 U	19			71/−58	+85	−59	-	>24 weeks
Botox 300 U	19			53/−54	+63	−56	-	>24 weeks
Cruz *et al.*/2011 [47]		121 SCI, 154 MS	Intravesical injection (trigone sparing)					
Placebo	92			7.6/−36	+3	+15	12	13.1 week
Botox 200 U	92			38.0/−67	+64	−55	30	42.1 week
Botox 300 U	91			39.6/−62	+64	−64	42	42.1 week
Herschorn *et al.*/2011 [49]		38 SCI, 19 MS	Intravesical injection (trigone sparing)					
Placebo	29			NA/0	−21.9	+4	-	NA
Botox 300 U	29			NA/−25	+21.5	+49.1	-	9 months
Ginsberg *et al.*/2012 [48]		189 SCI, 227 MS	Intravesical injection (trigone sparing)					
Placebo	149			NA/−31.1	+6.3	−4.7	10	92 days
Botox 200 U	135			NA/−65	+59.9	−68.4	35	256 days
Botox 300 U	132			NA/−73	+65.6	−70.7	42	254 days

Recently, a meta-analysis including the four RCTs was published [13]. It was revealed that BoNT/A resulted in changes of the mean number of UI per week ($SMD = -10.91$), MCC ($SMD = 146.09$), and maximum detrusor pressure ($SMD = -32.65$). Regardless of the doses of 200 U or 300 U, BoNT/A was more effective than placebo in treating patients with NDO.

4. Adverse Events

According the meta-analysis of BoNT/A in treating IDO patients, BoNT/A significantly increased PVR (32.77 *vs.* 2.01, $SMD = 31.73$), proportions of urinary tract infection (UTI) (19.69% and 5.94%, $OR = 3.89$), and proportions of CIC (8.41% and 0.46%, $OR = 13.39$) *versus* placebo [12]. In treating NDO patients, BoNT/A also led to a higher risk of UTI (relative risk [RR] = 1.48), hematuria ($RR = 1.81$), and urinary retention ($RR = 5.87$) requiring catheterization [13]. The effect of increased post-void residual volume (PVR) was dose dependent, and doses >150U was found to be more commonly associated with $PVR > 200$ mL [39,40]. It was reported that age >61 years, low maximum flow rate, low voiding efficiency (a percentage of the voided volume compared to the prevoid bladder volume <90%), and large PVR at baseline were risk factors for these adverse events [51]. The effect of increased PVR peaked by 2 weeks following BoNT/A injection, with a gradual decrease thereafter [39,49]. For urinary retention requiring catheterization, the duration was 6 weeks or less in more than half of the patients [12]. On the other hand, a meta-analysis showed there was no significant difference between trigonal and extratrigonal BoNT/A injection in terms of adverse events [52]. Kuo *et al.* demonstrated in a pilot study that intravesical instillation of liposome-encapsulated BoNT/A could effectively reduce the episodes of frequency and urgency in OAB patients without any increase in PVR or risk of UTI [53]. The promising role of liposome as vehicles delivering BoNT/A should be further validated. Finally, these results indicated that the adverse events of BoNT/A were primarily localized to the urinary tract, in contrast to the systemic effects of anticholinergic agents. Although muscle weakness or hyposthenia has been reported after BoNT/A injection, the incidence of systemic adverse events was rare and the duration was transient [54,55].

5. Conclusions

By blockade of neurotransmitter release and suburothelial sensory receptors expression, BoNT/A could cause chemical denervation of detrusor muscle. For patients with refractory OAB, BoNT/A offers an effective treatment option and the adverse events were primarily localized to the lower urinary tract.

Acknowledgments: This research received grant sponsor from China Medical University Hospital. Grant number was DMR-101-052.

Author Contributions: Po-Fan Hsieh drafted the manuscript. Hung-Chieh Chiu, Kuan-Chieh Chen, and Chao-Hsiang Chang revised the manuscript. Eric Chieh-Lung Chou supervised the drafting and revision.

Abbreviations

The following abbreviations are used in this manuscript:

OAB	overactive bladder
QOL	quality of life
DO	detrusor overactivity
BONT/A	botulinum toxin A
UUI	urgeny urinary incontinence
IDO	idiopathic detrusor overactivity
NDO	neurogenic detrusor overactivity
Ach	acetylcholine

MCC	maximum cystometric capacity
UI	urinary incontinence
HRQOL	health-related quality of life
CIC	clean intermittent catheterization
PVR	post-void residual volume
UTI	urinary tract infection

References

1. Abrams, P.; Cardozo, L.; Fall, M.; Griffiths, D.; Rosier, P.; Ulmsten, U.; van Kerrebroeck, P.; Victor, A.; Wein, A. The standardisation of terminology of lower urinary tract function: report for the Standardisation Sub-committee of the International Continence Society. *Neurourol. Urodynam.* **2002**, *21*, 167–178. [CrossRef] [PubMed]
2. Stewart, W.F.; van Rooyen, J.B.; Cundiff, G.W.; Abrams, P.; Herzog, A.R.; Corey, R.; Hunt, T.L.; Wein, A.J. Prevalence and burden of overactive bladder in the United States. *World J. Urol.* **2003**, *20*, 327–336. [PubMed]
3. Irwin, D.E.; Milsom, I.; Hunskaar, S.; Reilly, K.; Kopp, Z.; Herschorn, S.; Coyne, K.; Kelleher, C.; Hampel, C.; Artibani, W.; *et al.* Population-based survey of urinary incontinence, overactive bladder, and other lower urinary tract symptoms in five countries: results of the EPIC study. *Eur. Urol.* **2006**, *50*, 1306–1314. [CrossRef] [PubMed]
4. Lawrence, J.M.; Lukacz, E.S.; Nager, C.W.; Hsu, J.W.; Luber, K.M. Prevalence and co-occurrence of pelvic floor disorders in community-dwelling women. *Obstet. Gynecol.* **2008**, *111*, 678–685. [CrossRef] [PubMed]
5. Nitti, V.W. Clinical Impact of Overactive Bladder. *Rev. Urol.* **2002**, *4*, S2–S6. [PubMed]
6. Al-Ghazo, M.A.; Ghalayini, I.F.; Al-Azab, R.; Hani, O.B.; Matani, Y.S.; Haddad, Y. Urodynamic Detrusor Overactivity in Patients with Overactive Bladder Symptoms. *Int. Neurourol. J.* **2011**, *15*, 48–54. [CrossRef] [PubMed]
7. Gormley, E.A.; Lightner, D.J.; Faraday, M.; Vasavada, S.P.; American Urological Association; Society of Urodynamics, Female Pelvic Medicine. Diagnosis and treatment of overactive bladder (non-neurogenic) in adults: AUA/SUFU guideline amendment. *J. Urol.* **2015**, *193*, 1572–1580. [CrossRef] [PubMed]
8. Chapple, C.R.; Khullar, V.; Gabriel, Z.; Muston, D.; Bitoun, C.E.; Weinstein, D. The Effects of Antimuscarinic Treatments in Overactive Bladder: An Update of a Systematic Review and Meta-Analysis. *Eur. Urol.* **2008**, *54*, 543–562. [CrossRef] [PubMed]
9. Veenboer, P.W.; Bosch, J.L. Long-term adherence to antimuscarinic therapy in everyday practice: A systematic review. *J. Urol.* **2014**, *191*, 1003–1008. [CrossRef] [PubMed]
10. van Ermengem, E. Classics in infectious diseases. A new anaerobic bacillus and its relation to botulism. *Rev. Infect. Dis.* **1979**, *1*, 701–719. [CrossRef] [PubMed]
11. Ellsworth, P.; Travis, M. Onabotulinum toxin A: A therapeutic option for refractory neurogenic detrusor overactivity and idiopathic overactive bladder. *Urol. Nurs.* **2014**, *34*, 165–171. [PubMed]
12. Cui, Y.; Zhou, X.; Zong, H.; Yan, H.; Zhang, Y. The efficacy and safety of onabotulinumtoxinA in treating idiopathic OAB: A systematic review and meta-analysis. *Neurourol. Urodyn.* **2015**, *34*, 413–419. [CrossRef] [PubMed]
13. Zhou, X.; Yan, H.L.; Cui, Y.S.; Zong, H.T.; Zhang, Y. Efficacy and safety of onabotulinumtoxinA in treating neurogenic detrusor overactivity: A systematic review and meta-analysis. *Chin. Med. J. (Engl.)* **2015**, *128*, 963–968. [PubMed]
14. Lucas, M.G.; Bosch, R.J.; Burkhard, F.C.; Cruz, F.; Madden, T.B.; Nambiar, A.K.; Neisius, A.; de Ridder, D.J.; Tubaro, A.; Turner, W.H.; *et al.* EAU guidelines on surgical treatment of urinary incontinence. *Eur. Urol.* **2012**, *62*, 1118–1129. [CrossRef] [PubMed]
15. Li, B.; Peet, N.P.; Butler, M.M.; Burnett, J.C.; Moir, D.T.; Bowlin, T.L. Small molecule inhibitors as countermeasures for botulinum neurotoxin intoxication. *Molecules* **2010**, *16*, 202–220. [CrossRef] [PubMed]
16. Dong, M.; Yeh, F.; Tepp, W.H.; Dean, C.; Johnson, E.A.; Janz, R.; Chapman, E.R. SV2 is the protein receptor for botulinum neurotoxin A. *Science* **2006**, *28*, 592–596. [CrossRef] [PubMed]
17. Dolly, O. Synaptic transmission: inhibition of neurotransmitter release by Botulinum toxins. *Headache* **2003**, *43* (Suppl. 1), S16–S24. [CrossRef] [PubMed]

18. Yoshida, M.; Miyamae, K.; Iwashita, H.; Otani, M.; Inadome, A. Management of detrusor dysfunction in the elderly: Changes in acetylcholine and adenosine triphosphate release during aging. *Urology* **2004**, *63*, 17–23. [CrossRef] [PubMed]
19. Karsenty, G.; Denys, P.; Amarenco, G.; De Seze, M.; Gamé, X.; Haab, F.; Kerdraon, J.; Perrouin-Verbe, B.; Ruffion, A.; Saussine, C.; *et al.* Botulinum toxin A (Botox®) intradetrusor injections in adults with neurogenic detrusor overactivity/neurogenic overactive bladder: A systematic literature review. *Eur. Urol.* **2008**, *53*, 275–287. [CrossRef] [PubMed]
20. Atiemo, H.; Wynes, J.; Chuo, J.; Nipkow, L.; Sklar, G.N.; Chai, T.C. Effect of Botulinum toxin on detrusor overactivity induced by intravesical adenosine triphosphate and capsaicin in a rat model. *Urology* **2005**, *65*, 622–626. [CrossRef] [PubMed]
21. Brady, C.M.; Apostolidis, A.N.; Harper, M.; Yiangou, Y.; Beckett, A.; Jacques, T.S.; Freeman, A.; Scaravilli, F.; Fowler, C.J.; Anand, P. Parallel changes in bladder suburothelial vanilloid receptor TRPV1 (VR1) and pan-neuronal marker PGP9.5 immunoreactivity in patients with neurogenic detrusor overactivity (NDO) following intravesical resiniferatoxin treatment. *BJU Int.* **2004**, *93*, 770–776. [CrossRef] [PubMed]
22. Brady, C.; Apostolidis, A.; Yiangou, Y.; Baecker, P.A.; Ford, A.P.; Freeman, A.; Jacques, T.S.; Fowler, C.J.; Anand, P. P2X3-immunoreactive nerve fibres in neurogenic detrusor overactivity and the effect of intravesical resiniferatoxin (RTX). *Eur. Urol.* **2004**, *46*, 247–253. [CrossRef] [PubMed]
23. Apostolidis, A.; Popat, R.; Yiangou, Y.; Cockayne, D.; Ford, A.P.; Davis, J.B.; Dasgupta, P.; Fowler, C.J.; Anand, P. Decreased sensory receptors P2X3 and TRPV1 in suburothelial nerve fibers following intradetrusor injections of Botulinum toxin for human detrusor overactivity. *J. Urol.* **2005**, *174*, 977–983. [CrossRef] [PubMed]
24. Smet, P.J.; Moore, K.H.; Jonavicius, J. Distribution and colocalization of calcitonin gene-related peptide, tachykinins, and vasoactive intestinal peptide in normal and idiopathic unstable human urinary bladder. *Lab. Investig.* **1997**, *77*, 37–49. [PubMed]
25. Chuang, Y.C.; Yoshimura, N.; Huang, C.C.; Chiang, P.H.; Chancellor, M.B. Intravesical Botulinum toxin A administration produces analgesia against acetic acid induced bladder pain responses in rats. *J. Urol.* **2004**, *172*, 1529–1532. [CrossRef] [PubMed]
26. Lavin, S.T.; Southwell, B.R.; Murphy, R.; Jenkinson, K.M.; Furness, J.B. Activation of neurokinin 1 receptors on interstitial cells of Cajal of the guinea-pig small intestine by substance P. *Histochem. Cell Biol.* **1998**, *110*, 263–271. [CrossRef] [PubMed]
27. Giannantoni, A.; Di Stasi, S.M.; Nardicchi, V.; Zucchi, A.; Macchioni, L.; Bini, V.; Goracci, G.; Porena, M. Botulinum-A toxin injections into the detrusor muscle decrease nerve growth factor bladder tissue levels in patients with neurogenic detrusor overactivity. *J. Urol.* **2006**, *175*, 2341–2344. [CrossRef]
28. Liu, H.T.; Chancellor, M.B.; Kuo, H.C. Urinary nerve growth factor levels are elevated in patients with detrusor overactivity and decreased in responders to detrusor botulinum toxin-A injection. *Eur. Urol.* **2009**, *56*, 700–706. [CrossRef] [PubMed]
29. Papagiannopoulou, D.; Vardouli, L.; Dimitriadis, F.; Apostolidis, A. Retrograde transport of radiolabelled botulinum neurotoxin type A to the CNS after intradetrusor injection in rats. *BJU. Int.* **2015**, *24*. [CrossRef] [PubMed]
30. Wiseman, O.J.; Fowler, C.J.; Landon, D.N. The role of the human bladder lamina propria myofibroblast. *BJU Int.* **2003**, *91*, 89–93. [CrossRef] [PubMed]
31. Khullar, V.; Nadler, R.; Chaliha, C.; Yeo, L.; Underwood, J. Muscarinic type 2 receptors on bladder sensory nerves: A new site of drug action for detrusor overactivity? In Proceedings of the Abstracts of the 33rd Annual Meeting of the International Continence Society, Florence, Italy, 5–9 October 2003.
32. Radziszewski, P.; Dobronski, P. Treatment of the non-neurogenic storage and voiding disorders with the chemical denervation caused by botulinum toxin type A: A pilot study. *Neurourol. Urodyn.* **2001**, *20*, 410–412.
33. Sahai, A.; Khan, M.S.; Dasgupta, P. Efficacy of botulinum toxin-A for treating idiopathic detrusor overactivity: Results from a single center, randomized, double-blind, placebo controlled trial. *J. Urol.* **2007**, *177*, 2231–2236. [CrossRef] [PubMed]
34. Brubaker, L.; Richter, H.E.; Visco, A.; Mahajan, S.; Nygaard, I.; Braun, T.M.; Barber, M.D.; Menefee, S.; Schaffer, J.; Weber, A.M.; *et al.* Pelvic Floor Disorders Network. Refractory idiopathic urge urinary incontinence and botulinum A injection. *J. Urol.* **2008**, *180*, 217–222. [CrossRef] [PubMed]

35. Tincello, D.G.; Kenyon, S.; Abrams, K.R.; Mayne, C.; Toozs-Hobson, P.; Taylor, D.; Slack, M. Botulinum toxin a *versus* placebo for refractory detrusor overactivity in women: A randomised blinded placebo-controlled trial of 240 women (the RELAX study). *Eur. Urol.* **2012**, *62*, 507–514. [CrossRef] [PubMed]
36. Flynn, M.K.; Amundsen, C.L.; Perevich, M.; Liu, F.; Webster, G.D. Outcome of a randomized, double-blind, placebo controlled trial of botulinum A toxin for refractory overactive bladder. *J. Urol.* **2009**, *181*, 2608–2615. [CrossRef] [PubMed]
37. Dowson, C.; Sahai, A.; Watkins, J.; Dasgupta, P.; Khan, M.S. The safety and efficacy of botulinum toxin-A in the management of bladder oversensitivity: A randomised double-blind placebo-controlled trial. *Int. J. Clin. Pract.* **2011**, *65*, 698–704. [CrossRef] [PubMed]
38. Nitti, V.W.; Dmochowski, R.; Herschorn, S.; Sand, P.; Thompson, C.; Nardo, C.; Yan, X.; Haag-Molkenteller, C.; EMBARK Study Group. OnabotulinumtoxinA for the treatment of patients with overactive bladder and urinary incontinence: Results of a phase 3, randomized, placebo controlled trial. *J. Urol.* **2013**, *189*, 2186–2193. [CrossRef] [PubMed]
39. Dmochowski, R.; Chapple, C.; Nitti, V.W.; Chancellor, M.; Everaert, K.; Thompson, C.; Daniell, G.; Zhou, J.; Haag-Molkenteller, C. Efficacy and safety of onabotulinumtoxinA for idiopathic overactive bladder: A double-blind, placebo controlled, randomized, dose ranging trial. *J. Urol.* **2010**, *184*, 2416–2422. [CrossRef] [PubMed]
40. Rovner, E.; Kennelly, M.; Schulte-Baukloh, H.; Zhou, J.; Haag-Molkenteller, C.; Dasgupta, P. Urodynamic results and clinical outcomes with intradetrusor injections of onabotulinumtoxinA in a randomized, placebo-controlled dose-finding study in idiopathic overactive bladder. *Neurourol. Urodyn.* **2011**, *30*, 556–562. [CrossRef] [PubMed]
41. Fowler, C.J.; Auerbach, S.; Ginsberg, D.; Hale, D.; Radziszewski, P.; Rechberger, T.; Patel, V.D.; Zhou, J.; Thompson, C.; Kowalski, J.W. OnabotulinumtoxinA improves health-related quality of life in patients with urinary incontinence due to idiopathic overactive bladder: A 36-week, double-blind, placebo-controlled, randomized, dose-ranging trial. *Eur. Urol.* **2012**, *62*, 148–157. [CrossRef] [PubMed]
42. Denys, P.; Le Normand, L.; Ghout, I.; Costa, P.; Chartier-Kastler, E.; Grise, P.; Hermieu, J.F.; Amarenco, G.; Karsenty, G.; Saussine, C.; *et al.* Efficacy and safety of low doses of onabotulinumtoxinA for the treatment of refractory idiopathic overactive bladder: A multicentre, double-blind, randomised, placebo-controlled dose-ranging study. *Eur. Urol.* **2012**, *61*, 520–529. [CrossRef] [PubMed]
43. Chapple, C.; Sievert, K.D.; MacDiarmid, S.; Khullar, V.; Radziszewski, P.; Nardo, C.; Thompson, C.; Zhou, J.; Haag-Molkenteller, C. OnabotulinumtoxinA 100 U significantly improves all idiopathic overactive bladder symptoms and quality of life in patients with overactive bladder and urinary incontinence: A randomized double-blind placebo-controlled trial. *Eur. Urol.* **2013**, *64*, 249–256. [CrossRef] [PubMed]
44. Kuo, H.C. Bladder base/trigone injection is safe and as effective as bladder body injection of onabotulinumtoxinA for idiopathic detrusor overactivity refractory to antimuscarinics. *Neurourol. Urodyn.* **2011**, *30*, 1242–1248. [CrossRef] [PubMed]
45. Manecksha, R.P.; Cullen, I.M.; Ahmad, S.; McNeill, G.; Flynn, R.; McDermott, T.E.; Grainger, R.; Thornhill, J.A. Prospective randomised controlled trial comparing Trigone-sparing *versus* trigone-including intradetrusor injection of abobotulinumtoxinA for refractory idiopathic detrusor overactivity. *Eur. Urol.* **2012**, *61*, 928–935. [CrossRef] [PubMed]
46. Schurch, B.; Stöhrer, M.; Kramer, G.; Schmid, D.M.; Gaul, G.; Hauri, D. Botulinum-A toxin for treating detrusor hyperreflexia in spinal cord injured patients: A new alternative to anticholinergic drugs? Preliminary results. *J. Urol.* **2000**, *164*, 692–697. [CrossRef]
47. Schurch, B.; de Sèze, M.; Denys, P.; Chartier-Kastler, E.; Haab, F.; Everaert, K.; Plante, P.; Perrouin-Verbe, B.; Kumar, C.; Fraczek, S.; *et al.* Botulinum toxin type a is a safe and effective treatment for neurogenic urinary incontinence: results of a single treatment, randomized, placebo controlled 6-month study. *J. Urol.* **2005**, *174*, 196–200. [CrossRef] [PubMed]
48. Cruz, F.; Herschorn, S.; Aliotta, P.; Brin, M.; Thompson, C.; Lam, W.; Daniell, G.; Heesakkers, J.; Haag-Molkenteller, C. Efficacy and safety of onabotulinumtoxinA in patients with urinary incontinence due to neurogenic detrusor overactivity: A randomised, double-blind, placebo-controlled trial. *Eur. Urol.* **2011**, *60*, 742–750. [CrossRef] [PubMed]

49. Ginsberg, D.; Gousse, A.; Keppenne, V.; Sievert, K.D.; Thompson, C.; Lam, W.; Brin, M.F.; Jenkins, B.; Haag-Molkenteller, C. Phase 3 efficacy and tolerability study of onabotulinumtoxinA for urinary incontinence from neurogenic detrusor overactivity. *J. Urol.* **2012**, *187*, 2131–2139. [CrossRef] [PubMed]
50. Herschorn, S.; Gajewski, J.; Ethans, K.; Corcos, J.; Carlson, K.; Bailly, G.; Bard, R.; Valiquette, L.; Baverstock, R.; Carr, L.; *et al.* Efficacy of botulinum toxin A injection for neurogenic detrusor overactivity and urinary incontinence: A randomized, double-blind trial. *J. Urol.* **2011**, *185*, 2229–2235. [CrossRef] [PubMed]
51. Jiang, Y.H.; Ong, H.L.; Kuo, H.C. Predictive factors of adverse events after intravesical suburothelial onabotulinumtoxina injections for overactive bladder syndrome-A real-life practice of 290 cases in a single center. *Neurourol. Urodyn.* **2015**, *28*. [CrossRef] [PubMed]
52. Davis, N.F.; Burke, J.P.; Redmond, E.J.; Elamin, S.; Brady, C.M.; Flood, HD. Trigonal *versus* extratrigonal botulinum toxin-A: A systematic review and meta-analysis of efficacy and adverse events. *Int. Urogynecol. J.* **2015**, *26*, 313–389. [CrossRef] [PubMed]
53. Kuo, H.C.; Liu, H.T.; Chuang, Y.C.; Birder, L.A.; Chancellor, M.B. Pilot study of liposome-encapsulated onabotulinumtoxina for patients with overactive bladder: A single-center study. *Eur. Urol.* **2014**, *65*, 1117–1124. [CrossRef] [PubMed]
54. Grosse, J.; Kramer, G.; Stöhrer, M. Success of repeat detrusor injections of botulinum a toxin in patients with severe neurogenic detrusor overactivity and incontinence. *Eur. Urol.* **2005**, *47*, 653–659. [CrossRef] [PubMed]
55. Del Popolo, G.; Filocamo, M.T.; Li Marzi, V.; Macchiarella, A.; Cecconi, F.; Lombardi, G.; Nicita, G. Neurogenic detrusor overactivity treated with English botulinum toxin A: 8-year experience of one single centre. *Eur. Urol.* **2008**, *53*, 1013–1019. [CrossRef] [PubMed]

2

Efficacy and Safety of Intravesical OnabotulinumtoxinA Injection in Patients with Detrusor Hyperactivity and Impaired Contractility

Chung-Cheng Wang [1,2], Cheng-Ling Lee [3] and Hann-Chorng Kuo [3,*]

[1] Department of Urology, En Chu Kong Hospital, College of Medicine, National Taiwan University, Taipei 23702, Taiwan; ericwcc@ms27.hinet.net
[2] Department of Biomedical Engineering, Chung Yuan Christian University, Chung-Li 32023, Taiwan
[3] Department of Urology, Buddhist Tzu Chi General Hospital, and Tzu Chi University, Hualien 97002, Taiwan; chenglinglee@gmail.com
* Correspondence: hck@tzuchi.com.tw

Academic Editor: Joseph Jankovic

Abstract: We investigated the efficacy and safety of intravesical onabotulinumtoxinA injection in patients with detrusor hyperactivity and impaired contractility (DHIC). Twenty-one patients with urodynamically proven DHIC and 21 age-matched patients with overactive bladder (OAB) with urodynamic detrusor overactivity were treated with intravesical injections of 100 U of onabotulinumtoxinA. The overactive bladder symptom score, urgency severity score, patient perception of bladder condition, global response assessment, voiding diary, and procedure-related adverse events (AE) at baseline, two weeks, one, three, and six months after treatment were assessed. The results showed that the subjective symptom scores improved significantly in both groups, and the scores did not differ between the groups. The decrease in urgency episodes and urgency urinary incontinence were noted in OAB patients but not in DHIC patients. Although the incidence of AEs was comparable between the groups, the therapeutic efficacy lasted for a mean of 4.9 ± 4.8 months in DHIC patients and 7.2 ± 3.3 months in OAB patients ($p = 0.03$). We concluded that the efficacy of intravesical onabotulinumtoxinA injection for DHIC patients was limited and short-term. Nevertheless, AEs did not increase in DHIC. Intravesical onabotulinumtoxinA might not be a good indication in patients with DHIC and high post-voiding residual urine. Physicians should inform patients of the potential benefits and risks of onabotulinumtoxinA injection for treatment of DHIC.

Keywords: underactive detrusor; overactive bladder; onabotulinumtoxinA

1. Introduction

Overactive bladder (OAB) is a common condition in the community and is associated with substantial impairment of mental health and health-related quality of life [1]. Underactive bladder (UAB) is characterized by large post-void residual urine (PVR) volume and weak detrusor contractility [2]. Interestingly, some OAB patients have detrusor hyperactivity and impaired contractility (DHIC), resulting in urgency urinary incontinence and voiding difficulty [2]. The incidence of DHIC increases with age [3], but the underlying etiologies of DHIC remain complex. Chronic ischemia and inflammation of the bladder may contribute to DHIC in the elderly population [4]. Oshiro *et al.* have found that chronic urinary retention results in hypoxia and downregulation of connexin 43, a gap junction protein involved in intercellular communication, in the aged bladder that may reduce the contractility of the detrusor [5]. In addition, bladders in diabetic patients may undergo a transition from a compensated to a decompensated state, which means a transition from

OAB to UAB [6]. Though these studies provide possible explanation of the pathophysiology of DHIC, adequate treatment remains difficult.

In the last decade, intravesical injection of onabotulinumtoxinA has emerged as an effective and safe treatment for OAB in patients refractory or intolerable to antimuscarinic agents [7]. Several studies have proven that onabotulinumtoxinA significantly improved OAB symptoms and urodynamic parameters in OAB patients [7–11]. However, increased PVR volume and risk of urinary tract infection (UTI) after onabotulinumtoxinA treatment remain concerns among these patients [8]. Large PVR at baseline and low voiding efficiency (voided volume/bladder capacity, VE) (*i.e.*, VE < 67%) are significant predictors of developing adverse events (AE) after intravesical onabotulinumtoxinA injection for OAB treatment [9]. Therefore, onabotulinumtoxinA is not suggested for OAB patients with a PVR of more than 250 mL unless they are willing to accept the risk of acute urinary retention (AUR) and perform a clean intermittent catheterization.

Whether intravesical onabotulinumtoxinA injection for treatment of DHIC is safe and effective remains unknown. We hypothesized that patients with DHIC might have higher AE and poor therapeutic effectiveness after intravesical onabotulinumtoxinA injection. Thus, we investigated the therapeutic efficacy and safety of intravesical onabotulinumtoxinA (100 mL) in OAB patients who had a baseline PVR > 100 mL or VE < 67%. The results of the study might provide evidence for clinicians to select the appropriate DHIC patients for onabotulinumtoxinA treatment.

2. Results

2.1. Therapeutic Effectiveness

The mean ages of the DHIC and OAB patients were comparable (71.2 ± 8.2 *versus* 70.9 ± 14.1 years, $p = 0.35$). Table 1 lists the changes in the variables measured from baseline to six months for the two groups. The subjective symptom scores after onabotulinumtoxinA treatment, including the OAB Symptom Score, Urgency Severity Score, Patient perception of Bladder Condition, and Global Response Assessment all showed significantly improved in both groups. The findings did not differ between the groups. However, the decrease in the number of urgency episodes per three days after treatment occurred only in the OAB patients. Urgency urinary incontinence was significantly improved at three months and six months. Frequency episodes had significantly improved at four weeks and six months in OAB patients, but not in DHIC patients. There was no increase in voided volume in either group. Qmax showed no significant change after treatment in either group. PVR volume increased in DHIC patients at two and four weeks, but not at three and six months after onabotulinumtoxinA injection. However, in OAB patients, the significant increase in PVR volume occurred at two weeks after treatment and lasted for six months. VE showed similar changes to PVR in both groups. The decrease of VE after onabotulinumtoxinA injection was significantly greater in OAB compared to DHIC patients. Figure 1 shows the time-course changes of Qmax, volume, PVR and VE in DHIC and OAB patients.

Table 1. The parameters of patients with DHIC and OAB at baseline and two weeks, four weeks, three months, and six months after 100 U onabotulinumtoxinA injection.

Parameters		Baseline	2 Weeks	4 Weeks	3 Months	6 Months
OABSS	DHIC	12.3 ± 2.0	11.1 ± 2.56 *	10.1 ± 2.77 *	10.1 ± 3.80 *	9.61 ± 3.24 *
	OAB	11.2 ± 2.9	9.48 ± 3.2 *	9.52 ± 2.96 *	9.19 ± 2.87 *	8.06 ± 3.3 *
USS	DHIC	4.0 ± 0	3.48 ± 0.87 *	3.40 ± 0.88 *	3.7 ± 0.92	3.28 ± 0.96 *
	OAB	3.62 ± 0.74	3.14 ± 1.1 *	3.29 ± 1.01 *	3.10 ± 1.0 *	3.06 ± 1.06 *
GRA	DHIC	0	1.19 ± 1.33 *	1.30 ± 1.38 *	1.10 ± 1.74 *	1.50 ± 1.47 *
	OAB	0	0.95 ± 1.28 *	1.43 ± 1.12 *	1.52 ± 0.81 *	1.72 ± 0.96 *
PPBC	DHIC	4.67 ± 1.77	3.90 ± 1.70	3.25 ± 1.65 *	3.15 ± 1.76 *	2.89 ± 1.75 *
	OAB	4.52 ± 1.66	3.10 ± 1.61 *	2.48 ± 1.47 *	2.81 ± 1.63 *	2.56 ± 1.29 *

Table 1. *Cont.*

Parameters		Baseline	2 Weeks	4 Weeks	3 Months	6 Months
UUI/3 days	DHIC	7.44 ± 9.51	6.67 ± 11.1	5.84 ± 9.22	12.3 ± 20.9	9.53 ± 19.6
	OAB	6.0 ± 13.6	3.65 ± 7.39	4.70 ± 9.09	3.62 ± 8.13 *	2.88 ± 2.03 *
Urgency/3 days	DHIC	27.7 ± 17.7	27.9 ± 23.4	29.8 ± 30.2	27.5 ± 28.2	29.1 ± 33.5
	OAB	27.3 ± 15.0	22.4 ± 14.5 *	19.9 ± 15.7 *	26.9 ± 19.8	15.1 ± 11.9 *
Frequency/3 days	DHIC	26.6 ± 14.2	30.0 ± 14.4	31.1 ± 24.6	28.6 ± 22.4	29.7 ± 28.9
	OAB	38.0 ± 12.9	37.6 ± 22.5	31.5 ± 9.27 *	36.5 ± 19.8	31.4 ± 12.3 *
Nocturia/3 days	DHIC	10.5 ± 5.41	9.39 ± 3.29	8.16 ± 3.01	8.50 ± 2.09	7.59 ± 3.12 *
	OAB	11.4 ± 5.40	9.80 ± 4.57	8.55 ± 3.80 *	10.5 ± 5.0	9.44 ± 3.01
Qmax (mL/s)	DHIC	12.6 ± 10.7	8.43 ± 4.23	8.62 ± 3.34	10.1 ± 5.32	11.2 ± 6.33
	OAB	12.9 ± 7.1	10.9 ± 7.9	14.2 ± 7.02	14.5 ± 8.54	12.9 ± 8.2
Voided volume (mL)	DHIC	146 ± 69	146 ± 97	171 ± 99	171 ± 125	199 ± 126
	OAB	187 ± 106	164 ± 136	212 ± 93	205 ± 96	185 ± 106
PVR volume (mL)	DHIC	109 ± 149	199 ± 118 *	179 ± 93 *	194 ± 150	123 ± 79
	OAB	11 ± 15	158 ± 184 *	147 ± 123 *	81 ± 75 *	75 ± 72 *
VE (%)	DHIC	57.3 ± 24.8	42.3 ± 24.8 *	48.9 ± 19.8 *	46.8 ± 26.8	61.8 ± 20.1
	OAB	94.6 ± 7.9	50.9 ± 29.4 *	59.1 ± 21.8 *	71.6 ± 20.1 *	71.2 ± 22.4 *

DHIC: detrusor hyperactivity and impaired contractility; OAB: overactive bladder; OABSS: overactive bladder symptom score; USS: urgency severity score; GRA: global response assessment; PPBC: patient perception bladder condition; UUI: urgency urinary incontinence; Qmax: maximal urinary flow rate; PVR: post-void residual; VE: voiding efficacy. * Significantly different from baseline.

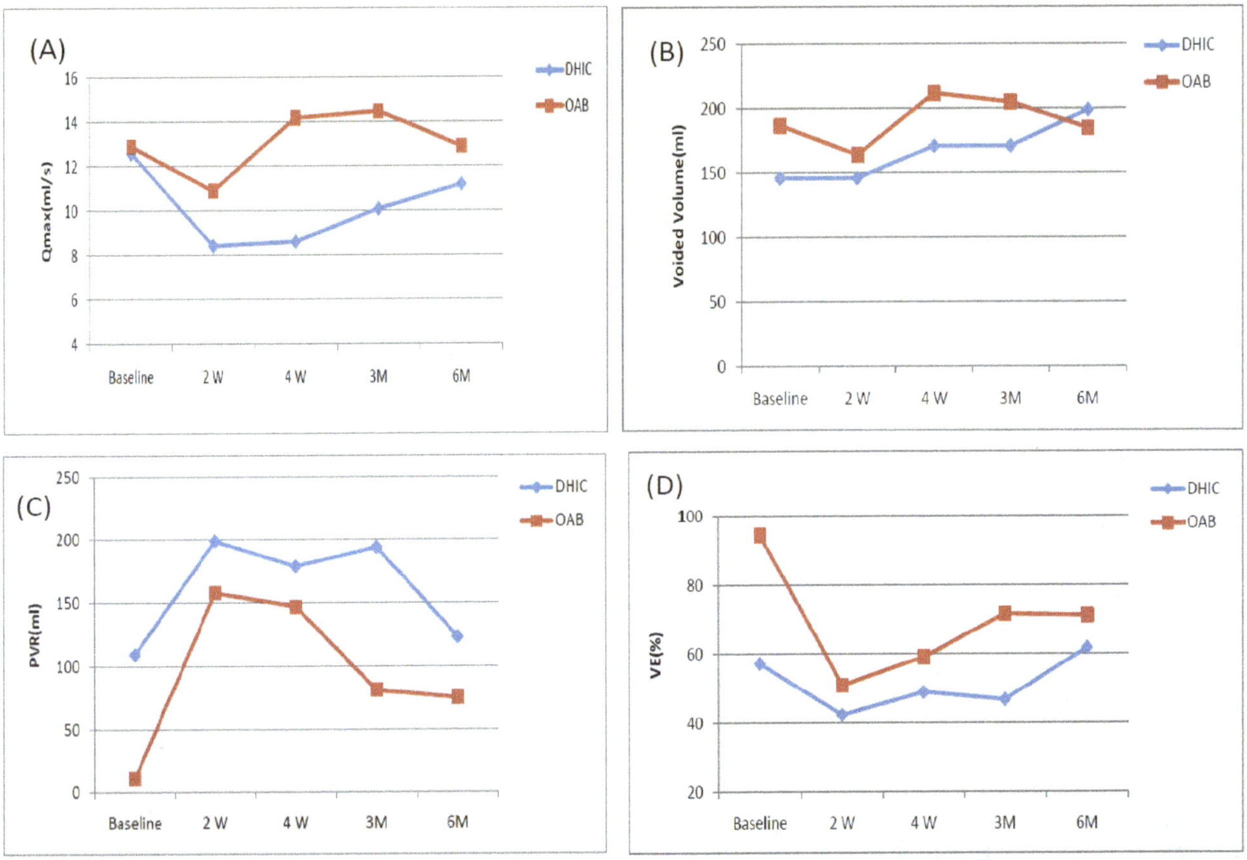

Figure 1. The changes of maximum flow rate (Qmax), voided volume (vol), post-void residual (PVR) volume, and voiding efficiency (VE) at different time-points in patients with detrusor hyperactivity and impaired contractility (DHIC) and overactive bladder (OAB) from baseline to six months. (**A**) Qmax; (**B**) Void volume; (**C**) PVR; (**D**) Voiding efficiency.

2.2. Adverse Events

Table 2 lists the incidence of AEs in DHIC and OAB patients. The incidence of AEs including AUR, PVR > 200 mL, UTI, gross hematuria and general weakness were all comparable in both groups. After onabotulinumtoxinA treatment, 7 (33.3%) DHIC patients and 16 (76.2%) OAB patients thought that the treatment improved their quality of life. The therapeutic efficacy lasted for a mean of 4.9 ± 4.8 months and 7.2 ± 3.3 months in DHIC and OAB patients ($p = 0.03$), respectively.

Table 2. Comparison of the adverse events and therapeutic duration in patients with DHIC and OAB after 100 U onabotulinumtoxinA injection.

Adverse Events	DHIC ($n = 21$)	OAB ($n = 21$)	p Value
AUR	7 (33.3%)	3 (14.3%)	0.277
PVR volume > 200 mL	12 (57.1%)	7 (33.3%)	0.215
UTI	8 (38.1%)	4 (19.0%)	0.306
Gross hematuria	0 (0%)	1 (4.8%)	1.000
General weakness	1 (4.8%)	0 (0%)	1.000
Therapeutic duration (months)	4.9 ± 4.8	7.2 ± 3.3	0.03

DHIC: detrusor hyperactivity and impaired contractility; OAB: overactive bladder; AUR: acute urinary retention; PVR: post-void residual volume; UTI: urinary tract infection.

3. Discussion

To our knowledge, this is the first study reporting the efficacy and safety of intravesical onabotulinumtoxinA injection for treatment of patients with DHIC. We found that patients with DHIC did not have a significantly increased risk of AEs after injection of 100 U of onabotulinumtoxinA compared to OAB patients. However, although the subjective urgency symptom score improved, the number of urgency episodes, frequency or urgency urinary incontinence did not change after onabotulinumtoxinA treatment in DHIC patients. The efficacy of onabotulinumtoxinA therapy declined significantly in DHIC patients compared to OAB patients.

The actual mechanism of DHIC, a paradoxical condition involving both the storage and voiding phases, is not well understood. Clinical observation shows DHIC is commonly associated with chronic bladder outlet obstruction (BOO), diabetes mellitus (DM), neurogenic diseases, and aging [10]. High voiding pressure due to BOO could initially induce OAB. However, chronic high pressure could cause subsequent bladder ischemia and reperfusion injury, which could trigger free radical production injuring the detrusor muscle or neurons [11]. Thus, some BOO patients manifest with DHIC during the transition from OAB to UAB. This phenomenon happens similarly in the DM bladders. Daneshgarin *et al.* have found that DM in the early stage causes compensated bladder function but DM in the late stage results in decompensated bladder function in diabetic animal models [6]. In clinical observations, men with type 2 DM aged <45 years had more OAB symptoms, but adequate voiding function [12]. Voiding dysfunction was commonly found in diabetic patients more than 60 years old, and the duration of diabetes was a risk factor for diabetic bladder dysfunction [13]. Based on these findings, the hypothesis that chronic untreated or treatment-refractory OAB progressed to DHIC and subsequently progressed to UAB with time was proposed [4].

The effective therapeutic choices for OAB include behavioral therapy, antimuscarinic agents, beta-3 agonists, intravesical onabotulinumtoxinA injection, and sacral neuromodulation [14]. However, compared to OAB patients, the treatment of patients with DHIC is often treated empirically, and these treatments often lacked efficacy. Impaired detrusor function limits the use of antimuscarinic agents while options to facilitate voiding function may potentially worsen OAB symptoms or incontinence. Liu *et al.* reported the pharmacotherapeutic outcomes in 43 DHIC patients [15]. Sixteen patients underwent anticholinergic treatment alone, and nine patients had symptomatic improvement. 6 of the 16 patients had symptomatic improvement after alpha-blockers alone. 4 of 5 patients had improvement after a combination of alpha-blockers and anticholinergics. One of the major drawbacks of this study was that the authors did not report how they chose the medication. Schulte-Baukloh H *et al.* reported the outcomes of onabotulinumtoxinA detrusor and external sphincter injection for treating OAB patients [16]. The additional injection of onabotulinumtoxinA into the sphincter reduced the potential risk of patients developing large PVR volumes after injection into the detrusor. This method of injecting both urethral sphincter and detrusor might be helpful for patients with DHIC.

Our study showed that compared to patients with OAB, patients with DHIC had worse therapeutic outcomes, which were proven by the lack of change in the parameters of the 3-day voiding diary. This finding is similar to a previous study of antimuscarinic agents for the treatment of OAB [17]. Hsiao *et al.* [17] showed that failure of the therapeutic efficacy of solifenacin was associated with a low Qmax at baseline and a large PVR volume, which may imply poor bladder emptying in these OAB patients. In a time-course study of diabetic animals, the gene expression of the M2 muscarinic receptors in the urothelium increased significantly by eight-fold at three-week streptozotocin-induced DM bladder and 14-fold at nine-week DM, but only four-fold at 20-week DM [18]. This trend might explain the transition from the compensated to the decompensated stage of bladder urothelial function. The changes in M2 muscarinic receptors in the different stages of DM could have modified urothelial cholinergic autocrine signaling and interrupted barrier function, which could have caused the various therapeutic outcomes found in the clinical studies, regardless of antimuscarinic or onabotulinumtoxinA treatment.

One interesting finding was that, compared with OAB patients, DHIC patients had no significant increase in PVR volumes and AEs after intravesical onabotulinumtoxinA injection. This finding seem different from our previous study showing that the male gender, the baseline PVR volume was $\geqslant$100 mL, comorbidities and onabotulinumtoxinA dose > 100 U were risk factors for increasing the incidence of AEs after intravesical onabotulinumtoxinA injection for DO patients [9]. In addition, Liao *et al.* reported an increased risk of large PVR volume and a lower long-term success rate in frail elderly patients with DO after intravesical onabotulinumtoxinA injection [8]. This discrepancy may be explained by our assumption that suburothelial injection of onabotulinumtoxinA might cause less detrusor contractility inhibition compared to detrusor injection and DHIC patients usually voided with abdominal straining. Thus although DHIC patients took more time to empty their bladders, the PVR and Qmax of DHIC could be similar with OAB patients after onabotulinumtoxinA injection. In addition, The VEs at two weeks after treatment (54.1% in OAB *vs.* 42.9% in DHIC) and four weeks post treatment (64.2% in OAB *vs.* 50.2% in DHIC) were comparable in both groups. VE may be an important factor predicting the occurrence of AEs such as AUR, UTI, and PVR volume > 200 mL. Comparable VEs in both groups could have resulted in similar AEs. In addition, we excluded the frail elderly patients from our study. Thus, the effect of the comorbidity on AEs could be decreased in this analysis.

The 2002 ICS standardization report defined detrusor underactivity (DU) as "a contraction of reduced strength and duration, resulting in prolonged bladder emptying and failure to achieve complete bladder emptying within a normal time span" [19]. However, the objective definition of DU based on pressure-flow analyses in clinical studies is not universal. Wang et al defined DU as PdetQmax < 30 cm H_2O and Qmax < 15 mL/s [20]. Nitti et al defined DU as a BOO index < 20 and a Qmax < 12 mL/s [21]. Jeong et al defined DU as bladder contractility index < 100 [22]. Using a simple method, Resnick *et al.* considered DHIC as involuntary detrusor contractility that emptied less than half of the volume instilled [23]. In this study, we arbitrarily defined DHIC as OAB patients with a baseline PVR > 100 mL or VE < 67%. The ambiguity of the different DHIC definitions requires discussion to achieve a global consensus in the future.

Our study had several limitations. First, the study was limited by its retrospective design and the lack of a placebo control. However, the main purpose of the study was to compare the efficacy and safety of onabotulinumtoxinA treatment in patients with OAB and DHIC. Secondly, the etiologies of patients with DHIC varied and different underlying pathophysiologies of DHIC could have affected the therapeutic outcomes. Finally, all of the OAB and DHIC patients were refractory to behavioral therapy and antimuscarinic agents before onabotulinumtoxinA treatment. The exact therapeutic results of treatment naïve OAB and DHIC patients are still unknown and should be investigated in the future.

4. Conclusions

The efficacy of onabotulinumtoxinA intradetrusor injection for treatment of DHIC was limited and short-term. Although the AEs did not significantly increase in DHIC patients, the relatively higher rates of AEs and shorter therapeutic duration still need attention when onabotulinumtoxinA therapy is recommended to patients with DHIC. Intravesical onabotulinumtoxinA might not be indicated in patients with DHIC and high PVR. Physicians should inform patients of the potential benefits and risks of onabotulinumtoxinA therapy for treatment of DHIC to reduce patients' over-expectations before treatment.

5. Materials and Methods

The institutional review board and ethics committee of the Tzu-Chi General hospital approved the study (IRB-094-08), approved 8 May 2014. All participants were informed about the possible AE after onabotulinumtoxinA injection and written informed consent was obtained from all patients before treatment. The clinical trial registration number was NCT-02135341.

A total of 21 patients with videourodynamically proven DHIC and 21 age-matched control OAB patients with urodynamic detrusor overactivity (DO) were retrospectively selected from patients who had participated in previous clinical trials at the authors' hospital from 2004 to 2009 [9,24,25]. Because this was a retrospective study, we could not reroll patients based on power calculation. Patients of either gender, aged $\geqslant$ 20 years of age with videourodynamic DO and, at least, one episode of urgency (urgency severity scale (USS) score $\geqslant$ 2) or urgency urinary incontinence per day, as recorded in a 3-day voiding diary, were enrolled. DHIC was defined as the presence of involuntary contraction during the filling phase and underactive detrusor function during voiding phase. Patients with underactive detrusor should fulfill these criteria including PVR > 100 mL, PdetQmax < $30H_2O$, Qmax <15 cm/s and relaxed sphincter EMG without outlet obstruction radiologically during videourodynamic study. We investigated patients with DHIC having a PVR of > 100 mL but < 250 mL or a VE of less than 67% at baseline. Patients with DO had a PVR < 50 mL and a VE > 67% at baseline.

All patients had tried behavioral modification and treatment with antimuscarinic agents for more than 3 months before enrollment. Antimuscarinic drugs were discontinued on the day of screening to wash out the residual effect and obtain a voiding diary that reflected the true bladder condition. Major exclusion criteria were overt neurogenic bladder dysfunction, urodynamically confirmed bladder outlet obstruction, prior pelvic surgery or radiation, malignant diseases of the pelvic organs, anti-incontinence surgery, urinary tract infection (UTI), and any other serious diseases making the patient unsuitable for the study, as considered by the investigator.

Patients were treated with suburothelial injections of 100 U of onabotulinumtoxinA (Allergan, Irvine, CA, USA) in 10 mL saline, 0.5 mL per injection in 20 injections in the bladder body, sparing the trigone. All procedures were performed transurethrally by a single urologist (HCK) under light intravenous general anesthesia in the operation room. Anticoagulant use was discontinued 1 week before onabotulinumtoxinA treatment. Bladder volume was maintained at 100–150 mL and blood vessels were avoided during the injections. The onabotulinumtoxinA solution was injected into the urothelium at the posterior and lateral walls of the bladder by using a 23-gauge needle and rigid cystoscopic injection instrument (22 Fr, Richard Wolf, Knittlingen, Germany). After the onabotulinumtoxinA injection, a 14-Fr urethral Foley catheter was inserted and left for one day. The patients were discharged on the following day. Broad-spectrum prophylactic antibiotics were administered postoperatively for 7 days.

All patients were evaluated at baseline, 2 weeks, and 1, 3, and 6 months after treatment. Treatment results were assessed using the Global Response Assessment, which is categorized as −3, −2, −1, 0, 1, 2, and 3 indicating markedly worse, moderately worse, mildly worse, no change, mildly improved, moderately improved, and markedly improved bladder symptoms, respectively. The OAB Symptom Score, Urgency Severity Score, Patient Perception of Bladder Condition, and voiding diary parameters including daytime frequency, nocturia, urgency, and urgency urinary incontinence episodes per 3 days (3 consecutive days within 7 days before the visit) were also evaluated. Additionally, uroflowmetry and PVR volume (Laborie®, Mississauga, Canada) were measured at each visit. The variables measured included maximum flow rate (Qmax), PVR volume, voided volume, and VE.

Procedure-related AEs were recorded during the 6-month follow-up period after onabotulinumtoxinA treatment. The common AEs included acute urinary retention (AUR) (severe difficulty urinating with a PVR volume >350 mL and necessitating the use of an indwelling catheter or clean intermittent catheterization); PVR volume > 200 mL (without requiring an indwelling catheter); gross hematuria; general weakness; and UTI (symptomatic or asymptomatic with a white blood cell count > 10/high-power field on urinalysis) during the follow-up period. Patients who developed AUR or PVR volumes > 350 mL were advised to perform clean intermittent catheterization to evacuate their bladders as needed.

Continuous variables were expressed as means ± standard deviations, and categorical data were expressed as numbers and percentages. Statistical comparisons between the groups were conducted using Fisher's exact test for categorical variables and analysis of variance test for continuous variables. The Wilcoxon matched-pair signed rank test was used to compare the parameters before and after treatment. All statistical assessments were two-sided and considered significant at a value of $p < 0.05$. The statistical analyses were performed using SPSS version 15.0 statistical software (SPSS Inc., Chicago, IL, USA, 2006).

Acknowledgments: We thanks support from the grant of En Chu Kong Hospital (grant number: ECK10502).

Author Contributions: Chung-Cheng Wang and Hann-Chorng Kuo conceived and designed the experiments; Cheng-Ling Lee and Hann-Chorng Kuo performed the experiments; Chung-Cheng Wang, Cheng-Ling Lee and Hann-Chorng Kuo analyzed the data; Hann-Chorng Kuo contributed reagents/materials/analysis tools; and Chung-Cheng Wang, Cheng-Ling Lee and Hann-Chorng Kuo wrote the paper.

Abbreviations

OAB	overactive bladder
UAB	underactive bladder
PVR	post-void residual urine
DHIC	detrusor hyperactivity and impaired contractility
VE	voiding efficiency
AE	adverse events
Qmax	maximal flow rate
Vol	voided volume
BOO	bladder outlet obstruction
DM	diabetes mellitus
DU	detrusor underactivity

References

1. Milsom, I.; Kaplan, S.A.; Coyne, K.S.; Sexton, C.C.; Kopp, Z.S. Effect of bothersome overactive bladder symptoms on health-related quality of life, anxiety, depression, and treatment seeking in the United States: Results from EpiLUTS. *Urology* **2012**, *80*, 90–96. [CrossRef] [PubMed]

2. Osman, N.I.; Chapple, C.R.; Abrams, P.; Dmochowski, R.; Haab, F.; Nitti, V.; Koelbl, H.; van Kerrebroeck, P.; Wein, A.J. Detrusor underactivity and the underactive bladder: A new clinical entity? A review of current terminology, definitions, epidemiology, aetiology, and diagnosis. *Eur. Urol.* **2014**, *65*, 389–398. [CrossRef] [PubMed]
3. Thomas, A.W.; Cannon, A.; Bartlett, E.; Ellis-Jones, J.; Abrams, P. The natural history of lower urinary tract dysfunction in men: Minimum 10-year urodynamic follow-up of untreated detrusor underactivity. *BJU Int.* **2005**, *96*, 1295–1300. [CrossRef] [PubMed]
4. Chancellor, M.B. The overactive bladder progression to underactive bladder hypothesis. *Int. Urol. Nephrol.* **2014**, *46* (Suppl. 1), S23–S27. [CrossRef] [PubMed]
5. Oshiro, T.; Miyazato, M.; Saito, S. Relationship between connexin43-derived gap junction proteins in the bladder and age-related detrusor underactivity in rats. *Life Sci.* **2014**, *116*, 37–42. [CrossRef] [PubMed]
6. Daneshgari, F. Diabetic bladder dysfunction: Current translational knowledge. *J. Urol.* **2009**, *182*, S18–S26. [CrossRef] [PubMed]
7. Kuo, Y.C.; Kuo, H.C. Botulinum toxin injection for lower urinary tract dysfunction. *Int. J. Urol.* **2013**, *20*, 40–55. [CrossRef] [PubMed]
8. Liao, C.H.; Kuo, H.C. Increased risk of large post-void residual urine and decreased long-term success rate after intravesical onabotulinumtoxinA injection for refractory idiopathic detrusor overactivity. *J. Urol.* **2013**, *189*, 1804–1810. [CrossRef] [PubMed]
9. Kuo, H.C. Urodynamic evidence of effectiveness of botulinum A toxin injection in treatment of detrusor overactivity refractory to anticholinergic agents. *Urology* **2004**, *63*, 868–872. [CrossRef] [PubMed]
10. Miyazato, M.; Yoshimura, N.; Chancellor, M.B. The other bladder syndrome: Underactive bladder. *Rev. Urol.* **2013**, *15*, 11–20. [PubMed]
11. Yildirim, A.; Onol, F.F.; Haklar, G.; Tarcan, T. The role of free radicals and nitric oxide in the ischemia-reperfusion injury mediated by acute bladder outlet obstruction. *Int. Urol. Nephrol.* **2008**, *40*, 71–77. [CrossRef] [PubMed]
12. Wang, C.C.; Chancellor, M.B.; Lin, J.M.; Hsieh, J.H.; Yu, H.J. Type 2 diabetes but not metabolic syndrome is associated with an increased risk of lower urinary tract symptoms and erectile dysfunction in men aged <45 years. *BJU Int.* **2010**, *105*, 1136–1140. [PubMed]
13. Yu, H.J.; Lee, W.C.; Liu, S.P.; Tai, T.Y.; Wu, H.P.; Chen, J. Unrecognized voiding difficulty in female type 2 diabetic patients in the diabetes clinic: A prospective case-control study. *Diabetes Care* **2004**, *27*, 988–989. [CrossRef] [PubMed]
14. Gormley, E.A.; Lightner, D.J.; Burgio, K.L.; Chai, T.C.; Clemens, J.Q.; Culkin, D.J.; Das, A.K.; Foster, H.E., Jr.; Scarpero, H.M.; Tessier, C.D.; *et al.* Diagnosis and treatment of overactive bladder (non-neurogenic) in adults: AUA/SUFU guideline. *J. Urol.* **2012**, *188* (Suppl. 6), 2455–2463. [CrossRef] [PubMed]
15. Liu, S.; Chan, L.; Tse, V. Clinical outcome in male patients with detrusor overactivity with impaired contractility. *Int. Neurourol. J.* **2014**, *18*, 133–137. [CrossRef] [PubMed]
16. Schulte-Baukloh, H.; Weiss, C.; Stolze, T.; Herholz, J.; Stürzebecher, B.; Miller, K.; Knispel, H.H. Botulinum-A toxin detrusor and sphincter injection in treatment of overactive bladder syndrome: Objective outcome and patient satisfaction. *Eur. Urol.* **2005**, *48*, 984–990. [CrossRef] [PubMed]
17. Hsiao, S.M.; Lin, H.H.; Kuo, H.C. Factors associated with a better therapeutic effect of solifenacin in patients with overactive bladder syndrome. *Neurourol. Urodyn.* **2014**, *33*, 331–334. [CrossRef] [PubMed]
18. Hanna-Mitchell, A.T.; Ruiz, G.W.; Daneshgari, F.; Liu, G.; Apodaca, G.; Birder, L.A. Impact of diabetes mellitus on bladder uroepithelial cells. *Am. J. Physiol. Regul. Integr. Comp. Physiol.* **2013**, *304*, R84–R93. [CrossRef] [PubMed]
19. Abrams, P.; Cardozo, L.; Fall, M.; Griffiths, D.; Rosier, P.; Ulmsten, U.; van Kerrebroeck, P.; Victor, A.; Wein, A.; Standardisation Sub-committee of the International Continence Society. The standardisation of terminology of lower urinary tract function: Report from the Standardisation Sub-committee of the International Continence Society. *Neurourol. Urodyn.* **2002**, *21*, 167–178. [CrossRef] [PubMed]
20. Wang, C.C.; Yang, S.S.; Chen, Y.T.; Hsieh, J.H. Videourodynamics identifies the causes of young men with lower urinary tract symptoms and low uroflow. *Eur. Urol.* **2003**, *4*, 386–390. [CrossRef]
21. Nitti, V.W.; Lefkowitz, G.; Ficazzola, M.; Dixon, C.M. Lower urinary tract symptoms in young men: Video urodynamic findings and correlation with noninvasive measures. *J. Urol.* **2002**, *168*, 135–138. [CrossRef]

22. Jeong, S.J.; Kim, H.J.; Lee, Y.J.; Lee, B.K.; Choo, Y.M.; Oh, J.J.; Lee, S.C.; Jeong, C.W.; Yoon, C.Y.; Hong, S.K.; *et al.* Prevalence and clinical features of detrusor underactivity among elderly with lower urinary tract symptoms: A comparison between men and women. *Korean J. Urol.* **2012**, *53*, 342–348. [CrossRef] [PubMed]
23. Resnick, N.M.; Yalla, S.V.; Laurino, E. The pathophysiology of urinary incontinence among institutionalized elderly persons. *N. Engl. J. Med.* **1989**, *320*, 1–7. [CrossRef] [PubMed]
24. Kuo, H.C.; Liao, C.H.; Chung, S.D. Adverse events of intravesical botulinum toxin A injections for idiopathic detrusor overactivity: Risk factors and influence on treatment outcome. *Eur. Urol.* **2010**, *58*, 919–926. [CrossRef] [PubMed]
25. Wang, C.C.; Liao, C.H.; Kuo, H.C. Diabetes mellitus does not affect the efficacy and safety of intravesical onabotulinumtoxinA injection in patients with refractory detrusor overactivity. *Neurourol. Urodyn.* **2014**, *33*, 1235–1239. [CrossRef] [PubMed]

3

Use of Botulinum Toxin A in the Treatment of Lower Urinary Tract Disorders

David C. Moore *, Joshua A. Cohn and Roger R. Dmochowski

Department of Urologic Surgery, Vanderbilt University Medical Center, Nashville, TN 37232-2765, USA; joshua.cohn@vanderbilt.edu (J.A.C.); roger.dmochowski@vanderbilt.edu (R.R.D.)

* Correspondence: david.c.moore@vanderbilt.edu

Academic Editor: Hann-Chorng Kuo

Abstract: Botulinum neurotoxin (BoNT) is used to treat a variety of ailments, and its therapeutic application in lower urinary tract disorders (LUTDs) is well studied. Robust evidence supporting the efficacy and tolerability of BoNT in the treatment of neurogenic detrusor overactivity (NDO) and non-neurogenic overactive bladder (OAB) has led to regulatory approval for these conditions. Use of BoNT in the treatment of interstitial cystitis/bladder pain syndrome, chronic pelvic pain, and detrusor sphincter dyssynergia has demonstrated some promise, but is still evolving and off-label for these indications. Trials to date do not support the use of BoNT for benign prostatic hyperplasia. This comprehensive review outlines the mechanisms of BoNT in the treatment of LUTDs in adults and presents background and updated data examining the efficacy and adverse events associated with the use of BoNT in common urologic applications.

Keywords: botulinum toxin; overactive bladder; neurogenic bladder; benign prostatic hyperplasia; detrusor sphincter dyssynergia; interstitial cystitis

---

1. Introduction

Botulinum neurotoxin (BoNT) is formed by the Gram-positive, anaerobic spore forming bacteria *Clostridium botulinum* and is responsible for human botulism. Clinical applications of BoNT injections include chronic migraines, chronic pain, head and neck dystonias, strabismus, hyperhidrosis, anal fissures, and many others [1]. Use of BoNT in lower urinary tract disorders (LUTDs) was first studied by Dykstra *et al.* in 1988 for the treatment of detrusor external sphincter dyssynergia (DSD) [2]. Following this, investigations into the multiple urologic applications of BoNT amplified. This comprehensive review will focus on the mechanism of action of BoNT, urologic administration, safety, and the data supporting its applications in LUTDs most relevant to practicing urologists.

2. Botulinum Toxin and Mechanism of Action

BoNT exerts its activity by prohibiting the release of neurotransmitters from autonomic and somatic nerve endings. BoNT is the most potent known neurotoxin as measured by LD_{50}, a product of its unique structure and specificity. If even 1 g of the purified toxin were evenly dispersed and inhaled, it could kill 1 million people [3]. The active 150 kDa polypeptide has three separate domains with distinct functions: (1) the *C*-terminus, which binds pre-synaptic membranes, (2) the *N*-terminus (L-chain), a specific zinc endopeptidase and (3) the middle domain, which facilitates translocation of the L-chain into the cytosol [4]. Translocation of the toxin is correlated with synaptic activity and, thus, the most active nerves are preferentially affected [1].

The seven identified sub-types (A–G) of the L-chain are specific intracellular proteases, with BoNT-A used most commonly for therapeutic applications. BoNT-A cleaves synaptosomal-associated protein (SNAP-25), which is necessary for fusion of synaptic vesicles at the cellular membrane, thus specifically preventing the SNARE-mediated release of neurotransmitters into the synaptic cleft [3]. BoNT-A prevents the release of several neurotransmitters (acetylcholine, adenosine triphosphate (ATP) substance P), as well as downregulates purinergic and capsaicin receptors on afferent neurons, all of which have been implicated in the pathophysiology of NDO and OAB [5,6].

BoNT-A binds with high affinity to synaptic vesicle protein 2 (SV2) and, thus, its activity is limited to cells that express this receptor. Immunofluorescent studies of the healthy human bladder have demonstrated SV2 expression in nearly all cholinergic parasympathetic fibers, half of sensory fibers, and none in urothelial or muscular cells [7]. Likewise, the effect of BoNT-A has been postulated to involve both efferent, parasympathetic pathways and afferent, nociceptive pathways. BoNT does not cause neuronal death, and the effect is temporary as the toxin is inactivated and degraded with time [8]. The commercially available BoNT-A preparations are Botox® (onabotulinumtoxin A, Allergan Pharmaceuticals, Parsippany-Troy Hills, NJ, USA), Dysport® (abobotulinumtoxinA, Ipson Biopharm, Paris, France), and Xeomin® (IncobotulinumtoxinA, Merz Pharmaceuticals, Frankfurt am Main, Germany). While no clinical dose conversion studies exist, it is generally accepted that one unit of onabotulinumtoxin A (onaBoNT-A) is equivalent to 3–5 units of abobotulinumtoxin A (aboBoNT-A) based on comparative effectiveness [9–11]. There are too few studies using incobotulinumtoxin A to speculate on dose equivalence.

3. Administration and Injection Technique

BoNT-A is administered via intradetrusor injection under local, regional or general anesthesia using a rigid or flexible cystoscope. This procedure can be completed safely in the clinical setting for most patients, although select patients, including those at risk for autonomic dysreflexia, should have closer monitoring in an operative suite. While no protocol regarding the location and number of injections is universally accepted, a technique using a flexible cystoscope with an ultrafine needle has been previously described and adopted by these authors and others [12–14]. Ten to thirty minutes prior to injection, 30 mg of 2% lidocaine are instilled into the bladder. For Food and Drug Administration approved indications, 100 U onaBoNT-A diluted in 10 mL preservative-free saline (OAB) or 200 U onaBoNT-A diluted in 20 mL preservative-free saline (NDO) are then injected 1 mL per site separated by a distance of 1 to 1.5 cm. Locations of injections for other indications are described separately.

The increasing evidence of BoNT-A effect on sensory nerves has led to increased focus on trigonal and suburothelial injections. Injections to the trigone have traditionally been spared out of concern for producing vesicoureteral reflux (VUR). Despite this, several studies have shown trigonal injections to be safe and effective without evidence of VUR [15,16]. However, a recent meta-analysis comparing trigonal and extratrigonal injection technique in patients with NDO and idiopathic detrusor overactivity (IDO) found no significant differences with regard to adverse effects or short-term efficacy, suggesting that patient-specific factors and dosing likely matter more for response to BoNT-A than location of injection [17].

As intravesical injection of BoNT-A is invasive and procedurally time-consuming, alternative strategies for topical administration of BoNT-A are being investigated [18]. Given the toxin's large size, topical application does not permit access to submucosal nerve endings. However, a recent double-blind, placebo-controlled, multicenter trial of liposome-encapsulated onaBoNT-A, an intravesical instillation, has shown statistically significant reductions in OAB symptom scores, micturition frequency, and urgency episodes at four weeks [19]. Such administration may reduce the risk of hematuria, pain, urinary retention, and urinary tract infection (UTI). While the depth of penetration of liposomal-encapsulated onaBoNT-A is yet unknown, this preparation is assumed to reach only the urothelium and suburothelium. Its efficacy supports the theory that BoNT-A does not solely block acetylcholine at parasympathetic nerve endings, and its action is at least partially mediated by urothelial cells or suburothelial afferent nerves [20].

4. Safety

Despite the incredible potency of BoNT, the toxin is highly specific for peripheral nerves and does not spread from its site of local injection in significant quantities to cause systemic symptoms [1]. Systemic BoNT toxicity is rare, often associated with higher doses or underlying disease [21]. Signs include impaired vision, extremity weakness, dry mouth, dysphagia, and constipation. Absolute contraindications to BoNT use include active urinary tract infection and hypersensitivity to the toxin or its components. Relative contraindications to BoNT injection include pregnancy, motor neuropathies, and concomitant use of drugs that affect the neuromuscular junction (*i.e.*, aminoglycosides). The most common adverse events (AEs) following BoNT injection in LUTD will be reviewed as relevant to each indication.

5. Neurogenic Detrusor Overactivity

Patients with NDO often have severe OAB symptoms with incontinence, and are at risk for elevated detrusor pressures and decreased compliance with associated potential for upper urinary tract deterioration. Ideal candidates for BoNT-A exhibit symptoms of OAB and urge urinary incontinence (UUI), are resistant to or intolerant of anticholinergics, are willing and able to perform clean intermittent catheterization (CIC), and do not have markedly elevated detrusor leak point pressures (DLPPs) or severely decreased detrusor compliance. The most robust data supporting the use of BoNT-A in NDO comes from two double-blind, placebo-controlled, phase-three studies, which were conducted after several phase-two studies demonstrated efficacy in this setting [22,23]. These two pivotal studies by Cruz *et al.* and Ginsberg *et al.* will be discussed together, as their data has previously been pooled for analysis [24–26].

A total of 691 patients with either multiple sclerosis (MS) or spinal cord injury (SCI) who had >14 episodes of urinary incontinence (UI) per week were included. Patients must have first experienced intolerance or inefficacy of an appropriately-dosed anticholinergic for >1 month duration. Patients on these medications were permitted to continue them at a constant dose, while those who had discontinued them remained off anticholinergic therapy. Patients were then randomized to receive 30 × 1 mL trigone-sparing injections of onaBoNT-A 200 U, 300 U, or placebo. The primary endpoint was change in UI episodes per week, and secondary outcomes included urodynamics (UDS) findings and Incontinence Quality of Life (I-QOL) score.

There were statistically significant decreases in UI episodes per week in the 200 U (−22.6 MS, −19.6 SCI) and 300 U (−24.0 MS, −18.2 SCI) groups when compared to placebo (−14.0 MS, −6.4 SCI). The percentage of patients who were dry at six weeks also increased with 200 U (41.5% MS, 30.9% SCI) and 300 U (44.2% MS, 35.9% SCI) when compared to placebo (10.7% MS, 7.3% SCI). There was also a reduction in the number of voluntary voids per week in the MS population who were not performing CIC prior to onaBoNT-A. Both MS and SCI patients noted significant increases in their I-QOL scores compared to placebo [26].

Repeat UDS studies were performed six weeks after injection, which are reported here as the range of values taken from both studies. Patients treated with 200 U and 300 U showed increased maximum cystometric capacity (MCC) compared to placebo (151 to 157 mL, 157.2 to 168 mL and 6.5 to 18 mL, respectively). Patients also experienced significant reductions in the number of involuntary detrusor contractions (IDC), and for those with IDO, the maximum detrusor pressure during first IDC ($P_{detmaxIDC}$) was reduced (−28.5 to −35.1 cm/H20, −26.9 to −33.3 cm/H20, −2.4 to 7.9 cm/H20 for 200 U, 300 U and placebo, respectively). Data regarding detrusor compliance were not available. These urodynamic findings were similar among both etiologies, although patients with SCI experienced a greater reduction in $P_{detmaxIDC}$ which is significant when considering long-term risk of upper urinary tract damage.

The most frequent AE was UTI across all patients, which was defined by positive urine culture; the authors did not differentiate asymptomatic bacteriuria from symptomatic infections. In SCI patients, the reported incidence of UTI was similar between onaBoNT-A and placebo (44.8% and 49.5%, respectively). However, among patients with MS there was a significantly increased rate of UTI in the treatment (53.5%) *versus* placebo (29.2%) groups. This difference is possibly secondary to increased rates of urinary retention among treated patients. Most patients with SCI already performed CIC prior to treatment. However, in MS patients, need for CIC after treatment was 40% with 200 U and 51% with 300 U, compared to 17% with placebo. Among those initiating CIC, average frequency was 2.5 times per day, and patient satisfaction was not impacted by need for CIC [26].

To evaluate long-term efficacy of onaBoNT-A injections for NDO, Kennely *et al.* conducted a three-year, prospective, multicenter extension study on 396 of the original study patients [27,28]. The extension study demonstrated sustained improvements in UI episodes per week and I-QOL score. The number of new patients initiating CIC decreased dramatically with each treatment; patients who did not require CIC after three treatments never went on CIC. Reported AEs and AE rates were similar, and no new safety concerns were raised. With 200 U dosing, the median duration of treatment effect was nine months. One small study evaluated 26 patients who had undergone a mean 7.1 BoNT-A injections and found that 26% went on to require definitive surgical treatment for their neurogenic bladder, suggesting that efficacy may decline with repeated injections [29].

Kennely, Cruz and Ginsberg found no statistically significant differences in efficacy between 200 U and 300 U onaBoNT-A, and a placebo-controlled, dose-response study in patients with 50, 100, and 200 U onaBoNT-A noted 200 U to be the most effective dose [30]. This has led to the approval of onaBoNT-A injections for NDO at a starting dose of 200 U by the FDA and similar recommendations by other international consensus agencies [31]. The majority of studies, thus far, have focused on onaBoNT-A; however, limited randomized, placebo-controlled, double-blind studies utilizing aboBoNT-A have demonstrated efficacy with this preparation as well [32,33].

6. Non-Neurozgenic Overactive Bladder

Non-neurogenic Overactive Bladder is a symptom complex defined by "urinary urgency, usually accompanied by frequency and nocturia, with or without urgency urinary incontinence, in the absence of UTI or other obvious pathology" [34,35]. While not life-threatening, OAB is a chronic condition and can have a profound impacts on health-related quality of life [36]. First line treatment is behavioral therapy, and second line treatment options include a multitude of anti-muscarinics and β_3 adrenoceptor agonists [35]. BoNT-A is considered third line therapy, reserved for patients with moderate to severe OAB symptoms who fail first and second line therapies and are willing to tolerate the risk of having to perform CIC.

Initial efficacy of BoNT-A in the treatment of OAB was demonstrated by several randomized, multi-center, double-blinded trials [37–39]. The largest of these, a phase-two dose-ranging study by Dmochowski *et al.* [38], compared 50 U, 100 U, 150 U, 200 U, and 300 U onaBoNT-A to placebo. Doses of 100 U or greater resulted in durable improvements in UUI episodes per week, as well as other OAB symptoms. Doses of 150 U or greater did not result in differences in efficacy relative to 100 U dosing and were associated with dose-dependent increases in post-void residual (PVR) up to 200 U. A PVR of 200 mL or greater seemed to be highly correlated with need for CIC, as well as AEs including UTI and urinary retention.

Phase-two trials demonstrating the efficacy and tolerability of 100 U onaBoNT-A subsequently led to two large, double-blind, placebo-controlled, phase-three studies. Results from these two pivotal studies by Chapple *et al.* and Nitti *et al.* were subsequently pooled for analysis [40–42]. A total of 1097 patients with $\geqslant$3 UUI episodes per three days and $\geqslant$8 micturitions per day were randomized to receive 20 $\times$ 0.5 mL trigone sparing injections of onaBoNT-A 100 U or placebo into the detrusor. All patients had failed anticholinergic therapy, with the majority of patients (82.2%) demonstrating inadequate efficacy and a smaller percentage suffering intolerable side effects. OAB symptoms were recorded in patient diaries, and perceptions of treatment benefit were rated on the Treatment Benefit Scale (TBS) at follow-up.

At 12 weeks, the onaBoNT-A arm demonstrated significant improvements in UUI episodes per day relative to placebo (−2.80 *vs.* −0.95; $p < 0.001$). Additionally, 60.5% of patients experienced >50% improvement in UUI, and 27.1% achieved 100% improvement (continence). Positive response on the TBS was significantly higher after treatment when compared to placebo (61.8% *vs.* 28.0%; $p < 0.001$). Patients on active treatment also experienced significant improvements relative to placebo in daily episodes of urgency and frequency. On sub-group analysis, these effects persisted despite the number of prior anticholinergics used or the reason for discontinuation of medical therapy [42]. The median duration of effect among treated patients was 24 weeks.

The most common AE was UTI (25.5% onaBoNT-A *vs.* 9.6% placebo), defined by a positive urine culture (10^5 cfu/mL), regardless of symptoms. Other significant AEs were dysuria (10.9% onaBoNT-A *vs.* 7.0% placebo), bacteruria (8.0% *vs.* 3.5%) and urinary retention (5.8% *vs.* 0.4%), which was defined as a PVR ⩾200 mL. Patients were started on CIC for PVR ⩾ 200 mL with symptoms or PVR > 350 mL regardless of symptoms.. Overall, rates of CIC were low (6.5% onaBoNT-A *vs.* 0.4% placebo), with similar numbers requiring CIC for ⩽6 weeks and >12 weeks (2.5% and 2.7%, respectively).

A separate dose ranging, randomized controlled trial (RCT) by Rovner *et al.* obtained baseline UDS in all patients followed by repeat measurements at 12 and 36 weeks post treatment [43]. 76.0% of enrolled patients had demonstrable detrusor overactivity (DO) on baseline UDS. Relative to placebo, patients treated with 100 U onaBoNT-A showed increased MCC at 12 weeks (+71.0 mL *vs.* 49.5 mL). Significant increases in detrusor compliance at MCC or prior to terminal IDC were noted at week 12 (+63.0 *vs.* −22.8 mL/cm H_2O). No difference in efficacy was noted between patients who had demonstrated DO on UDS *vs.* those who did not. In patients with urodynamic DO, there were similar reductions in proportion with demonstrable DO at week 12 between patients on treatment *vs.* placebo (34.9% *vs.* 31.4%). Similar results were observed with regard to detrusor pressure at first IDC. Thus, while some UDS parameters are improved following onaBoNT-A treatment for OAB, the clinical utility of these findings is unclear. Consequently, routine UDS testing in patients with OAB is not required prior to treatment with BoNT-A.

To determine the difference in efficacy between therapies, Visco *et al.* conducted a double-blind, double-placebo-controlled RCT comparing anticholinergic therapy (AT) to BoNT-A injections [44]. 249 women with an average 5.0 UUI episodes/3 day were randomized to receive oral AT + intravesical placebo injections or 100 U onaBoNT-A + oral placebo. Episodes of UUI improved in both AT and onaBoNT-A groups (3.4 *vs.* 3.3 per day, respectively) as did QOL. More patients treated with BoNT-A experienced resolution of UUI (27% *vs.* 13%, $p = 0.003$). At six months, the majority of patients in both arms had adequate control of symptoms (71% AT *vs.* 70% onaBoNT-A). When comparing adverse events, AT patients were more likely to experience dry mouth (46% *vs.* 31%), but less likely to experience UTI (13% *vs.* 33%) and require CIC (0% *vs.* 5%). Thus, 100 U onaBoNT-A has comparable efficacy to AT in the treatment of OAB, albeit with higher rates of complete continence.

To evaluate long-term efficacy of onaBoNT-A injections for OAB, Mohee *et al.* conducted a seven-year retrospective evaluation of 137 patients treated with onaBoNT-A at a single center [45]. Patients were initially treated with 200 U, which was subsequently lowered as guidelines emerged. The mean re-treatment interval was eight months, but the majority of patients (61.3%) discontinued treatment at 36 months. The principal reason for discontinuing treatment were intolerance of side effects (need for CIC, urinary retention, UTIs). Younger patients and those with persistent incontinence were more likely to discontinue treatment. In small retrospective series, Smits *et al.* evaluated patients who had failed BoNT-A treatment for OAB referred for sacral neuromodulation (SNM) and noted treatment efficacy of SNM in 70% (14/20) of patients, suggesting a role for SNM in patients who are unable or do not wish to continue therapy with BoNT-A [46].

These data demonstrate conclusive efficacy for onaBoNT-A as a treatment option for refractory OAB. While the longevity of treatment response may be limited, it does not appear to compromise success of neuromodulation. While most studies, thus far, have focused on onaBoNT-A, one small study does demonstrate efficacy of aboBoNT-A [47]. Taken together, these findings have led to FDA approval of onaBoNT-A injections for patients with OAB who have failed second line therapy at a starting dose of 100 U, with similar recommendations by other international consensus agencies [31,35].

7. Benign Prostatic Hyperplasia

Use of BoNT-A for benign prostatic hyperplasia (BPH) was first investigated by Maria *et al.* in 2003 [48]. This placebo-controlled RCT compared 30 patients receiving 200 U onaBoNT-A or saline via perineal intraprostatic injection. The authors noted a statistically significant 65% reduction in American Urological Association symptom score (AUA-SS) and 51% reduction in PSA values in the treatment group. Several other small studies reported improvements in symptom scores and flow rates [49–51]. Crawford *et al.* subsequently conducted a double-blinded RCT comparing 100 U to 300 U onaBoNT-A injected transrectally under ultrasound guidance [52]. None of the 134 patients randomized were on medical therapy at time of treatment; both doses demonstrated significant improvements in AUA-SS and flow rates.

As a follow-up to these initial investigations, Marberger *et al.* and McVary *et al.* conducted two large randomized, placebo-controlled trials on 492 total patients with peak flow rates <15 mL/s and International Prostate Symptom Score (IPSS) >12 [53,54]. Marberger compared 100 U, 200 U, and 300 U onaBoNT-A via perineal or transrectal administration, whereas McVary administered 200 U under transrectal guidance. The procedure was well tolerated, with the most common AEs being hematuria and hematospermia.

Both studies reported significant improvement in symptom scores and flow rates from baseline after injection; however, there were no differences between the treatment and placebo arms. A recent meta-analysis of the three placebo controlled trials also corroborated this profound placebo effect, asserting no benefit for onaBoNT-A in the treatment of BPH [55]. Thus, studies to date do not support the use of onaBoNT-A as first-line treatment for BPH, and it is not included in the most updated AUA guidelines [56]. Nevertheless, small separate sub-analyses did demonstrate improvement in flow rates in patients on concurrent medical therapy (McVary), and improvements in symptom scores in patients who had been treated previously with alpha-blockers (Marberger). Consequently, there may yet be a subset of patients on maximal medical management and poor candidates for surgical intervention who may benefit from intraprostatic onaBoNT-A injection. An ongoing RCT comparing onaBoNT-A to optimized medical therapy (the PROTOX study) may provide additional details [57].

8. Interstitial Cystitis/Bladder Pain Syndrome

The Interstitial Cystitis/Bladder Pain Syndrome (IC/BPS) complex is defined as "an unpleasant sensation (pain, pressure, discomfort) perceived to be related to the urinary bladder, associated with lower urinary tract symptoms of more than six weeks duration, in the absence of infection or other identifiable causes" [58]. No standardized treatment regimen exists, as patient response is highly variable to a multitude of therapies, including behavioral modification, physical therapy, pharmacologic agents, and surgical treatments such as cystoscopy with hydrodistention (HD) or fulguration of Hunner's lesions, sacral neuromodulation and cystectomy. BoNT-A injections were first used after several observational studies reported efficacy in this patient population [59–61]. Several follow-up prospective studies reported efficacy of onaBoNT-A, often in conjunction with hydrodistention, for the treatment of IC/BPS [62–65]. As these studies varied in their injection locations and inclusion criteria, consensus opinion remained elusive.

Two RCTs were subsequently conducted to further delineate which patients might benefit from BoNT-A. The first by Kuo and Chancellor compared onaBoNT-A injections to the posterior and lateral bladder walls + HD two weeks later at doses of 100 U and 200 U to HD alone [66]. Enrolled patients ($N = 67$) had failed conventional treatments and remained on pentosan sulfate throughout the trial. Success of onaBoNT-A + HD based on global response assessment (GRA) at three months was 80% in the 200 U arm and 72% in the 100 U arm, compared to 48% for HD alone. Only patients treated with onaBoNT-A demonstrated improvements in bladder pain visual analog scale (VAS) and MCC.

These effects diminished by 12 and 24 months. Importantly, rates of AEs (dysuria, elevated PVRs) were higher in the 200 U group, despite no significant difference in efficacy.

Kuo *et al.* followed this study with a double-blind, placebo-controlled multicenter trial randomizing 60 patients to 20 × 0.5 mL suburothelial injections to the posterior and lateral bladder wall of either 100 U onaBoNT-A or saline immediately followed by HD [67]. All patients had failed six months of conventional therapy, and ulcerative forms of IC/PBS were excluded. At 8 weeks, the onaBoNT-A group demonstrated a significant reduction in VAS compared to placebo (−2.6 *vs.* −0.9; $p = 0.02$). MCC was also increased in onaBoNT-A treated patients (+67.8 *vs.* −45.4; $p = 0.020$), however, other UDS metrics as well as GRA and subjective symptoms of frequency/nocturia did not differ between treatment arms. The most common AEs were dysuria (40%), UTI (5%) and urinary retention (2.5%). This AE profile, including the uncommon need for CIC, is corroborated by other studies [62,64,68]. While larger placebo-controlled trials will be required for FDA approval, these early trials suggest potential efficacy of 100 U onaBoNT-A for the treatment of IC/BPS. Subsequently, the AUA recommends onaBoNT-A at a starting dose of 100 U as a fourth-line treatment option for IC/BPS in patients willing to CIC and refractory to other treatment modalities [69]. As IC/BPS is widely varied in its presentation and symptomatology, it would follow that certain patients would be more likely to respond to BoNT-A therapy. This should be a focus of future studies.

9. Chronic Pelvic Pain

Chronic pelvic pain (CPP) in men and women is defined by chronic or persistent pain for at least six months duration perceived to originate in the organs of the pelvis [70]. Chronic prostatitis/chronic pelvic pain syndrome (CP/CPPS) and IC/BPS all fall within the spectrum of CPP, each defined by pain referred specifically to the respective organs. Treatment is varied and includes psychological counseling, multimodal pharmacologic analgesia, biofeedback and pelvic floor physiotherapy, among others. The pathophysiology of CPP is unclear but likely involves pelvic floor muscle (PFM) tenderness and spasm, as well as chronic central nervous system hypersensitivity and neurogenic inflammation [71–73]. Consequently, BoNT-A has been investigated as a treatment modality given its unique ability to target these pathways.

Efficacy of BoNT-A in the treatment of CP/CPPS was first investigated in small studies reporting relief of prostate pain and urethral hyperalgesia after transurethral perisphincteric injection of 200 U onaBoNT-A [74]. Later, a small placebo controlled RCT showed modest improvements in pain scores after injection of 100 U onaBoNT-A into the perineal body and bulbospongiosus muscle [75]. Subsequently, a double-blind, placebo-controlled RCT was conducted to evaluate BoNT use in men with CP/CPS refractory to 4–6 weeks of conventional medical therapy [76]. Enrolled patients ($N = 60$) were randomized to receive transurethral intraprostatic injection of 100 U onaBoNT-A or saline. Treated patients demonstrated significant improvements in National Institutes of Health Chronic Prostatitis Symptom Index (NIH-CPSI) total and subscale scores, AUA-SS, QOL scores, urinary frequency and nocturia compared to placebo. Most notably at six months, marked improvement in VAS scores (82.2% lower *vs.* 2.4% higher) and NIH-CPSI pain scores (79.97% lower *vs.* 4.7% higher) were seen in patients receiving onaBoNT-A compared to placebo, respectively. No major AEs were observed, with transient hematuria noted in only two patients. Another small uncontrolled randomized trial recently showed improved efficacy with transrectal ultrasound guided BoNT-A injection compared to transurethral injection [77]. A phase-two study of 40 men with CP/CPS is currently underway comparing 300 U onaBoNT-A to 1% lidocaine (ClinicalTrials.gov identifier: NCT00529386).

BoNT-A use in the treatment of CPP in women, specifically PFM spasm, has received limited study. Jarvis *et al.* first reported efficacy of 40 U onaBoNT-A injected into the puborectalis and pubococcygeus muscles under conscious sedation in 12 women with CPP [78]. Subsequently, Abott *et al.* conducted a double-blind, placebo-controlled RCT in women with CPP >2 years duration and evidence of pelvic muscle spasm [79]. Patients ($N = 60$) were randomized to receive 80 U onaBoNT-A (20 U/mL) or saline in four 1 mL injections to PFMs as described previously. Treated patients showed improvements in dyspareunia and nonmenstrual pelvic pain, whereas the placebo arm showed only improvement in dyspareunia. Patients treated with onaBoNT-A demonstrated a larger decrease in pelvic floor pressure compared to placebo. Two patients developed incontinence after treatment, and no AEs were observed in the placebo arm.

More recently, an open-label, prospective pilot study investigated electromyography (EMG) guided onaBoNT-A injections in 21 women with CPP [80]. Using this technique, a needle attached to an EMG electrode is used to localize spastic PFMs and target these sites for injection, potentially using up to 300 U onaBoNT-A in total. The majority of patients noted improvement in QOL scores, and 83.3% reported improvement in dyspareunia at 24 weeks. Resting vaginal pressures also decreased, and less point tenderness was noted on physical exam of the PFMs. Significant AEs were constipation (28.6%), UI (4.8%) and fecal incontinence (4.8%). A systemic review of these studies and others also reported benefit of onaBoNT-A in patients with CPP related to PFM spasm [81].

While small in number, these preliminary studies suggest efficacy of BoNT-A injections for the treatment of CPP. As this is a heterogenous condition, it is not surprising that reported injection locations, methods and dosages are highly variable. Larger RCTs are needed to standardize treatments for these various indications. Further research will elucidate which pathophysiologic parameters are being affected by BoNT-A injection and identify subsets of patients most likely to benefit from therapy.

10. Detrusor Sphincter Dyssynergia

Detrusor Sphincter Dyssynergia (DSD) refers to spastic and uncoordinated contraction of the external sphincter upon voiding seen in many patients with SCI and MS. Dysfunctional voiding can lead to incomplete emptying, thus increasing the risks of UTI and upper urinary tract damage. While often managed with CIC and less commonly sphincterotomy, BoNT-A injection into the external sphincter was one of the earliest urologic indications evaluated [2,82,83]. Subsequently, multiple small observational studies demonstrated efficacy of 100 U onaBoNT-A for treatment of DSD when injected via transurethral, transrectal or transperineal routes [84–87]. An small RCT (N = 13) comparing 100 U onaBoNT-A to lidocaine in SCI patients with DSD showed improvements in PVR at 30 days after treatment (−159.4 mL after onaBoNT-A *vs.* −49.8 mL after lidocaine), although mean post-treatment PVR remained elevated at 105 mL [88]. The authors noted improvements in mean urethral pressure (MUP) and other objective measurements of DSD. A recent meta-analysis of these studies in patients with SCI noted a mean PVR decrease from 251.8 to 153.0 mL after treatment with BoNT-A lasting up to six months, as well as a reduction in UTIs and CIC in some series [89]. AEs described in these studies have been minimal.

Similarly, Gallien *et al.* conducted a multi-center, double-blind RCT comparing 100 U onaBoNT-A to placebo via single transperineal injection in patients with MS [90]. Enrolled patients (N = 86) had MS with DSD and elevated PVRs (100–500 mL). At 30 days, there was no difference in PVR between treatment and placebo, but those treated with onaBoNT-A did demonstrate increased voiding volume (+54%, p = 0.02), pre-micturition P_{det} (229%, p = 0.02) and maximal P_{det} (221%, p = 0.02). Several heterogenous small studies have demonstrated efficacy of onaBoNT-A injections in reducing PVR in patients with SCI and DSD, an effect that was not observed in patients with MS. This may be explained by differences in study design, pathophysiology of these disease states, and/or the sex distribution of patients with these conditions (*i.e.*, SCI patients are majority male, MS majority female). Although quality data are lacking, onaBoNT-A injections to the external sphincter appear to be a reasonable short-term treatment option for patients with DSD [91]. Further research is needed before more definitive recommendations can be made.

11. Conclusions

Evidence for the use of BoNT-A, specifically onaBoNT-A, in the treatment of LUTDs continues to accumulate. Multiple robust, well-designed trials have demonstrated clear efficacy of BoNT-A in the treatment of NDO and OAB, subsequently leading to FDA approval of onaBoNT-A for these conditions and widespread clinical use. Studies to date do not support the use of BoNT-A in the treatment of BPH. Although evidence is limited, existing data suggest BoNT-A may be a promising option for some patients with CPP and IC/BPS. Similarly, small studies demonstrate safety and efficacy of BoNT-A use in the treatment of DSD, but certainly larger, well-designed RCTs are needed. As this field rapidly evolves, future research will focus on efficacy in non-approved indications, alternative delivery systems, and elucidating the histophysiologic changes in LUTDs in relation to the BoNT-A mechanism of action.

Author Contributions: Roger R. Dmochowski conceived of the project. David C. Moore, Joshua A. Cohn and Roger R. Dmochowski wrote the paper.

Abbreviations

The following abbreviations are used in this manuscript:

aboBoNT-A	abobotulinumtoxin A
AE	adverse event
AT	anticholinergic therapy
AUA-SS	American Urologic Association symptom scores
BoNT	Botulinum neurotoxin
BPH	benign prostatic hyperplasia
CIC	clean intermittent catheterization
CP/CPPS	chronic prostatitis/chronic pelvic pain syndrome
CPP	chronic pelvic pain
DLPPs	Detrusor leak point pressures
DO	detrusor overactivity
DSD	Detrusor Sphincter Dyssynergia
EMG	electromyography
GRA	global response assessment
HD	hydrodistention
I-QOL	Incontinence Quality of Life
IC/BPS	Interstitial Cystitis/Bladder Pain Syndrome
IDC	involuntary detrusor contractions
IDO	idiopathic detrusor overactivity
IPSS	International Prostate Symptom Score
LUTDs	lower urinary tract disorders
MCC	maximum cystometric capacity
MS	multiple sclerosis
MUP	mean urethral pressure
NDO	neuropathic detrusor overactivity
NIH-CPSI	National Institutes of Health Chronic Prostatitis Symptom Index
onaBoNT-A	onabotulinumtoxin A
$P_{detmaxIDC}$	maximum detrusor pressure during first IDC
PFM	pelvic floor muscle
PVR	post void residual
RCT	randomized controlled trial
SCI	spinal cord injury
SNM	sacral neuromodulation
SV2	synaptic vesicle protein 2

TBS	Treatment Benefit Scale
UDS	urodynamics
UI	urinary incontinence
UTI	urinary tract infection
UUI	urge urinary incontinence
VAS	visual analog scale
VUR	vesicoureteral reflux

References

1. Montecucco, C.; Molgó, J. Botulinal neurotoxins: Revival of an old killer. *Curr. Opin. Pharmacol.* **2005**, *5*, 274–279. [CrossRef] [PubMed]
2. Dykstra, D.D.; Sidi, A.A.; Scott, A.B.; Pagel, J.M.; Goldish, G.D. Effects of botulinum A toxin on detrusor-sphincter dyssynergia in spinal cord injury patients. *J. Urol.* **1988**, *139*, 919–922. [PubMed]
3. Harper, M.; Fowler, C.J.; Dasgupta, P. Botulinum toxin and its applications in the lower urinary tract. *BJU Int.* **2004**, *93*, 702–706. [CrossRef] [PubMed]
4. Simpson, L.L. Molecular pharmacology of botulinum toxin and tetanus toxin. *Ann. Rev. Pharmacol. Toxicol.* **1986**, *26*, 427–453. [CrossRef] [PubMed]
5. Yoshimura, N. Bladder afferent pathway and spinal cord injury: Possible mechanisms inducing hyperreflexia of the urinary bladder. *Prog. Neurobiol.* **1999**, *57*, 583–606. [CrossRef]
6. Chapple, C.; Patel, A. Botulinum toxin—New mechanisms, new therapeutic directions? *Eur. Urol.* **2006**, *49*, 606–608. [CrossRef] [PubMed]
7. Coelho, A.; Dinis, P.; Pinto, R.; Gorgal, T.; Silva, C.; Silva, A.; Silva, J.; Cruz, C.D.; Cruz, F.; Avelino, A. Distribution of the high-affinity binding site and intracellular target of botulinum toxin type A in the human bladder. *Eur. Urol.* **2010**, *57*, 884–890. [CrossRef] [PubMed]
8. Mangera, A.; Andersson, K.E.; Apostolidis, A.; Chapple, C.; Dasgupta, P.; Giannantoni, A.; Gravas, S.; Madersbacher, S. Contemporary management of lower urinary tract disease with botulinum toxin A: A systematic review of botox (onabotulinumtoxinA) and dysport (abobotulinumtoxinA). *Eur. Urol.* **2011**, *60*, 784–795. [CrossRef] [PubMed]
9. Sampaio, C.; Ferreira, J.J.; Simões, F.; Rosas, M.J.; Magalhães, M.; Correia, A.P.; Bastos-Lima, A.; Martins, R.; Castro-Caldas, A. DYSBOT: A single-blind, randomized parallel study to determine whether any differences can be detected in the efficacy and tolerability of two formulations of botulinum toxin type A—Dysport and Botox—Assuming a ratio of 4:1. *Mov. Disord.* **1997**, *12*, 1013–1018. [CrossRef] [PubMed]
10. Odergren, T.; Hjaltason, H.; Kaakkola, S.; Solders, G.; Hanko, J.; Fehling, C.; Marttila, R.J.; Lundh, H.; Gedin, S.; Westergren, I.; *et al.* A double blind, randomised, parallel group study to investigate the dose equivalence of Dysport and Botox in the treatment of cervical dystonia. *J. Neurol. Neurosurg. Psychiatr.* **1998**, *64*, 6–12. [CrossRef] [PubMed]
11. Ranoux, D.; Gury, C.; Fondarai, J.; Mas, J.L.; Zuber, M. Respective potencies of Botox and Dysport: A double blind, randomised, crossover study in cervical dystonia. *J. Neurol. Neurosurg. Psychiatry* **2002**, *72*, 459–462. [PubMed]
12. Smith, C.P.; Chancellor, M.B. Simplified bladder botulinum-toxin delivery technique using flexible cystoscope and 10 sites of injection. *J. Endourol.* **2005**, *19*, 880–882. [CrossRef] [PubMed]
13. Popat, R.; Apostolidis, A.; Kalsi, V.; Gonzales, G.; Fowler, C.J.; Dasgupta, P. A comparison between the response of patients with idiopathic detrusor overactivity and neurogenic detrusor overactivity to the first intradetrusor injection of botulinum-A toxin. *J. Urol.* **2005**, *174*, 984–989. [CrossRef] [PubMed]
14. Apostolidis, A.; Dasgupta, P.; Denys, P.; Elneil, S. Recommendations on the use of botulinum toxin in the treatment of lower urinary tract disorders and pelvic floor dysfunctions: A european consensus report. *Eur. Urol.* **2009**, *55*, 100–120. [CrossRef] [PubMed]
15. Kuo, H.-C. Comparison of effectiveness of detrusor, suburothelial and bladder base injections of botulinum toxin A for idiopathic detrusor overactivity. *J. Urol.* **2007**, *178*, 1359–1363. [CrossRef] [PubMed]

16. Karsenty, G.; Elzayat, E.; Delapparent, T.; St-Denis, B. Botulinum toxin type a injections into the trigone to treat idiopathic overactive bladder do not induce vesicoureteral reflux. *J. Urol.* **2007**, *177*, 1011–1014. [CrossRef] [PubMed]
17. Davis, N.F.; Burke, J.P.; Redmond, E.J.; Elamin, S.; Brady, C.M.; Flood, H.D. Trigonal *versus* extratrigonal botulinum toxin-A: A systematic review and meta-analysis of efficacy and adverse events. *Int. Urogynecol. J.* **2015**, *26*, 313–319. [CrossRef] [PubMed]
18. Kuo, H.C.; Liu, H.T.; Chuang, Y.C.; Birder, L.A.; Chancellor, M.B. Pilot study of liposome-encapsulated onabotulinumtoxina for patients with overactive bladder: A single-center study. *Eur. Urol.* **2014**, *65*, 1117–1124. [CrossRef] [PubMed]
19. Chuang, Y.C.; Kaufmann, J.H.; Chancellor, D.D.; Chancellor, M.B.; Kuo, H.C. Bladder instillation of liposome encapsulated onabotulinumtoxina improves overactive bladder symptoms: A prospective, multicenter, double-blind, randomized trial. *J. Urol.* **2014**, *192*, 1743–1749. [CrossRef] [PubMed]
20. Michel, M.C. OnabotulinumtoxinA: How deep will it go? *Eur. Urol.* **2014**, *65*, 1125–1127. [CrossRef] [PubMed]
21. Nuanthaisong, U.; Abraham, N.; Goldman, H.B. Incidence of adverse events after high doses of onabotulinumtoxinA for multiple indications. *Urology* **2014**, *84*, 1044–1048. [CrossRef] [PubMed]
22. Schurch, B.; de Sèze, M.; Denys, P.; Chartier-Kastler, E.; Haab, F.; Everaert, K.; Plante, P.; Perrouin-Verbe, B.; Kumar, C.; Fraczek, S.; *et al.* Botox detrusor hyperreflexia study team botulinum toxin type a is a safe and effective treatment for neurogenic urinary incontinence: Results of a single treatment, randomized, placebo controlled 6-month study. *J. Urol.* **2005**, *174*, 196–200. [CrossRef] [PubMed]
23. Schurch, B.; Denys, P.; Kozma, C.M.; Reese, P.R.; Slaton, T.; Barron, R.L. Botulinum toxin A improves the quality of life of patients with neurogenic urinary incontinence. *Eur. Urol.* **2007**, *52*, 850–858. [CrossRef] [PubMed]
24. Cruz, F.; Herschorn, S.; Aliotta, P.; Brin, M.; Thompson, C.; Lam, W.; Daniell, G.; Heesakkers, J.; Haag-Molkenteller, C. Efficacy and safety of onabotulinumtoxinA in patients with urinary incontinence due to neurogenic detrusor overactivity: A randomised, double-blind, placebo-controlled trial. *Eur. Urol.* **2011**, *60*, 742–750. [CrossRef] [PubMed]
25. Ginsberg, D.; Gousse, A.; Keppenne, V.; Sievert, K.D.; Thompson, C.; Lam, W.; Brin, M.F.; Jenkins, B.; Haag-Molkenteller, C. Phase 3 efficacy and tolerability study of onabotulinumtoxinA for urinary incontinence from neurogenic detrusor overactivity. *J. Urol.* **2012**, *187*, 2131–2139. [CrossRef] [PubMed]
26. Ginsberg, D.; Cruz, F.; Herschorn, S.; Gousse, A.; Keppenne, V.; Aliotta, P.; Sievert, K.D.; Brin, M.F.; Jenkins, B.; Thompson, C.; *et al.* OnabotulinumtoxinA is effective in patients with urinary incontinence due to neurogenic detrusor overactivity regardless of concomitant anticholinergic use or neurologic etiology. *Adv. Ther.* **2013**, *30*, 819–833. [CrossRef] [PubMed]
27. Kennelly, M.; Dmochowski, R.; Ethans, K.; Karsenty, G.; Schulte-Baukloh, H.; Jenkins, B.; Thompson, C.; Li, D.; Haag-Molkenteller, C. Long-term efficacy and safety of onabotulinumtoxinA in patients with urinary incontinence due to neurogenic detrusor overactivity: An interim analysis. *Urology* **2013**, *81*, 491–497. [CrossRef] [PubMed]
28. Kennelly, M.; Dmochowski, R.; Schulte-Baukloh, H.; Ethans, K.; del Popolo, G.; Moore, C.; Jenkins, B.; Guard, S.; Zheng, Y.; Karsenty, G. Efficacy and safety of onabotulinumtoxinA therapy are sustained over 4 years of treatment in patients with neurogenic detrusor overactivity: Final results of a long-term extension study. *Neurourol. Urodyn.* **2015**. [CrossRef] [PubMed]
29. Pannek, J.; Göcking, K.; Bersch, U. Long-term effects of repeated intradetrusor botulinum neurotoxin A injections on detrusor function in patients with neurogenic bladder dysfunction. *BJU Int.* **2009**, *104*, 1246–1250. [CrossRef] [PubMed]
30. Apostolidis, A.; Thompson, C.; Yan, X.; Mourad, S. An exploratory, placebo-controlled, dose-response study of the efficacy and safety of onabotulinumtoxinA in spinal cord injury patients with urinary incontinence due to neurogenic detrusor overactivity. *World J. Urol.* **2013**, *31*, 1469–1474. [CrossRef] [PubMed]
31. Nambiar, A.; Lucas, M. Chapter 4: Guidelines for the diagnosis and treatment of overactive bladder (OAB) and neurogenic detrusor overactivity (NDO). *Neurourol. Urodyn.* **2014**, *33* (Suppl. S3), S21–S25. [CrossRef] [PubMed]

32. Ehren, I.; Volz, D.; Farrelly, E.; Berglund, L.; Brundin, L.; Hultling, C.; Lafolie, P. Efficacy and impact of botulinum toxin A on quality of life in patients with neurogenic detrusor overactivity: A randomised, placebo-controlled, double-blind study. *Scand. J. Urol. Nephrol.* **2007**, *41*, 335–340. [CrossRef] [PubMed]
33. Mangera, A.; Apostolidis, A.; Andersson, K.E.; Dasgupta, P.; Giannantoni, A.; Roehrborn, C.; Novara, G.; Chapple, C. An updated systematic review and statistical comparison of standardised mean outcomes for the use of botulinum toxin in the management of lower urinary tract disorders. *Eur. Urol.* **2014**, *65*, 981–990. [CrossRef] [PubMed]
34. Haylen, B.T.; de Ridder, D.; Freeman, R.M.; Swift, S.E.; Berghmans, B.; Lee, J.; Monga, A.; Petri, E.; Rizk, D.E.; Sand, P.K.; *et al.* International urogynecological association; international continence society an international urogynecological association (IUGA)/international continence society (ICS) joint report on the terminology for female pelvic floor dysfunction. *Neurourol. Urodyn.* **2010**, *29*, 4–20. [PubMed]
35. Gormley, E.A.; Lightner, D.J.; Burgio, K.L.; Chai, T.C.; Clemens, J.Q.; Culkin, D.J.; Das, A.K.; Foster, H.E.; Scarpero, H.M.; Tessier, C.D.; *et al.* American urological association; society of urodynamics, female pelvic medicine & urogenital reconstruction diagnosis and treatment of overactive bladder (non-neurogenic) in adults: AUA/SUFU guideline. *J. Urol.* **2012**, *188*, 2455–2463. [PubMed]
36. Coyne, K.S.; Payne, C.; Bhattacharyya, S.K.; Revicki, D.A.; Thompson, C.; Corey, R.; Hunt, T.L. The impact of urinary urgency and frequency on health-related quality of life in overactive bladder: Results from a national community survey. *Value Health* **2004**, *7*, 455–463. [CrossRef] [PubMed]
37. Denys, P.; le Normand, L.; Ghout, I.; Costa, P.; Chartier-Kastler, E.; Grise, P.; Hermieu, J.F.; Amarenco, G.; Karsenty, G.; Saussine, C.; *et al.* VESITOX study group in France efficacy and safety of low doses of onabotulinumtoxinA for the treatment of refractory idiopathic overactive bladder: A multicentre, double-blind, randomised, placebo-controlled dose-ranging study. *Eur. Urol.* **2012**, *61*, 520–529. [CrossRef] [PubMed]
38. Dmochowski, R.; Chapple, C.; Nitti, V.W.; Chancellor, M.; Everaert, K.; Thompson, C.; Daniell, G.; Zhou, J.; Haag-Molkenteller, C. Efficacy and safety of onabotulinumtoxinA for idiopathic overactive bladder: A double-blind, placebo controlled, randomized, dose ranging trial. *J. Urol.* **2010**, *184*, 2416–2422. [CrossRef] [PubMed]
39. Tincello, D.G.; Kenyon, S.; Abrams, K.R.; Mayne, C.; Toozs-Hobson, P.; Taylor, D.; Slack, M. Botulinum toxin A *versus* placebo for refractory detrusor overactivity in women: A randomised blinded placebo-controlled trial of 240 women (the RELAX study). *Eur. Urol.* **2012**, *62*, 507–514. [CrossRef] [PubMed]
40. Chapple, C.; Sievert, K.D.; MacDiarmid, S.; Khullar, V.; Radziszewski, P.; Nardo, C.; Thompson, C.; Zhou, J.; Haag-Molkenteller, C. OnabotulinumtoxinA 100 U significantly improves all idiopathic overactive bladder symptoms and quality of life in patients with overactive bladder and urinary incontinence: A randomised, double-blind, placebo-controlled trial. *Eur. Urol.* **2013**, *64*, 249–256. [CrossRef] [PubMed]
41. Nitti, V.W.; Dmochowski, R.; Herschorn, S.; Sand, P.; Thompson, C.; Nardo, C.; Yan, X.; Haag-Molkenteller, C.; EMBARK study group. OnabotulinumtoxinA for the treatment of patients with overactive bladder and urinary incontinence: Results of a phase 3, randomized, placebo controlled trial. *J. Urol.* **2013**, *189*, 2186–2193. [CrossRef] [PubMed]
42. Sievert, K.D.; Chapple, C.; Herschorn, S.; Joshi, M.; Zhou, J.; Nardo, C.; Nitti, V.W. OnabotulinumtoxinA 100 U provides significant improvements in overactive bladder symptoms in patients with urinary incontinence regardless of the number of anticholinergic therapies used or reason for inadequate management of overactive bladder. *Int. J. Clin. Pract.* **2014**, *68*, 1246–1256. [CrossRef] [PubMed]
43. Rovner, E.; Kennelly, M.; Schulte-Baukloh, H.; Zhou, J.; Haag-Molkenteller, C.; Dasgupta, P. Urodynamic results and clinical outcomes with intradetrusor injections of onabotulinumtoxinA in a randomized, placebo-controlled dose-finding study in idiopathic overactive bladder. *Neurourol. Urodyn.* **2011**, *30*, 556–562. [CrossRef] [PubMed]
44. Visco, A.G.; Brubaker, L.; Richter, H.E.; Nygaard, I.; Paraiso, M.F.R.; Menefee, S.A.; Schaffer, J.; Lowder, J.; Khandwala, S.; Sirls, L.; *et al.* Pelvic floor disorders network anticholinergic therapy *vs.* onabotulinumtoxina for urgency urinary incontinence. *N. Engl. J. Med.* **2012**, *367*, 1803–1813. [CrossRef] [PubMed]
45. Mohee, A.; Khan, A.; Harris, N.; Eardley, I. Long-term outcome of the use of intravesical botulinum toxin for the treatment of overactive bladder (OAB). *BJU Int.* **2013**, *111*, 106–113. [CrossRef] [PubMed]

46. Smits, M.A.C.; Oerlemans, D.; Marcelissen, T.A.T.; van Kerrebroeck, P.E.V.; de Wachter, S.G.G. Sacral neuromodulation in patients with idiopathic overactive bladder after initial botulinum toxin therapy. *J. Urol.* **2013**, *190*, 2148–2152. [CrossRef] [PubMed]
47. Jeffery, S.; Fynes, M.; Lee, F.; Wang, K.; Williams, L.; Morley, R. Efficacy and complications of intradetrusor injection with botulinum toxin A in patients with refractory idiopathic detrusor overactivity. *BJU Int.* **2007**, *100*, 1302–1306. [CrossRef] [PubMed]
48. Maria, G.; Brisinda, G.; Civello, I.M.; Bentivoglio, A.R.; Sganga, G.; Albanese, A. Relief by botulinum toxin of voiding dysfunction due to benign prostatic hyperplasia: Results of a randomized, placebo-controlled study. *Urology* **2003**, *62*, 259–264. [CrossRef]
49. Kuo, H.-C.; Liu, H.-T. Therapeutic effects of add-on botulinum toxin A on patients with large benign prostatic hyperplasia and unsatisfactory response to combined medical therapy. *Scand. J. Urol. Nephrol.* **2009**, *43*, 206–211. [CrossRef] [PubMed]
50. Chuang, Y.C.; Chiang, P.H.; Huang, C.C.; Yoshimura, N.; Chancellor, M.B. Botulinum toxin type A improves benign prostatic hyperplasia symptoms in patients with small prostates. *Urology* **2005**, *66*, 775–779. [CrossRef] [PubMed]
51. Brisinda, G.; Cadeddu, F.; Vanella, S.; Mazzeo, P.; Marniga, G.; Maria, G. Relief by botulinum toxin of lower urinary tract symptoms owing to benign prostatic hyperplasia: Early and long-term results. *Urology* **2009**, *73*, 90–94. [CrossRef] [PubMed]
52. Crawford, E.D.; Hirst, K.; Kusek, J.W.; Donnell, R.F.; Kaplan, S.A.; McVary, K.T.; Mynderse, L.A.; Roehrborn, C.G.; Smith, C.P.; Bruskewitz, R. Effects of 100 and 300 units of onabotulinum toxin A on lower urinary tract symptoms of benign prostatic hyperplasia: A phase II randomized clinical trial. *J. Urol.* **2011**, *186*, 965–970. [CrossRef] [PubMed]
53. Marberger, M.; Chartier-Kastler, E.; Egerdie, B.; Lee, K.S.; Grosse, J.; Bugarin, D.; Zhou, J.; Patel, A.; Haag-Molkenteller, C. A randomized double-blind placebo-controlled phase 2 dose-ranging study of onabotulinumtoxinA in men with benign prostatic hyperplasia. *Eur. Urol.* **2013**, *63*, 496–503. [CrossRef] [PubMed]
54. McVary, K.T.; Roehrborn, C.G.; Chartier-Kastler, E.; Efros, M.; Bugarin, D.; Chen, R.; Patel, A.; Haag-Molkenteller, C. A multicenter, randomized, double-blind, placebo controlled study of onabotulinumtoxinA 200 U to treat lower urinary tract symptoms in men with benign prostatic hyperplasia. *J. Urol.* **2014**, *192*, 150–156. [CrossRef] [PubMed]
55. Shim, S.R.; Cho, Y.J.; Shin, I.S.; Kim, J.H. Efficacy and safety of botulinum toxin injection for benign prostatic hyperplasia: A systematic review and meta-analysis. *Int. Urol. Nephrol.* **2016**, *48*, 19–30. [CrossRef] [PubMed]
56. McVary, K.T.; Roehrborn, C.G.; Avins, A.L.; Barry, M.J.; Bruskewitz, R.C.; Donnell, R.F.; Foster, H.E.; Gonzalez, C.M.; Kaplan, S.A.; Penson, D.F.; *et al.* Update on AUA guideline on the management of benign prostatic hyperplasia. *J. Urol.* **2011**, *185*, 1793–1803. [CrossRef] [PubMed]
57. Robert, G.; Descazeaud, A.; Benard, A.; Delongchamps, N. 685 A randomised clinical trial comparing prostatic injection of botulinum neurotoxin type A (Botox®) to optimized medical therapy in the treatment of LUTS related to BPH: The PROTOX study. *Eur. Urol. Suppl.* **2015**, *14*. [CrossRef]
58. Hanno, P.; Dmochowski, R. Status of international consensus on interstitial cystitis/bladder pain syndrome/painful bladder syndrome: 2008 snapshot. *Neurourol. Urodyn.* **2009**, *28*, 274–286. [CrossRef] [PubMed]
59. Liu, H.T.; Kuo, H.C. Intravesical botulinum toxin A injections plus hydrodistension can reduce nerve growth factor production and control bladder pain in interstitial cystitis. *Urology* **2007**, *70*, 463–468. [CrossRef] [PubMed]
60. Giannantoni, A.; Costantini, E.; di Stasi, S.M.; Tascini, M.C.; Bini, V.; Porena, M. Botulinum A toxin intravesical injections in the treatment of painful bladder syndrome: A pilot study. *Eur. Urol.* **2006**, *49*, 704–709. [CrossRef] [PubMed]
61. Ramsay, A.K.; Small, D.R.; Conn, I.G. Intravesical botulinum toxin type A in chronic interstitial cystitis: Results of a pilot study. *Surgeon* **2007**, *5*, 331–333. [CrossRef]
62. Pinto, R.; Lopes, T.; Frias, B.; Silva, A.; Silva, J.A.; Silva, C.M. Trigonal injection of botulinum toxin A in patients with refractory bladder pain syndrome/interstitial cystitis. *Eur. Urol.* **2010**, *58*, 360–365. [CrossRef] [PubMed]

63. Lee, C.L.; Kuo, H.C. Intravesical botulinum toxin a injections do not benefit patients with ulcer type interstitial cystitis. *Pain Physician* **2013**, *16*, 109–116. [PubMed]
64. Pinto, R.; Lopes, T.; Costa, D.; Barros, S.; Silva, J.; Silva, C.; Cruz, C.; Dinis, P.; Cruz, F. Ulcerative and nonulcerative forms of bladder pain syndrome/interstitial cystitis do not differ in symptom intensity or response to onabotulinum toxin A. *Urology* **2014**, *83*, 1030–1034. [CrossRef] [PubMed]
65. Kuo, H.C. Repeated onabotulinumtoxin-a injections provide better results than single injection in treatment of painful bladder syndrome. *Pain Physician* **2013**, *16*, E15–E23. [PubMed]
66. Kuo, H.C.; Chancellor, M.B. Comparison of intravesical botulinum toxin type A injections plus hydrodistention with hydrodistention alone for the treatment of refractory interstitial cystitis/painful bladder syndrome. *BJU Int.* **2009**, *104*, 657–661. [CrossRef] [PubMed]
67. Kuo, H.C.; Jiang, Y.H.; Tsai, Y.C. Intravesical botulinum toxin-A injections reduce bladder pain of interstitial cystitis/bladder pain syndrome refractory to conventional treatment—A prospective, multicenter, randomized, double-blind, placebo-controlled clinical trial. *Neurourol. Urodyn.* **2015**. [CrossRef] [PubMed]
68. Chung, S.D.; Kuo, Y.C.; Kuo, H.C. Intravesical onabotulinumtoxinA injections for refractory painful bladder syndrome. *Pain Physician* **2012**, *15*, 197–202. [PubMed]
69. Hanno, P.M.; Erickson, D.; Moldwin, R.; Faraday, M.M.; American Urological Association. Diagnosis and treatment of interstitial cystitis/bladder pain syndrome: AUA guideline amendment. *J. Urol.* **2015**, *193*, 1545–1553. [CrossRef] [PubMed]
70. Fall, M.; Baranowski, A.P.; Elneil, S.; Engeler, D.; Hughes, J.; Messelink, E.J.; Oberpenning, F.; de Williams, A.C.; European Association of Urology. EAU guidelines on chronic pelvic pain. *Eur. Urol.* **2010**, *57*, 35–48. [CrossRef] [PubMed]
71. Montenegro, M.L.; Mateus-Vasconcelos, E.C.; Rosa e Silva, J.C.; Nogueira, A.A.; dos Reis, F.J.; Poli Neto, O.B. Importance of pelvic muscle tenderness evaluation in women with chronic pelvic pain. *Pain Med.* **2010**, *11*, 224–228. [CrossRef] [PubMed]
72. Kaya, S.; Hermans, L.; Willems, T.; Roussel, N.; Meeus, M. Central sensitization in urogynecological chronic pelvic pain: A systematic literature review. *Pain Physician* **2013**, *16*, 291–308. [PubMed]
73. Graziottin, A.; Skaper, S.D.; Fusco, M. Mast cells in chronic inflammation, pelvic pain and depression in women. *Gynecol. Endocrinol.* **2014**, *30*, 472–477. [CrossRef] [PubMed]
74. Zermann, D.H.; Ishigooka, M.; Schubert, J.; Schmidt, R.A. Perisphincteric injection of botulinum toxin type A. A treatment option for patients with chronic prostatic pain? *Eur. Urol.* **2000**, *38*, 393–399. [CrossRef] [PubMed]
75. Gottsch, H.P.; Yang, C.C.; Berger, R.E. A pilot study of botulinum toxin A for male chronic pelvic pain syndrome. *Scand. J. Urol. Nephrol.* **2011**, *45*, 72–76. [CrossRef] [PubMed]
76. Falahatkar, S.; Shahab, E.; Moghaddam, K.G.; Kazemnezhad, E. Transurethral intraprostatic injection of botulinum neurotoxin type A for the treatment of chronic prostatitis/chronic pelvic pain syndrome: Results of a prospective pilot double-blind and randomized placebo-controlled study. *BJU Int.* **2015**, *116*, 641–649. [CrossRef] [PubMed]
77. El-Enen, M.A.; Abou-Farha, M.; El-Abd, A.; El-Tatawy, H.; Tawfik, A.; El-Abd, S.; Rashed, M.; El-Sharaby, M. Intraprostatic injection of botulinum toxin-A in patients with refractory chronic pelvic pain syndrome: The transurethral *vs.* transrectal approach. *Arab. J. Urol.* **2015**, *13*, 94–99. [CrossRef] [PubMed]
78. Jarvis, S.K.; Abbott, J.A.; Lenart, M.B.; Steensma, A.; Vancaillie, T.G. Pilot study of botulinum toxin type A in the treatment of chronic pelvic pain associated with spasm of the levator ani muscles. *Aust. New Zealand J. Obstet. Gynaecol.* **2004**, *44*, 46–50. [CrossRef] [PubMed]
79. Abbott, J.A.; Jarvis, S.K.; Lyons, S.D.; Thomson, A. Botulinum toxin type A for chronic pain and pelvic floor spasm in women: A randomized controlled trial. *Obstet. Gynecol.* **2006**, *108*, 915–923. [CrossRef] [PubMed]
80. Morrissey, D.; El-Khawand, D.; Ginzburg, N.; Wehbe, S.; O'Hare, P.; Whitmore, K. Botulinum toxin A injections into pelvic floor muscles under electromyographic guidance for women with refractory high-tone pelvic floor dysfunction: A 6-month prospective pilot study. *Female Pelvic Med. Reconstr. Surg.* **2015**, *21*, 277–282. [CrossRef] [PubMed]
81. Bhide, A.A.; Puccini, F.; Khullar, V.; Elneil, S. Botulinum neurotoxin type A injection of the pelvic floor muscle in pain due to spasticity: A review of the current literature. *Int. Urogynecol. J.* **2013**, *24*, 1429–1434. [CrossRef] [PubMed]

82. Petit, H.; Wiart, L.; Gaujard, E.; le Breton, F.; Ferrière, J.M.; Lagueny, A.; Joseph, P.A.; Barat, M. Botulinum A toxin treatment for detrusor-sphincter dyssynergia in spinal cord disease. *Spinal Cord* **1998**, *36*, 91–94. [CrossRef] [PubMed]
83. Gallien, P.; Robineau, S.; Verin, M.; le Bot, M.P.; Nicolas, B.; Brissot, R. Treatment of detrusor sphincter dyssynergia by transperineal injection of botulinum toxin. *Arch. Phys. Med. Rehabil.* **1998**, *79*, 715–717. [CrossRef]
84. Tsai, S.J.; Ying, T.H.; Huang, Y.H.; Cheng, J.W.; Bih, L.I.; Lew, H.L. Transperineal injection of botulinum toxin A for treatment of detrusor sphincter dyssynergia: Localization with combined fluoroscopic and electromyographic guidance. *Arch. Phys. Med. Rehabil.* **2009**, *90*, 832–836. [CrossRef] [PubMed]
85. Kuo, H.C. Satisfaction with urethral injection of botulinum toxin A for detrusor sphincter dyssynergia in patients with spinal cord lesion. *Neurourol. Urodyn.* **2008**, *27*, 793–796. [CrossRef] [PubMed]
86. Chen, S.L.; Bih, L.I.; Chen, G.D.; Huang, Y.H.; You, Y.H.; Lew, H.L. Transrectal ultrasound-guided transperineal botulinum toxin A injection to the external urethral sphincter for treatment of detrusor external sphincter dyssynergia in patients with spinal cord injury. *Arch. Phys. Med. Rehabil.* **2010**, *91*, 340–344. [CrossRef] [PubMed]
87. Chen, S.L.; Bih, L.I.; Huang, Y.H.; Tsai, S.J.; Lin, T.B.; Kao, Y.L. Effect of single botulinum toxin A injection to the external urethral sphincter for treating detrusor external sphincter dyssynergia in spinal cord injury. *J. Rehabil. Med.* **2008**, *40*, 744–748. [CrossRef] [PubMed]
88. De Seze, M.; Petit, H.; Gallien, P.; de Sèze, M.P.; Joseph, P.A. Botulinum A toxin and detrusor sphincter dyssynergia: A double-blind lidocaine-controlled study in 13 patients with spinal cord disease. *Eur. Urol.* **2002**, *42*, 56–62. [CrossRef]
89. Mehta, S.; Hill, D.; Foley, N.; Hsieh, J.; Ethans, K. A meta-analysis of botulinum toxin sphincteric injections in the treatment of incomplete voiding after spinal cord injury. *Arch. Phys. Med. Rehabil.* **2012**, *93*, 597–603. [CrossRef] [PubMed]
90. Gallien, P.; Reymann, J.M.; Amarenco, G.; Nicolas, B.; de Seze, M.; Bellissant, E. Placebo controlled, randomised, double blind study of the effects of botulinum A toxin on detrusor sphincter dyssynergia in multiple sclerosis patients. *J. Neurol. Neurosurg. Psychiatry* **2005**, *76*, 1670–1676. [CrossRef] [PubMed]
91. Groen, J.; Pannek, J.; Diaz, D.C.; del Popolo, G.; Gross, T.; Hamid, R.; Karsenty, G.; Kessler, T.M.; Schneider, M.; Hoen, L.; *et al.* Summary of European Association of Urology (EAU) guidelines on neuro-urology. *Eur Urol.* **2016**, *69*, 324–333. [CrossRef] [PubMed]

4

Botulinum Toxin A and Lower Urinary Tract Dysfunction: Pathophysiology and Mechanisms of Action

Jia-Fong Jhang and Hann-Chorng Kuo *

Department of Urology, Buddhist Tzu Chi General Hospital, Tzu Chi University, 707 Chung-Yang Road, Section 3, Hualien 970, Taiwan; alur1984@tzuchi.com.tw
* Correspondence: hck@tzuchi.com.tw

Academic Editor: Joseph Jankovic

Abstract: The use of onabotulinumtoxinA (BoNT-A) for the treatment of lower urinary tract diseases (LUTD) has increased markedly in recent years. The indications for BoNT-A treatment of LUTD now include neurogenic or idiopathic detrusor overactivity, interstitial cystitis/bladder pain syndrome and voiding dysfunction. The mechanisms of BoNT-A action on LUTDs affect many different aspects. Traditionally, the effects of BoNT-A were believed to be attributable to inhibition of acetylcholine release from the presynaptic efferent nerves at the neuromuscular junctions in the detrusor or urethral sphincter. BoNT-A injection in the bladder also regulated sensory nerve function by blocking neurotransmitter release and reducing receptor expression in the urothelium. In addition, recent studies revealed an anti-inflammatory effect for BoNT-A. Substance P and nerve growth factor in the urine and bladder tissue decreased after BoNT-A injection. Mast cell activation in the bladder also decreased. BoNT-A-induced improvement of urothelium function plays an important mitigating role in bladder dysfunction. Vascular endothelial growth factor expression in urothelium decreased after BoNT-A injection, as did apoptosis. Studies also revealed increased apoptosis in the prostate after BoNT-A injection. Although BoNT-A injection has been widely used to treat different LUTDs refractory to conventional treatment, currently, onabotulinumtoxinA has been proven effective only on urinary incontinence due to IDO and NDO in several large-scale clinical trials. The effects of onabotulinumtoxinA on other LUTDs such as interstitial cystitis, benign prostatic hyperplasia, dysfunctional voiding or detrusor sphincter dyssynergia have not been well demonstrated.

Keywords: interstitial cystitis; overactive bladder; treatment

---

1. Introduction

Normal lower urinary tract function promotes efficient voluntary urine emptying and low-pressure urine storage, which contribute to continence [1]. The symptoms of dysuria, urinary frequency, and incontinence are signs of lower urinary tract diseases (LUTD) [2]. LUTD is a common health problem and its prevalence increases with age. A recent cross-sectional study revealed 61.2% of men and 61.1% of women reported LUTD [3]. The pathophysiology of LUTD is usually complicated, and the same symptom in different patients may have a different pathogenesis. Conventionally, LUTD is classified as originating from the bladder or bladder outlet. Oral medications such as alpha-adrenergic blockers and anti-muscarinic agents are effective first-line treatments for LUTD in many patients. However, some patients with LUTD are refractory to these conventional drugs.

Botulinum toxin (BoNT) is a potent neurotoxin produced by the bacterium *Clostridium botulinum*. It inhibits the release of the neurotransmitter acetylcholine from nerve fibers, thereby inhibiting muscle contractions. Because of these toxic effects, BoNT is widely used in medical practice [4]. Therapeutic onabotulinumtoxinA was first injected to correct strabismus in 1983 [5]. Currently, it is broadly applied to treat many neuromuscular and neuropathic pain diseases that are difficult to treat with conventional drugs [6,7]. The first application of onabotulinumtoxinA for the treatment of LUTD was in patients with spinal cord injury (SCI) and detrusor sphincter dyssynergia (DSD). Nowadays, onabotulinumtoxinA is used to treat urinary incontinence due to detrusor overactivity (DO). OnabotulinumtoxinA injection into the bladder wall (detrusor muscle) has been a breakthrough in treating refractory DO. The United States Food and Drug Administration approved this indication in 2013 [8,9]. The advantages of onabotulinumtoxinA injection are not only minimal invasiveness, but also provide an opportunity for the patients with LUTD in which conventional treatment has failed. Even with such widespread use, the mechanisms of onabotulinumtoxinA action in treating LUTDs remain unclear and involve many different pathways. Thus, the aim of this review is to introduce the pathophysiology of LUTD and describe the mechanisms of onabotulinumtoxinA effects in the treatment of LUTD.

2. Mechanism and Biology of OnabotulinumtoxinA

BoNT is the most potent biological toxin, and it was first isolated more than 100 years ago [10]. Seven different strains of *Clostridium botulinum* produce seven immunologically distinct neurotoxins (types A to G) [11], and the most common medically used type is BoNT-A. BoNT-A is a protein consisting of a 50-kDa light chain and a 100-kDa heavy chain connected by a disulfide bond [12]. In the presynaptic nerve membrane, the *C*-terminal of the heavy chain of BoNT-A binds to synaptic vesicle protein 2 (SV2), and then BoNT-A is taken into the nerve terminal by endocytosis [13]. In the endosomal vesicle, the light chain and heavy chain separate. The *N*-terminal of the heavy chain binds to the endosomal membrane where it induces the light chain to be transported from the endosome to the cytosol [14]. The light chain is the biologically active moiety of BoNT-A.

In the presynaptic nerve terminal, neurotransmitters are released by exocytosis and mediated by soluble *N*-ethylmaleimide-sensitive factor attachment receptor protein complexes that consist of synaptobrevin, syntaxin and synaptosome-associated protein 25 (SNAP-25) [15]. The light chain of BoNT-A cleaves SNAP-25, inhibiting the release of the neurotransmitter acetylcholine by disrupting the fusion of vesicles with the neuron cell membrane, finally causing the flaccid paralysis of muscles [16]. In addition, studies also revealed BoNT-A blocks noxious neurotransmitter release, including substance P, calcitonin gene-related peptide and adenosine triphosphate (ATP) [17,18]. Recently, many clinical studies have proven the efficacy of BoNT-A in treating different neuropathic pain disorders, such as post herpetic neuralgia, trigeminal neuralgia and post-traumatic neuralgia [19].

BoNT-A injection has been widely used to treat different LUTDs refractory to conventional treatment. Currently, onabotulinumtoxinA has been proven effective only on urinary incontinence due to IDO and NDO in several large-scale clinical trials. The effects of onabotulinumtoxinA on other LUTDs such as IC/BPS, BPH, DV, DSD have not been well demonstrated.

3. Mechanism Action of BoNT-A on Bladder Disease

Symptoms only are not a reliable tool for diagnosis of LUTD. Symptoms, such as a weak urine stream, could be the result of diseases originating from the bladder or bladder outlet. Further examinations, such as uroflowmetry or bladder sonography, are usually necessary to confirm the diagnosis [20]. LUTDs originating from the bladder include DO, interstitial cystitis/bladder pain syndrome (IC/BPS) and hypersensitive bladder. Even today, the details of the complete pathogenesis of many LUTDs remain an enigma, and this is why these diseases are sometimes difficult to treat successfully.

3.1. *Pathophysiology and Mechanism of BoNT-A in DO*

The International Continence Society defines DO as an urodynamic observation characterized by involuntary detrusor contractions during the bladder-filling phase that may be spontaneous or provoked [2]. Patients with DO usually suffer from symptoms of urgency, which is defined as a complaint of sudden, compelling desire to pass urine that is difficult to defer [21]. Disturbances in or injury to nerves, the detrusor muscle or urothelium can cause DO [22]. Clinically, the cause is classified as neurogenic (NDO) in patients with the relevant neurological conditions or idiopathic (IDO) in patients without definitive cause [21]. Bladder contraction is mediated by the parasympathetic nervous system via the release of predominantly acetylcholine, which interacts with muscarinic receptors on the detrusor muscle [22]. Parasympathetic nerves also release adenosine triphosphate (ATP) and stimulate the purinergic receptors (P2X) in the detrusor to induce contraction [23].

In central nervous system (CNS), detrusor contraction may be inhibited by the prefrontal cerebral cortex, the L-region of the pontine micturition center and the lumbar spinal cord [22]. These inhibitory neurons in the CNS release gamma-aminobutyric acid and glycine, inhibiting detrusor contraction [24]. A lesion above the lumbosacral cord level interrupts voluntary control of micturition and results in NDO due to dysfunction of the inhibitory pathway. In addition, a sacral spinal reflex, which is mediated by formerly silent capsaicin-sensitive unmyelinated C-fibers is also active in patients with SCI [24]. This reflex also plays a significant role in NDO. On the other hand, the pathogenesis of IDO is more complicated. Although the patients with IDO do not have any specific disease of the central or peripheral nervous systems, recent studies revealed neurologic dysfunction involving afferent pathways that contributed to the pathogenesis of IDO [24]. The bladder afferent pathways consist of mechanosensitive myelinated A fibers and chemosensitive unmyelinated C fibers [25]. Urothelial dysfunction could increase the afferent stimulation produced by bladder fullness and contribute to the perception of urgency, thereby contributing to activation of the abnormal detrusor contractions [26]. Increased expression of urothelium receptors such as P2X2, transient receptor potential cation channel subfamily V member 1 (TRPV1) and muscarinic receptors is associated with IDO in the human bladder [27].

Since Schurch first used intravesical BoNT-A injection in patients with SCI and NDO in 2000, many studies had proven its efficacy in reducing urgency and urgency incontinence [28]. In the efferent nerves of the bladder, BoNT-A injection blocks the release of acetylcholine from both preganglionic and postganglionic parasympathetic nerves by cleaving SNAP-25, thereby temporarily inhibiting detrusor muscle contraction [29]. Studies also showed that vesicular noradrenaline release was inhibited after BoNT-A injection in the bladder wall [30]. BoNT-A not only blocked neurotransmitter release after injection into the detrusor muscle but also reduced muscarinic receptor M2 in the nerve terminal [31]. An animal study also revealed BoNT-A block ATP release from purinergic efferent nerves in the detrusor muscle, which may have contributed to the effectiveness of BoNT-A in treating DO [32].

In addition to efferent nerve signals, increased afferent nerve signals are believed to be central to the pathophysiology of IDO and the generation of urgency [27]. When the urothelium is stretching, both acetylcholine and ATP are released from the basal lateral surface of the urothelium. This activates afferent nerves in the suburothelial layer and induces the micturition reflex [33]. Recently, increasing evidence suggests that BoNT-A blocks afferent signaling in the bladder [34]. In a study of the bladders of patients with SCI, onabotulinumtoxinA injection markedly reduced urothelial ATP release by 53% [35]. Valerie *et al.* also reported that onabotulinumtoxinA injection attenuated ATP release in the bladder with physiological and supra-physiological distension pressures [36]. Nitric oxide (NO) also inhibits afferent nerve conduction in the bladder detrusor, with increased NO release from the urothelium after onabotulinumtoxinA injection [36]. However, in the study by Valerie *et al.*, acetylcholine release from urothelium was not significantly decreased [36].

Evidence also shows that afferent nerve receptors in the suburothelium are regulated after onabotulinumtoxinA injection into the urothelium. A study of patients with DO revealed decreased expression of P2X3 in the bladder mucosa within four weeks after onabotulinumtoxinA injection [37]. Additionally, the decline in P2X3 receptors was significantly correlated with the reduction of urgency episodes four and 16 weeks after onabotulinumtoxinA injection. In another single-blind study of children with NDO, the purinergic receptors P2X2 and P2X3 in urothelium reached significant reductions ($p < 0.05$) after onabotulinumtoxinA injection [38]. Increased urothelial TRPV1 in patients with NDO may also play a role in the pathophysiology [39]. After onabotulinumtoxinA injection, a significant reduction of TRPV-1 in the suburothelial nerve fibers was reported [37]. In summary, the effect of BoNT-A in patients with DO involves efferent and afferent nerve pathways. Table 1 summarizes the primary mechanisms of action of BoNT-A on neurotransmitters (acetylcholine, ATP and NO) and receptors (M2, M3, P2X2, P2X3, and TRPV-1).

Table 1. Mechanism of botulinum toxin A action on detrusor overactivity.

Nerve System of Botulinum Toxin A Action	Evidence of BoNT-A Effects in the Bladder	
	Changes of Neurotransmitters	Changes of Receptors
Efferent nerve system	Decreased Ach and ATP release in efferent nerve endings	Decreased M2 receptor in the detrusor muscle
Sensory nerve system	Decrease ATP and increased NO release from urothelium	Decreased P2X2, P2X3, and TRPV1 receptor in the urothelium

Ach: acetylcholine; ATP: adenosine triphosphate; NO: nitric oxide; TRPV1: transient receptor potential cation channel subfamily V member 1.

3.2. Pathophysiology and Mechanism of BoNT-A on IC/BPS

The clinical characteristics of IC/BPS are severe bladder pain associated with urgency, frequency, nocturia, dysuria and sterile urine [40]. Although many studies have focused on the pathophysiology of IC/BPS, it is still is a mystery in urology. Previously infection, autoimmune, central sensitization and urine abnormalities have been considered as etiologies of IC/BPS [41]. Recently, urothelial dysfunction and neurogenic inflammation have attracted great interest. A urothelial defect of surface glycosaminoglycan and associated changes in epithelial permeability are associated with the pathogenesis of IC/BPS [42,43]. Furthermore, as with DO, bladders affected with IC/BPS also had up-regulation of P2X3 receptors and increasing ATP release in the urothelium [44,45]. TRPV1 is the receptor of capsaicin stimulation and detects pain in the bladder [46]. The expression of TRPV1 in humans with IC/BPS is up-regulated and could be involved in the pathogenesis of IC/BPS [47]. The cell tight junction protein zonula occludens-1 (ZO-1) and adhesive junction protein E-cadherin are significantly decreased in the bladders of patients with IC/BPS but not in patients with DO [48]. Many studies revealed an increase in mast cell infiltration in the bladders of IC/BPS patients, which could play a central role in the pathogenesis of IC/BPS [49]. Substance P is a neurotransmitter secreted from the sensory nerve endings and is associated with inflammatory processes and pain [50]. Pang *et al.* reported significantly increased numbers of substance P-positive nerve fibers in the bladder submucosa of patients with IC/BPS [51]. Neurokinin-1 receptors, the high-affinity binding sites of substance P, were also upregulated in the bladders of patients with IC/BPS [52]. Substance P and mast cells play a pivotal role in the neurogenic inflammation of IC/BPS and induce inflammation in the bladder by the release of histamine and tumor necrosis factor alpha [51,53]. Nerve growth factor (NGF) is a neuropeptide involved in the regulation of growth; it is released by mast cells in the inflammation process NGF induces axonal outgrowth in pain neurons and leads to increased pain perception [54]. Increased NGF is found in the bladder mucosa, urine, and serum of patients with IC/BPS and is likely involved in the pathogenesis of IC/BPS [55,56].

OnabotulinumtoxinA injections in the bladder urothelium have been used in treating IC/BPS since 2004 [57]. A recent randomized, double-blind, placebo-controlled clinical trial revealed that intravesical injections of 100 U of onabotulinumtoxinA effectively reduced bladder pain symptoms in patients with IC/BPS [58]. Currently, the American Urology Association recommends intradetrusor onabotulinumtoxinA injections for treatment of IC/BPS in patients for whom conventional treatments failed [59]. BoNT-A injections improve urothelial function in patients with IC/BPS by decreasing P2X3 and TRPV1 receptor expression in the urothelium, which is a likely mechanism reducing pain in patients with IC/BPS [60]. Additionally, BoNT-A inhibits sensory neurotransmitter release further reducing pain sensation. CGRP is a potent peptide vasodilator that functions in the transmission of pain [61]. A study in rats revealed that BoNT-A injection into the bladder inhibited the evoked release of CGRP from afferent nerve terminals in the bladder, reducing pain [62]. In another study of acute and chronic rat bladder inflammation, BoNT-A injection also significantly inhibited the release of substance P and CGRP [63]. OnabotulinumtoxinA decreased NGF mRNA expression in the bladder mucosa of IC/BPS patients who responded to intravesical onabotulinumtoxinA injection [64]. The level of urinary NGF also decreased in these patients [65]. Pinto *et al.* also reported decreased urinary NGF after onabotulinumtoxinA injection into the trigone, even in patients with ulcerative IC/BPS [66]. Recent evidence also suggests onabotulinumtoxinA injections reduce bladder inflammation. Immunohistochemical studies reveal decreased tryptase expression in the urothelium after repeated injections, which suggests a reduction in active mast cells in the bladders of IC/BPS patients [67]. OnabotulinumtoxinA decreases the expression of vascular endothelial growth factor in the bladders of patients with IC/BPS and indicates attenuation of vasculogenesis in these patients [68]. Urothelial apoptosis is also declined after onabotulinumtoxinA injection. The expression of apoptosis regulation protein bcl-2-like protein 4 in the urothelium decreased within six months after onabotulinumtoxinA injection [68]. Additionally, the evidence of apoptotic signaling cascades also decreased [67,68]. Moreover, recent studies revealed peripheral BoNT-A injection has antinociceptive activity via CNS regulation [69] BoNT-A reaches the CNS by retrograde transport and blocks CNS synaptic transmission of glutamate, dopamine, ATP and gamma-aminobutyric acid [69]. Table 2 provides a summary of mechanisms of BoNT-A action in IC/BPS.

Table 2. Mechanism of botulinum toxin A action on interstitial cystitis/bladder pain syndrome.

Mechanisms of Botulinum Toxin A Action	Evidence of BoNT-A Effects in the Bladder	
	Changes of Neurotransmitters	**Changes of Receptors**
Sensory nerve system	Decrease CGRP, ATP, and substance P release from urothelium	Decreased P2X3 and TRPV1 receptor in urothelium
Central nerve system	Inhibit glutamate, dopamine, ATP, gamma-aminobutyric acid	
Anti-inflammatory effect	Decreased active mast cell Decreased substance P, NGF, and VEGF	
Improve urothelium dysfunction	Decreased apoptosis in the urothelium	

CGRP: calcitonin gene-related peptide; ATP: adenosine triphosphate; TRPV1: transient receptor potential cation channel subfamily V member 1; NGF: nerve growth factor; VEGF: vascular endothelial growth factor.

4. Mechanism Action of BoNT-A on Bladder Outlet Dysfunction

The main symptoms of bladder outlet obstruction are incomplete bladder emptying, diminished urinary stream, and post voiding urinary dribbling, which manifest in DSD, bladder neck dysfunction and benign prostatic obstruction (BPO) [70]. The anatomic structures of the bladder outlet include the bladder neck, urethral sphincter and prostate in men. Both the anatomic or functional obstruction of these structures results in slow urinary flow and an increase in intravesical pressure [70]. Anatomic disorders of bladder outlet obstruction such as BPO may be managed well with medical treatment or surgical intervention, such as resection of the prostate. However, the functional problems including DSD in patients with SCI, dysfunctional voiding (DV) or poor relaxation of the external urethral sphincter can be troublesome when conventional treatments fail [70].

DSD is characterized by involuntary contractions of the external urethral sphincter during a detrusor contraction caused by CNS injury between the pontine micturition center and the sacral spinal cord [71]. Transperineal onabotulinumtoxinA injection under electromyographic control was first used to treat such patients with SCI and DSD in 1997 [72]. Most urologists now use a rigid cystoscope with an injection needle to inject onabotulinumtoxinA directly into the urethral sphincter [73]. Although a large, randomized controlled trial is lacking, several preliminary studies suggest onabotulinumtoxinA injection for treatment of DSD due to SCI could result in higher voided urine volumes and lower voiding detrusor pressures [73]. In an earlier study of SCI with DSD, the amplitude of bulbosphincteric reflexes were decreased after urethral sphincter onabotulinumtoxinA injection and the latency also became normal [74]. An electromyographic study revealed static and dynamic urethral pressure in the patients with severe spasticity of the urethral sphincter decreased significantly after onabotulinumtoxinA injection [75]. When the bladder outlet resistance stemming from the urethral sphincter decreased, the voiding efficiency in the patients with DSD improved. The effect of BoNT-A on DSD is thought to be attributable to blocking acetylcholine release from presynaptic vesicles at the neuromuscular junction. This temporary, reversible chemo-denervation by BoNT-A relaxes the spastic external urethral sphincter in SCI patients with DSD [76]. Laboratory evidence confirming this mechanism of action of BoNT-A is needed.

DV is characterized by an intermittent or fluctuating urine flow rate due to intermittent, involuntary contractions of the periurethral striated muscle during voiding in neurologically normal individuals [2]. Traditionally, DV has been considered a learned chronic disorder of childhood, presumably because the misguided habit of contracting the external urethral sphincter rather than relaxing it during voiding [77]. However, many adult patients with DV completely deny the existence of any voiding symptoms during their childhood [78]. Fowler *et al.* reported DV patients presenting with urinary retention, and the urethral sphincter electromyography of these patients demonstrated unexpected decelerating bursts and complex repetitive discharges [79]. On the other hand, some patients without such strong electromyographic activity might also have similar symptoms of DV due to poor relaxation of the pelvic floor muscle and urethral sphincter [80]. Relaxation of the bladder neck also is an important step of micturition. Bladder neck dysfunction leads to a weak urine stream and increases residual urine volume [80]. In the past, treating these voiding problems was difficult. However, recent studies suggest onabotulinumtoxinA injections in the external urethral sphincter, bladder neck or pelvic floor muscle offer promising prospects for improving DV symptoms [81–83]. OnabotulinumtoxinA injection into the rat urethral sphincter significantly inhibited acetylcholine and norepinephrine release caused by high-frequency electrical stimulation and decreasing urethral resistance and bladder outlet obstruction [84]. In another study, a significant reduction in pelvic floor pressure after onabotulinumtoxinA injection was reported in which relaxation of the pelvic floor also decreased bladder outlet resistance, especially in female patients [83]. Further laboratory evidence is necessary to clarify the mechanism of BoNT-A action in DV.

BPO is a term used to describe bladder outlet obstruction secondary to hyperplasia of the prostate (adenoma). It is the most common cause of bladder outlet obstruction in elderly men [85]. Traditionally, the growth of the prostate gland was believed to be associated with testosterone, but recently inflammation, infection, and metabolic disorders are considered possible etiologies [86]. Several clinical trials suggested transurethral intraprostatic onabotulinumtoxinA injection may be an effective treatment for patients with symptomatic BPO [87–89]. The prostate gland is innervated by sympathetic and parasympathetic nerves, and the parasympathetic nerves interact with the sympathetic nerves and influence secretions and contraction of the prostate [90]. Cholinergic nerves and muscarinic receptors are expressed in the prostate fibromuscular stroma, playing a role in the cell growth of the prostate tissue [91]. Therefore, blocking acetylcholine release from cholinergic nerves by BoNT-A may disrupt the neural control of the prostate, inhibit prostate contraction and growth, and bring symptomatic relief in men with BPO [92]. In a study of onabotulinumtoxinA injections in dog prostates, atrophy and increased apoptosis were observed on hematoxylin and eosin and TUNEL stains at one and three months after treatment [93]. The prostate weight, tyrosine hydroxylase-positive sympathetic nerve fibers, and synaptophysin-positive cells in the epithelium were decreased in rat prostates after onabotulinumtoxinA injection [94,95]. Although pilot studies of onabotulinumtoxinA treatment on BPO seem promising, the studies did not consistently show the same results [96,97]. A high placebo effect was noted in a double-blind, placebo-controlled phase II trial that could have contributed to the improvement of symptom scores after treatment [98]. Because the high placebo effect, BoNT-A seems not a good indication for treatment of BPO.

5. Conclusions

The mechanism of BoNT-A action involves the motor nervous system including the inhibition of neuromuscular junctions by blocking acetylcholine release. Desensitization of sensory nerves by reducing neurotransmitter release of ATP, substance P, and CGRP also plays a significant role. Laboratory evidence also proved BoNT-A injection regulates abnormal neurogenic inflammation and apoptosis in the bladder. Understanding of pathogenesis of LUTDs and the mechanisms of action of BoNT-A injection on these LUTDs helps clinicians properly select patients to receive BoNT-A treatment. However, not all LUTDs refractory to conventional therapy, such as BPH, IC/BPS, DV, and DSD, can benefit from BoNT-A treatment, possibly because the underlying pathophysiology of these LUTDs has not been completely elucidated. The only LUTD that can be effectively treated by BoNT-A injection is urinary incontinence due to IDO and NDO.

References

1. Alan, J.W. Pathophysiology and classification of lower urinary tract dysfunction: Overview. In *Campbell Walsh Urology*, 10th ed.; Louis, R.K., Andrew, C.N., Eds.; Elsevier: Philadelphia, PA, USA, 2012; Volume 3, p. 1834.
2. Abrams, P.; Cardozo, L.; Fall, M.; Griffiths, D.; Rosier, P.; Ulmsten, U.; van Kerrebroeck, P.; Victor, A.; Wein, A. The standardisation of terminology of lower urinary tract function: Report from the standardisation sub-committee of the international continence society. *Neurourol. Urodyn.* **2002**, *21*, 167–178. [CrossRef] [PubMed]
3. Wang, Y.; Hu, H.; Xu, K.; Wang, X.; Na, Y.; Kang, X. Prevalence, risk factors and the bother of lower urinary tract symptoms in China: A population-based survey. *Int. Urogynecol. J.* **2015**, *26*, 911–919. [CrossRef] [PubMed]
4. Dressler, D.; AdibSaberi, F. Botulinum toxin: Mechanisms of action. *Eur. Neurol.* **2005**, *53*, 3–9. [CrossRef] [PubMed]
5. Scott, A.B. Botulinum toxin injection of eye muscles to correct strabismus. *Trans. Am. Ophthalmol. Soc.* **1981**, *79*, 734–770. [PubMed]
6. Brown, E.A.; Schütz, S.G.; Simpson, D.M. Botulinum toxin for neuropathic pain and spasticity: An overview. *Pain Manag.* **2014**, *4*, 129–151. [CrossRef] [PubMed]
7. Kharkar, S.; Ambady, P.; Venkatesh, Y.; Schwartzman, R.J. Intramuscular botulinum toxin in complex regional pain syndrome: Case series and literature review. *Pain Phys.* **2011**, *14*, 419–424.
8. U.S. Food and Drug Administration. FDA Approves Botox to Treat Specific Form of Urinary Incontinence. Available online: http://www.fda.gov/NewsEvents/Newsroom/PressAnnouncements/ucm269509.htm (accessed on 25 August 2011).
9. U.S. Food and Drug Administration. FDA Approves Botox to Treat Overactive Bladder. Available online: http://www.fda.gov/newsevents/newsroom/pressannouncements/ucm336101.htm (accessed on 18 January 2013).
10. Schiavo, G.; Santucci, A.; DasGupta, B.R.; Mehta, P.P.; Jontes, J.; Benfenati, F.; Wilson, M.C.; Montecucco, C. Botulinum neurotoxins serotypes A and E cleave Snap-25 at distinct COOH-terminal peptide bonds. *FEBS Lett.* **1993**, *335*, 99. [CrossRef]
11. Franciosa, G.; Floridi, F.; Maugliani, A.; Aureli, P. Differentiation of the gene clusters encoding botulinum neurotoxin type A complexes in *Clostridium botulinum* type A, Ab, and A(B) Strains. *Appl. Environ. Microbiol.* **2004**, *70*, 7192–7199. [CrossRef] [PubMed]
12. Dolly, J.O.; Oonnell, M.A. Neurotherapeutics to inhibit exocytosis from sensory neurons for the control of chronic pain. *Curr. Opin. Pharmacol.* **2012**, *12*, 100–108. [CrossRef] [PubMed]
13. Rummel, A. The long journey of botulinum neurotoxins into the synapse. *Toxicon* **2015**, in press. [CrossRef] [PubMed]
14. Singh, B.R. Intimate details of the most poisonous poison. *Nat. Struct. Biol.* **2000**, *7*, 617–619. [CrossRef] [PubMed]

15. Fdez, E.; Thomas, A.J.; Wang, M.-C.; Rajebhosale, M.; Foster, K.; Bella, J.; Baldock, C.; Philip, G.W.; Hilfiker, S. A role for soluble *N*-ethylmaleimide-sensitive factor attachment protein receptor complex dimerization during neurosecretion. *MolBiol. Cell* **2008**, *19*, 3379–3389. [CrossRef] [PubMed]
16. Dong, M.; Yeh, F.; Tepp, W.H.; Dean, C.; Johnson, E.A.; Janz, R.; Chapman, E.R. SV2 is the protein receptor for botulinum neurotoxin A. *Science* **2006**, *312*, 592–596. [CrossRef] [PubMed]
17. Kaya, S.; Hermans, L.; Willems, T.; Roussel, N.; Meeus, M. Central sensitization in urogynecological chronic pelvic pain: A systematic literature review. *Pain Phys.* **2013**, *16*, 291–308.
18. Aoki, K.R. Evidence for antinociceptive activity of botulinum toxin type A in pain management. *Headache* **2003**, *43*, 9–15. [CrossRef] [PubMed]
19. Oh, H.M.; Chung, M.E. Botulinum toxin for neuropathic pain: A review of the literature. *Toxins (Basel)* **2015**, *7*, 3127–3154. [CrossRef] [PubMed]
20. Singla, S.; Garg, R.; Singla, A.; Sharma, S.; Singh, J.; Sethi, P. Experience with uroflowmetry in evaluation of lower urinary tract symptoms in patients with benign prostatic hyperplasia. *J. Clin. Diagn. Res.* **2014**, *8*, NC01–NC03. [PubMed]
21. Wein, A. Symptom-based diagnosis of overactive bladder: An overview. *Can Urol Assoc J.* **2011**, *5*, S135–S136. [CrossRef] [PubMed]
22. Steers, W.D. Pathophysiology of overactive bladder and urge urinary incontinence. *Rev. Urol.* **2002**, *4*, S7–S18. [PubMed]
23. Yokoyama, O.; Yoshiyama, M.; Namiki, M.; de Groat, W.C. Glutamatergic and dopaminergic contributions to rat bladder hyperactivity after cerebral artery occlusion. *Am. J. Physiol.* **1999**, *276*, 935–942.
24. Andersson, K.E.; Pehrson, R. CNS involvement in overactive bladder: Pathophysiology and opportunities for pharmacological intervention. *Drugs* **2003**, *63*, 2595–2611. [CrossRef] [PubMed]
25. Banakhar, M.A.; Al-Shaiji, T.F.; Hassouna, M.M. Pathophysiology of overactive bladder. *Int. Urogynecol. J.* **2012**, *23*, 975–982. [CrossRef] [PubMed]
26. McMurray, G.; Dass, N.; Brading, A.F. Purinoceptor subtypes mediating contraction and relaxation of marmoset urinary bladder smooth muscle. *Br. J. Pharmacol.* **1998**, *123*, 1579–1586. [CrossRef] [PubMed]
27. Birder, L.A.; de Groat, W.C. Mechanisms of disease: Involvement of the urothelium in bladder dysfunction. *Nat. Clin. Pract. Urol.* **2007**, *4*, 46–54. [CrossRef] [PubMed]
28. Schurch, B.; Stohrer, M.; Kramer, G.; Griffiths, D.; Rosier, P.; Ulmsten, U.; van Kerrebroeck, P.; Victor, A.; Wein, A. Botulinum-A toxin for treating detrusor hyperreflexia in spinal cord injured patients: A new alternative to anticholinergic drugs? Preliminary results. *J. Urol.* **2000**, *164*, 692–697. [CrossRef]
29. Cruz, F. Targets for botulinum toxin in the lower urinary tract. *Neurourol. Urodyn.* **2014**, *33*, 31–38. [CrossRef] [PubMed]
30. Andersson, K.E.; Arner, A. Urinary bladder contraction and relaxation: Physiology and pathophysiology. *Physiol. Rev.* **2004**, *84*, 935–986. [CrossRef] [PubMed]
31. Schulte-Baukloh, H.; Priefert, J.; Knispel, H.H.; Lawrence, G.W.; Miller, K.; Neuhaus, J. Botulinum toxin A detrusor injections reduce postsynaptic muscular M2, M3, P2X2, and P2X3 receptors in children and adolescents who have neurogenic detrusor overactivity: A single-blind study. *Urology* **2013**, *81*, 1052–1057. [CrossRef] [PubMed]
32. Lawrence, G.W.; Aoki, K.R.; Dolly, J.O. Excitatory cholinergic and purinergic signaling in bladder are equally susceptible to botulinum neurotoxin a consistent with co-release of transmitters from efferent fibers. *J. Pharmacol. Exp. Ther.* **2010**, *334*, 1080–1086. [CrossRef] [PubMed]
33. Fowler, C.J.; Griffiths, D.; de Groat, W.C. The neural control of micturition. *Nat. Rev. Neurosci.* **2008**, *9*, 453–466. [CrossRef] [PubMed]
34. Ikeda, Y.; Zabbarova, I.V.; Birder, L.A.; de Groat, W.C.; McCarthy, C.J.; Hanna-Mitchell, A.T.; Kanai, A.J. Botulinum neurotoxin serotype A suppresses neurotransmitter release from afferent as well as efferent nerves in the urinary bladder. *Eur. Urol.* **2012**, *62*, 1157–1164. [CrossRef] [PubMed]
35. Khera, M.; Somogyi, G.T.; Kiss, S.; Boone, T.B.; Smith, C.P. Botulinum toxin A inhibits ATP release from bladder urothelium after chronic spinal cord injury. *Neurochem. Int.* **2004**, *45*, 987–993. [CrossRef] [PubMed]
36. Collins, V.M.; Daly, D.M.; Liaskos, M.; McKay, N.G.; Sellers, D.; Chapple, C.; Grundy, D. OnabotulinumtoxinA significantly attenuates bladder afferent nerve firing and inhibits ATP release from the urothelium. *BJU Int.* **2013**, *112*, 1018–1026. [CrossRef] [PubMed]

37. Apostolidis, A.; Popat, R.; Yiangou, Y.; Cockayne, D.; Ford, A.P.; Davis, J.B.; Dasgupta, P.; Fowler, C.J.; Anand, P. Decreased sensory receptors P2X3 and TRPV1 in suburothelial nerve fibers following intradetrusor injections of botulinum toxin for human detrusor overactivity. *J. Urol.* **2005**, *174*, 977–982. [CrossRef] [PubMed]
38. Soljanik, I. Efficacy and safety of botulinum toxin A intradetrusor injections in adults with neurogenic detrusor overactivity/neurogenic overactive bladder: A systematic review. *Drugs* **2013**, *73*, 1055–1066. [CrossRef] [PubMed]
39. Apostolidis, A.; Brady, C.M.; Yiangou, Y.; Davis, J.; Fowler, C.J.; Anand, P. Capsaicin receptor TRPV1 in urothelium of neurogenic human bladders and effect of intravesical resiniferatoxin. *Urology* **2005**, *65*, 400–405. [CrossRef] [PubMed]
40. Hanno, P.; Lin, A.; Nordling, J.; Nyberg, L.; van Ophoven, A.; Ueda, T.; Wein, A. Bladder pain syndrome committee of the international consultation on incontinence. *Neurourol. Urodyn.* **2010**, *29*, 191–198. [CrossRef] [PubMed]
41. Hanno, P.M. Bladder pain syndrome (interstitial cystitis) and related disorders. In *Campbell Walsh Urology*, 10th ed.; Louis, R.K., Andrew, C.N., Eds.; Elsevier: Philadelphia, PA, USA, 2012; Volume 1, p. 357.
42. Graham, E.; Chai, T.C. Dysfunction of bladder urothelium and bladder urothelial cells in interstitial cystitis. *Curr. Urol. Rep.* **2006**, *7*, 440–446. [CrossRef] [PubMed]
43. Nickel, J.C.; Emerson, L.; Cornish, J. The bladder mucus (glycosaminoglycan) layer in interstitial cystitis. *J. Urol.* **1993**, *149*, 716–718.
44. Sun, Y.; Chai, T.C. Up-regulation of P2X3 receptor during stretch of bladder urothelial cells from patients with interstitial cystitis. *J. Urol.* **2004**, *171*, 448–452. [CrossRef] [PubMed]
45. Sun, Y.; Keay, S.; Lehrfeld, T.J.; Chai, T.C. Changes in adenosine triphosphate-stimulated ATP release suggest association between cytokine and purinergic signaling in bladder urothelial cells. *Urology* **2009**, *74*, 1163–1168. [CrossRef] [PubMed]
46. Lazzeri, M.; Costantini, E.; Porena, M. TRP family proteins in the lower urinary tract: Translating basic science into new clinical prospective. *Ther. Adv. Urol.* **2009**, *1*, 33–42. [CrossRef] [PubMed]
47. Liu, B.L.; Yang, F.; Zhan, H.L.; Feng, Z.Y.; Zhang, Z.G.; Li, W.B.; Zhou, X.F. Increased severity of inflammation correlates with elevated expression of TRPV1 nerve fibers and nerve growth factor on interstitial cystitis/bladder pain syndrome. *Urol. Int.* **2014**, *92*, 202–208. [CrossRef] [PubMed]
48. Liu, H.T.; Shie, J.H.; Chen, S.H.; Wang, Y.S.; Kuo, H.C. Differences in mast cell infiltration, E-cadherin, and zonula occludens-1 expression between patients with overactive bladder and interstitial cystitis/bladder pain syndrome. *Urology* **2012**, *80*. [CrossRef] [PubMed]
49. Sant, G.R.; Kempuraj, D.; Marchand, J.E.; Theoharides, T.C. The mast cell in interstitial cystitis: Role in pathophysiology and pathogenesis. *Urology* **2007**, *69*, 34–40. [CrossRef] [PubMed]
50. O'Connor, T.M.; O'Connell, J.; O'Brien, D.I.; Goode, T.; Bredin, C.P.; Shanahan, F. The role of substance P in inflammatory disease. *J. Cell Physiol.* **2004**, *201*, 167–180. [CrossRef] [PubMed]
51. Pang, X.; Marchand, J.; Sant, G.R.; Kream, R.M.; Theoharides, T.C. Increased number of substance P positive nerve fibres in interstitial cystitis. *Br. J. Urol.* **1995**, *75*, 744–750. [CrossRef] [PubMed]
52. Buffington, C.A.; Wolfe, S.A., Jr. High-affinity binding sites for [3*H*]substance P in urinary bladders of cats with interstitial cystitis. *J. Urol.* **1998**, *160*, 605–611. [CrossRef]
53. Rudick, C.N.; Bryce, P.J.; Guichelaar, L.A.; Berry, R.E.; Klumpp, D.J. Mast cell-derived histamine mediates cystitis pain. *PLoS ONE* **2008**, *7*, e2096. [CrossRef]
54. McMahon, S.B. NGF as a mediator of inflammatory pain. *Philos. Trans. R Soc. Lond. B Biol. Sci.* **1996**, *351*, 431–440. [CrossRef] [PubMed]
55. Cruz, C.D. Neurotrophins in bladder function: what do we know and where do we go from here? *Neurourol. Urodyn.* **2014**, *33*, 39–45. [CrossRef] [PubMed]
56. Liu, H.T.; Kuo, H.C. Increased urine and serum nerve growth factor levels in interstitial cystitis suggest chronic inflammation is involved in the pathogenesis of disease. *PLoS ONE* **2012**, *7*, e44687. [CrossRef] [PubMed]
57. Smith, C.P.; Radziszewski, P.; Borkowski, A.; Somogyi, G.T.; Boone, T.B.; Chancellor, M.B. Botulinum toxin A has antinociceptive effects in treating interstitial cystitis. *Urology* **2004**, *64*, 871–875. [CrossRef] [PubMed]

58. Kuo, H.C.; Jiang, Y.H.; Tsai, Y.C.; Kuo, Y.C. Intravesical botulinum toxin-A injections reduce bladder pain of interstitial cystitis/bladder pain syndrome refractory to conventional treatment—A prospective, multicenter, randomized, double-blind, placebo-controlled clinical trial. *Neurourol. Urodyn.* **2015**. in press. [CrossRef] [PubMed]
59. Hanno, P.M.; Erickson, D.; Moldwin, R.; Faraday, M.M.; American Urological Association. Diagnosis and treatment of interstitial cystitis/bladder pain syndrome: AUA guideline amendment. *J. Urol.* **2015**, *193*, 1545–1553. [CrossRef] [PubMed]
60. Apostolidis, A.; Dasgupta, P.; Fowler, C.J. Proposed mechanism for the efficacy of injected botulinum toxin in the treatment of human detrusor overactivity. *Eur. Urol.* **2006**, *49*, 644–650. [CrossRef] [PubMed]
61. Brain, S.D.; Williams, T.J.; Tippins, J.R.; Morris, H.R.; MacIntyre, I. Calcitonin gene-related peptide is a potent vasodilator. *Nature* **1985**, *313*, 54–56. [CrossRef] [PubMed]
62. Rapp, D.E.; Turk, K.W.; Bales, G.T.; Cook, S.P. Botulinum toxin type A inhibits calcitonin gene-related peptide release from isolated rat bladder. *J. Urol.* **2006**, *175*, 1138–1142. [CrossRef]
63. Lucioni, A.; Bales, G.T.; Lotan, T.L.; McGehee, D.S.; Cook, S.P.; Rapp, D.E. Botulinum toxin type A inhibits sensory neuropeptide release in rat bladder models of acute injury and chronic inflammation. *BJU Int.* **2008**, *101*, 366–370. [CrossRef] [PubMed]
64. Liu, H.T.; Kuo, H.C. Intravesical botulinum toxin A injections plus hydrodistension can reduce nerve growth factor production and control bladder pain in interstitial cystitis. *Urology* **2007**, *70*, 463–468. [CrossRef] [PubMed]
65. Liu, H.T.; Tyagi, P.; Chancellor, M.B.; Kuo, H.C. Urinary nerve growth factor level is increased in patients with interstitial cystitis/bladder pain syndrome and decreased in responders to treatment. *BJU Int.* **2009**, *104*, 1476–1481. [CrossRef] [PubMed]
66. Pinto, R.; Lopes, T.; Costa, D.; Barros, S.; Silva, J.; Silva, C.; Cruz, C.; Dinis, P.; Cruz, F. Ulcerative and nonulcerative forms of bladder pain syndrome/interstitial cystitis do not differ in symptom intensity or response to onabotulinum toxin A. *Urology* **2014**, *83*, 1030–1034. [CrossRef] [PubMed]
67. Shie, J.H.; Liu, H.T.; Wang, Y.S.; Kuo, H.C. Immunohistochemical evidence suggests repeated intravesical application of botulinum toxin A injections may improve treatment efficacy of interstitial cystitis/bladder pain syndrome. *BJU Int.* **2013**, *111*, 638–646. [CrossRef] [PubMed]
68. Peng, C.H.; Jhang, J.F.; Shie, J.H.; Kuo, H.C. Down-regulation of vascular endothelial growth factor is associated with decreased inflammation after intravesical OnabotulinumtoxinA injections combined with hydrodistention for patients with interstitial cystitis-clinical results and immunohistochemistry analysis. *Urology* **2013**, *82*, e1–e6. [PubMed]
69. Akaike, N.; Shin, M.C.; Wakita, M.; Torii, Y.; Harakawa, T.; Ginnaga, A.; Kato, K.; Kaji, R.; Kozaki, S. Trans synaptic inhibition of spinal transmission by A2 botulinum toxin. *J. Physiol.* **2013**, *15*, 1031–1043. [CrossRef] [PubMed]
70. Dmochowski, R.R. Bladder outlet obstruction: Etiology and evaluation. *Rev. Urol.* **2005**, *7*, S3–S13. [PubMed]
71. Chancellor, M.B.; Kaplan, S.A.; Blaivas, J.G. Detrusor-external sphincter dyssynergia. *Ciba. Found Symp.* **1990**, *151*, 195–206. [PubMed]
72. Schurch, B.; Hodler, J.; Rodic, B. Botulinum A toxin as a treatment of detrusor-sphincter dyssynergia in patients with spinal cord injury: MRI controlled transperineal injections. *J. Neurol. Neurosurg. Psychiatry* **1997**, *63*, 474–476. [CrossRef] [PubMed]
73. Utomo, E.; Groen, J.; Blok, B.F. Surgical management of functional bladder outlet obstruction in adults with neurogenic bladder dysfunction. *Cochrane Database Syst. Rev.* **2014**, *24*, CD004927.
74. Dykstra, D.D.; Sidi, A.A.; Scott, A.B.; Pagel, J.M.; Goldish, G.D. Effects of botulinum A toxin on detrusor-sphincter dyssynergia in spinal cord injury patients. *J. Urol.* **1988**, *139*, 919–922. [PubMed]
75. Chen, S.L.; Bih, L.I.; Huang, Y.H.; Tsai, S.J.; Lin, T.B.; Kao, Y.L. Effect of single botulinum toxin A injection to the external urethral sphincter for treating detrusor external sphincter dyssynergia in spinal cord injury. *J. Rehabil. Med.* **2008**, *40*, 744–748. [CrossRef] [PubMed]
76. Mahfouz, W.; Corcos, J. Management of detrusor external sphincter dyssynergia in neurogenic bladder. *Eur. J. Phys. Rehabil. Med.* **2011**, *47*, 639–650. [PubMed]
77. Sinha, S. Dysfunctional voiding: A review of the terminology, presentation, evaluation and management in children and adults. *Indian J. Urol.* **2011**, *27*, 437–447. [CrossRef] [PubMed]

78. Groutz, A.; Blaivas, J.G.; Pies, C.; Sassone, A.M. Learned voiding dysfunction (non-neurogenic, neurogenic bladder) among adults. *Neurourol. Urodyn.* **2001**, *20*, 259–268. [CrossRef] [PubMed]
79. Fowler, C.J.; Christmas, T.J.; Chapple, C.R.; Parkhouse, H.F.; Kirby, R.S.; Jacobs, H.S. Abnormalel ectromyographic activity of the urethral sphincter, voiding dysfunction, and polycystic ovaries: A new syndrome? *Br. Med. J.* **1988**, *297*, 1436–1438. [CrossRef]
80. Kuo, H.C. Videourodynamic characteristics and lower urinary tract symptoms of female bladder outlet obstruction. *Urology* **2005**, *66*, 1005–1009. [CrossRef] [PubMed]
81. Franco, I.; Landau-Dyer, L.; Isom-Batz, G.; Collett, T.; Reda, E.F. The use of botulinum toxin A injection for the management of external sphincter dyssynergia in neurologically normal children. *J. Urol.* **2007**, *178*, 1775–1779. [CrossRef] [PubMed]
82. Sacco, E.; Tienforti, D.; Bientinesi, R.; D'Addessi, A.; Racioppi, M.; Pinto, F.; Totaro, A.; Vittori, M.; D'Agostino, D.; Bassi, P. OnabotulinumtoxinA injection therapy in men with LUTS due to primary bladder-neck dysfunction: Objective and patient-reported outcomes. *Neurourol. Urodyn.* **2014**, *33*, 142–146. [CrossRef] [PubMed]
83. Abbott, J.A.; Jarvis, S.K.; Lyons, S.D.; Thomson, A.; Vancaille, T.G. Botulinum toxin type A for chronic pain and pelvic floor spasm in women: A randomized controlled trial. *Obstet. Gynecol.* **2006**, *108*, 915–923. [CrossRef] [PubMed]
84. Smith, C.P.; Franks, M.E.; McNeil, B.K.; Ghosh, R.; de Groat, W.C.; Chancellor, M.B.; Somogyi, G.T. Effect of botulinum toxin A on the autonomic nervous system of the rat lower urinary tract. *J. Urol.* **2003**, *169*, 1896–1900. [CrossRef] [PubMed]
85. Abrams, P. LUTS, BPH, BPE, BPO: A plea for the logical use of correct terms. *Rev. Urol.* **1999**, *1*, 65. [PubMed]
86. Isaacs, J.T. Etiology of benign prostatic hyperplasia. *Eur. Urol.* **1994**, *25*, 6–9. [PubMed]
87. Brisinda, G.; Cadeddu, F.; Vanella, S.; Mazzeo, P.; Marniga, G.; Maria, G. Relief by botulinum toxin of lower urinary tract symptoms owing to benign prostatic hyperplasia: Early and long-term results. *Urology* **2009**, *73*, 90–94. [CrossRef] [PubMed]
88. HamidiMadani, A.; Enshaei, A.; Heidarzadeh, A.; Mokhtari, G.; Farzan, A.; Asli, M.M.; Esmaeili, S. Transurethral intraprostatic Botulinum toxin-A injection: A novel treatment for BPH refractory to current medical therapy in poor surgical candidates. *World J. Urol.* **2013**, *31*, 235–239. [CrossRef] [PubMed]
89. Sacco, E.; Bientinesi, R.; Marangi, F.; Totaro, A.; D'Addessi, A.; Racioppi, M.; Pinto, F.; Vittori, M.; Bassi, P. Patient-reported outcomes in men with lower urinary tract symptoms (LUTS) due to benign prostatic hyperplasia (BPH) treated with intraprostatic OnabotulinumtoxinA: 3-month results of a prospective single-armed cohort study. *BJU Int.* **2012**, *110*, E837–E844. [CrossRef] [PubMed]
90. Rusnack, S.R.; Kaplan, S.A. The use of botulinum toxin in men with benign prostatic hyperplasia. *Rev. Urol.* **2005**, *7*, 234–236. [PubMed]
91. Ruggieri, M.R.; Colton, M.D.; Wang, P.; Wang, J.; Smyth, R.J.; Pontari, M.A.; Luthin, G.R. Human prostate muscarinic receptor subtypes. *J. Pharmacol. Exp. Ther.* **1995**, *274*, 976–982. [PubMed]
92. Doggweiler, R.; Zermann, D.; Ishigooka, M.; Schmidt, R.A. Botox-induced prostatic involution. *Prostate* **1998**, *37*, 44–50. [CrossRef]
93. Chuang, Y.C.; Tu, C.H.; Huang, C.C.; Lin, H.J.; Chiang, P.H.; Yoshimura, N.; Chancellor, M.B. Intraprostatic injection of botulinum toxin type-A relieves bladder outlet obstruction in human and induces prostate apoptosis in dogs. *BMC Urol.* **2006**, *18*. [CrossRef]
94. Silva, J.; Pinto, R.; Carvallho, T.; Coelho, A.; Avelino, A.; Dinis, P.; Cruz, F. Mechanisms of prostate atrophy after glandular botulinum neurotoxin type A injection: An experimental study in the rat. *Eur. Urol.* **2009**, *56*, 134–140. [CrossRef] [PubMed]
95. Nishiyama, Y.; Yokoyama, T.; Tomizawa, K.; Okamura, K.; Yamamoto, Y.; Matsui, H.; Oguma, K.; Nagai, A.; Kumon, H. Effects of purified newly developed botulinum neurotoxin type A in rat prostate. *Urology* **2009**, *74*, 436–439. [CrossRef] [PubMed]
96. Kuo, H.C.; Liu, H.T. Therapeutic effects of add-on botulinum toxin A on patients with large benign prostatic hyperplasia and unsatisfactory response to combined medical therapy. *Scand. J. Urol. Nephrol.* **2009**, *43*, 206–211. [CrossRef] [PubMed]

97. De Kort, L.M.; Kok, E.T.; Jonges, T.N.; Rosier, P.F.; Bosch, J.L. Urodynamic effects of transrectal intraprostatic Ona botulinum toxin A injections for symptomatic benign prostatic hyperplasia. *Urology* **2012**, *80*, 889–893. [CrossRef] [PubMed]
98. Marberger, M.; Chartier-Kastler, E.; Egerdie, B.; Lee, K.S.; Grosse, J.; Bugarin, D.; Zhou, J.; Patel, A.; Haag-Molkenteller, C. A randomized, double-blind, placebo-controlled, phase 2 dose-ranging study of onabotulinumtoxinA in men with benign prostatic hyperplasia. *Eur. Urol.* **2013**, *63*, 496–503. [CrossRef] [PubMed]

5

Clinical Efficacy and Changes of Urothelial Dysfunction after Repeated Detrusor Botulinum Toxin A Injections in Chronic Spinal Cord-Injured Bladder

Sheng-Fu Chen, Chia-Hwei Chang and Hann-Chorng Kuo *

Department of Urology, Buddhist Tzu Chi General Hospital and Tzu Chi University, 707, Section 3, Chung Yang Road, Hualian 970, Taiwan; madaux@yahoo.com.tw (S.-F.C.); cha615@tzuchi.com.tw (C.-H.C.)
* Correspondence: ck@tzuchi.com.tw

Academic Editor: Flaminia Pavone

Abstract: Chornic spinal cord injury (SCI) will induce bladder urothelium dysfunction. This study investigated the therapeutic effects on urothelial dysfunction after repeated detrusor injections of onabotulinumtoxinA (BoNT-A) in SCI patients with neurogenic detrusor overactivity (NDO). Twenty chronic suprasacral SCI patients with NDO were enrolled. The patients received 300 U BoNT-A injection into the detrusor every six months. The urothelium was assessed by cystoscopic biopsy at baseline and six months after each BoNT-A treatment. Immunofluorescence staining for urothelial dysfunction, including E-cadherin, zonula occludens-1 (ZO-1), tryptase for mast cell activity, and urothelial apoptosis were investigated. The outcome of urothelial dysfunction parameters after BoNT-A injection were compared between baseline and six months after each treatment. Repeated 300 U BoNT-A injections showed a sustained decrease of detrusor pressure compared with baseline. After three repeated BoNT-A detrusor injections, significantly greater distributions of E-cadherin ($p = 0.042$) and ZO-1 ($p = 0.003$) expressions, but no significant changes, of urothelial apoptosis and mast cell activation were found after repeated BoNT-A therapy. Urothelial dysfunction, such as adhesive and junction protein concentrations in SCI patients' bladders, recovered after three repeated cycles of BoNT-A treatment. The therapeutic effects sustained. However, urothelial inflammation and apoptosis after SCI were not significantly improved after three repeated BoNT-A injections.

Keywords: botulinum toxin A; urothelial dysfunction; spinal cord injury

---

1. Introduction

Spinal cord injury (SCI) is a significant cause of morbidity and mortality in developing countries, with the worldwide incidence of SCI reported in the literature ranges from 12.1 to 57.8 per million [1]. In chronic SCI patients, the main problems of neurogenic lower urinary tract dysfunction (NLUTD) are failure to store due to detrusor overactivity (DO), or urethral incompetence. Another problem is failure to empty due to detrusor areflexia, bladder neck dysfunction, or detrusor sphincter dyssynergia (DSD), and a usually-combined failure to store and empty, such as due to DSD or DO and impaired contractility [2]. If not well managed, high intravesical pressure may damage the upper urinary tract, causing renal scarring and chronic renal insufficiency, which greatly impairs the quality of life [3]. SCI also leads to rapid disruption of the uroepithelial barrier. This manifests in a loss of cell–cell interactions, decrease in transepithelial resistance, and increases in water and urea permeability [4]. Disruption of the urothelial barrier initiates a cascade of bladder dysfunction events, leading to suburothelial inflammation and vulnerability to chronic or recurrent cystitis or infection, or both. Suburothelial inflammation might also affect urothelial function, leading to a vicious cycle.

Our previous study had shown decreased expression of urothelial adhesive and junction proteins and increased suburothelial inflammation and apoptosis in patients with chronic SCI, regardless of injury level [5]. OnabotulinumtoxinA (BoNT-A) has been proved useful in the treatment of NDO in SCI patients in a large phase-three clinical trial [6].

BoNT-A is one of the most powerful neurotoxins; it inhibits the release of neurotransmitters from the nerve fibers and urothelium [7]. It is possible to stem the disruption of the uroepithelium by modulating the release of neurotransmitters and inflammatory mediators. BoNT-A injection decreases bladder nerve growth factor (NGF) production and urinary NGF levels, suggesting an anti-inflammatory response can be achieved after intravesical BoNT-A treatment [8]. In our recent study, the urothelial dysfunction and adhesive and junction protein concentrations in SCI patients' bladders recovered after BoNT-A treatment after a single injection [9].

Repeated BoNT-A detrusor injection has been shown to have good results and safety for control of NDO in chronic SCI bladders [10,11]. However, there is insufficient data to definitively determine whether repeated BoNT-A injection into the detrusor has a sustained improvement in the urothelial dysfunction. This study investigated the therapeutic effects of repeated detrusor injection of BoNT-A on urothelial dysfunction in SCI bladders.

2. Results

A total of 20 patients with chronic SCI and 10 controls were enrolled in this study. The SCI patients included 11 men and nine women with a mean age of 48.2 ± 18.41 years. Among them, 15 had complete injuries while five had incomplete injuries. The injury level was at cervical spinal cord in seven patients, thoracic cord in 11, and lumbar cord in two. Among the SCI patients, 16 patients had DSD. No patient having an indwelling catheter or cystostomy was enrolled in this study. The control group included 10 women with stress urinary incontinence with a mean age of 52.40 ± 10.51 years.

The changes in urodynamic parameters after repeated BoNT-A injections are shown in Table 1. Significant increases in cystometric bladder capacity (CBC) and post-void residual (PVR) volume, and a significant decrease in detrusor pressure at Qmax (Pdet.Qmax) were noted six months after each BoNT-A injection. The therapeutic effects of repeated injections on the objective measures of Video-urodynamic study (VUDS) were consistent throughout the treatment course until the end of the study. The Pdet.Qmax decreased to less than 25 cmH_2O, which was considered a level safe enough to prevent upper urinary tract damage. Not surprisingly, the PVR volume also increased along with the incremental CBC increase.

Table 1. Changes of the urodynamic parameters at 6 months after each set of 300 U BoNT-A detrusor injection compared with baseline and the control.

Videourodynamic Parameter	Control	Baseline 1st BoNt-A	1st BoNT-A + 6 M	2nd BoNt-A + 6 M	3rd BoNT-A + 6 M
CBC (mL)	364 ± 196	163 ± 97.7 *	223 ± 150 **	245 ± 137 **	239 ± 118 **
Pdet(cmH_2O)	25.2 ± 14.5	42.7 ± 12.5 *	33.2 ± 28.6 **	22.8 ± 16.9 **	22.2 ± 19.1 **
Qmax (mL/s)	11.9 ± 6.25	6.9 ± 6.27 *	2.61 ± 3.50 **	2.75 ± 4.89 **	3.15 ± 4.97 **
Volume (mL)	302 ± 154	91.4 ± 99.2 *	34.9 ± 51.3 **	38.6 ± 71.5 **	57.7 ± 82.6 **
PVR (mL)	93.3 ± 107	118 ± 90.7 *	245 ± 179 **	343 ± 190 **	329 ± 170 **
Compliance (mL/cmH_2O)	86.3 ± 38.0	25.6 ± 28.3 *	30.0 ± 35.1	36.7 ± 32.5	44.5 ± 56.2

CBC: cystometric bladder capacity; Pdet: detrusor pressure at Qmax; Qmax: maximum flow rate; PVR: post-void residual volume; BoNT-A: OnabotulinumtoxinA. Data are expressed as mean ± standard deviation. * Indicates significantly different between control and the baseline before BoNT-A treatment of SCI bladders; ** Indicates significant difference between six months after each BoNT-A treatment compared with baseline.

Table 2 showed the changes of the urothelial dysfunction at baseline and six months after each set of 300 U BoNT-A detrusor injections and the control. At baseline, the expression of E-cadherin, ZO-1 in the SCI patients decreased significantly, compared with the controls ($p < 0.01$). A significant increase in urothelial cell apoptosis was also observed in the bladder specimens from SCI patients ($p = 0.047$). Figure 1 shows the significantly lower expressions of E-cadherin and ZO-1 in the SCI bladders compared with the corresponding expressions in the control bladders ($p < 0.001$).

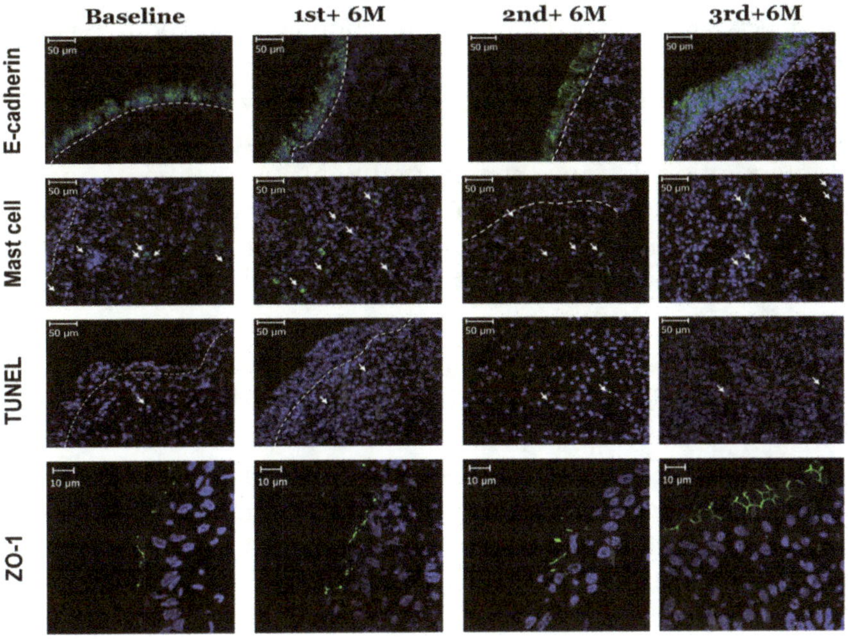

Figure 1. Shows the significantly lower expressions of E-cadherin and zonula occludens-1 (ZO-1) in the spinal cord injury (SCI) bladders compared with the corresponding expressions in the control bladders. The target cells are labelled in green (as the arrows indicate) and the white dotted lines indicate the boundary between the urothelium and suburothelium.

Table 2. Changes of the urothelial dysfunction parameters at baseline and 6 months after each set of 300 U BoNT-A detrusor injections and compared with control.

Urothelial Dysfunction Parameter	Control	Baseline 1st BoNT-A	1st BoNT-A + 6 M	2nd BoNT-A + 6 M	3rd BoNT-A + 6 M
E-cadherin	41.3 ± 8.40	25.6 ± 21.4 *	29.5 ± 28.4	30.9 ± 32.8	42.4 ± 27.0 #
Mast cell	5.89 ± 4.92	7.51 ± 6.60	9.61 ± 6.92	7.47 ± 6.22	9.87 ± 7.29
TUNEL	1.00 ± 1.35	2.40 ± 4.67 *	2.59 ± 2.11 *	2.23 ± 1.31 *	2.42 ± 2.45 *
ZO-1	6.37 ± 1.72	2.77 ± 3.24 *	5.08 ± 6.09	6.86 ± 7.25 #	8.32 ± 6.78 #

TUNEL: the terminal deoxynucleotidyl transferase dUTP nick end labelling; ZO-1: zonula occludens-1. Data are expressed as mean ± standard deviation. * Indicates significantly different ($p < 0.05$) between each BoNT-A treatment compared with control group; # Indicates significantly different ($p < 0.05$) 6 months after each BoNT-A treatment compared with baseline.

At six months after each BoNT-A injection, persistent improvements of E-cadherin and ZO-1 expressions were noted compared with the baseline. After the third BoNT-A injection, the distribution of E-cadherin expression was significantly higher compared with baseline (42.4 ± 27.0 *vs.* 25.6 ± 21.4 fluorescence intensity units per 4 μm^2, $p = 0.004$). The same trend was also noted in ZO-1 expression. A significantly higher distribution of ZO-1 after repeated second and third BoNT-A injection compared with baseline was noted (6.86 ± 7.25 *vs.* 2.77 ± 3.24, $p = 0.008$, and 8.32 ± 6.78 *vs.* 2.77 ± 3.24, $p = 0.003$, respectively). However, the mast cell activity showed no significant difference between baseline and six months after each injections, nor did urothelial cell apoptosis differ significantly after repeated BoNT-A treatment compared with baseline (Table 2).

When we compared the urothelial dysfunction parameters after repeated BoNT-A injection with the controls the distribution of E-cadherin expression improved to non-significant difference from the control after the first and second BoNT-A injections, and sustained at six months after the third BoNT-A injection. ($p = 0.187$, $p = 0.403$, $p = 0.812$, respectively). The same finding was also noted in ZO-1 expression ($p = 0.11$, $p = 0.965$, $p = 0.373$, respectively). On the other hand, the urothelial cell apoptosis did not decrease after each BoNT-A injection and showed persistently greater than the control ($p = 0.03$, $p = 0.03$, $p = 0.04$, respectively).

No severe adverse events such as general weakness or severe autonomic dysreflexia occurred after BoNT-A injection. Five patients had slight hematuria which was spontaneously resolved within three days without intervention. During the repeated BoNT-A treatment course, one-third patients suffered from symptomatic urinary tract infection (UTI) (febrile or micturition pain with pyuria and positive urine culture), which were carefully controlled by antibiotic treatment. The rate of satisfactory dryness reported by patients was 60%.

3. Discussion

This study shows that impaired expression of the adhesive protein E-cadherin and tight junction protein ZO-1 and significantly higher apoptosis in the urothelium of patients with chronic SCI and NDO. After repeated detrusor BoNT-A injections, E-cadherin, and ZO-1 expressions were recovered, and the effects sustained up to 6 months after the third treatment. However, the chronic inflammation and urothelial apoptosis did not improve after repeated BoNT-A injections.

To our knowledge, there is limited data focus on urothelial dysfunction after repeated detrusor BoNT-A injections for SCI patients with NDO. This study provides evidence that repeated detrusor BoNT-A injections improve the impaired adhesive and junction proteins of urothelium in SCI patients. Lower urinary tract dysfunction and complications are major concerns in the management of SCI patients. Apodaca *et al.* found that SCI also led to rapid disruption of the uroepithelial barrier [4]. The impaired urothelium in SCI bladders may cause chronic infammation and easy to induce UTI. SCI is associated with a number of changes in the urothelium, including both structural changes and defects in urothelial signaling changes [12]. Our previous study showed increased urothelial cell apoptosis and chronic inflammation are associated with recurrent UTI [13]. The asymptomatic bacteriuria might result in increased excitability of suburothelial sensory fibers and induce DO at a small bladder volume. Cruz *et al.* recently proposed that the changes in the urothelium after SCI might play a role in the pathophysiology of NDO [14].

Since 2000, minimally invasive BoNT-A injections into the detrusor have been reported to improve clinical and urodynamic parameters and quality of life in patients with refractory NDO in several open-label studies [15–19]. In our previous study, the success rate was 73.3% in SCI patients with NDO who received a single detrusor injection of 200 U BoNT-A, and the therapeutic effect lasted for 3 to 9 months (mean, 5.3 months) [20]. Based on that study, the injection protocol in this study was designed as repeated injections every six months in order to observe the consistency of therapeutic effects of the repeated BoNT-A injections.

BoNT-A can inhibit adenosin triphosphate release from the urothelium [7]. BoNT-A treatment not only inhibits transmitter release from efferent nerve endings but also sensory nerve terminals and urothelium [7]. In humans with NDO the expressions of bladder muscarinic receptors M2 and M3 and purinergic receptors $P2X_2$ and $P2X_3$ are reduced after detrusor BoNT-A injections, suggesting that BoNT-A inhibits DO by acting through inhibition of both the sensory and motor arms of the micturition reflex [21–24].

E-cadherin is a calcium-dependent glycoprotein, which plays a critical role in cell-to-cell adhesion. Loss of E-cadherin function can trigger cancer progression and metastasis [21]. ZO-1 is a tight junction protein that maintains the highly resistant urothelial barrier [25]. Previous study has also established a molecular connection between E-cadherin and transient receptor potential vanilloid 4 channel (TRPV4), suggesting that E-cadherin is also associated with bladder sensation and barrier function [26]. Our previous study showed decreased expression of E-cadherin and junction protein ZO-1 in patients with chronic SCI, regardless of injury level [5]. In the current study, the urothelial barrier function recovered after BoNT-A injections by improving the adhesive and tight junction protein levels. This result might, in part, explain the mechanism of decrease of the hyperexcitability of C-fiber bladder afferents, thereby reducing NDO. Our recent study reported the urothelial dysfunction improved at short-term but not persistent in a single BoNT-A injection [9]. This study further provides evidence that repeated BoNT-A injections can have a sustained therapeutic effect on NDO in SCI patients.

The mast cells degranulate and release pre-formed mediators of inflammation including histamine, heparin, and tryptase [27]. Apoptosis is a stepwise process characterized by a series of stereotypical morphological changes that eventually lead to cell death. Urothelial cell apoptosis in patients with interstitial cystitis/bladder pain syndrome resulted from upregulation of the inflammatory signals, including p38 mitogen-activated protein kinase and tumor necrosis factor-α [28]. In the present study, we showed that the apoptotic process was highly activated in the bladders of patients with SCI compared to the control group. After repeated BoNT-A injections, the urothelial apoptosis and mast cell activity were persistently higher than controls, which suggested that the neurogenic inflammation of SCI bladders cannot be inhibited by BoNT-A treatments. One possible cause for this result is the presence of asymptomatic UTI in one third of patients during the BoNT-A treatment course. Despite of this, the barrier function improvement could prevent the vicious cycle which might lead to end-stage bladder dysfunction.

In addition to the benefit of decreased detrusor pressure to prevent renal damage, BoNT-A injection for SCI with NDO significantly improves quality of life [29]. In the past 10 years, most study used 300 U of BoNT-A for treatment of NDO, usually as 30 injections of 10 U/mL in the bladder (excluding the trigone) under cystoscopic guidance and with different types of anesthesia [16]. Several phase-three multicenter trials were conducted to investigate the efficacy and safety of detrusor BoNT-A injections in patients with NDO due to SCI or multiple sclerosis. BoNT-A 200 U or 300 U injection significantly reduced urinary incontinence episodes compared with placebo. The effects were equally observed in both SCI and multiple sclerosis patients, and less side effects occurred in 200 U treatment group [6]. This study shows that BoNT-A injection improves NDO in SCI bladders not only by anticholinergic effect, but also by the improvement of the urothelium function after treatment.

Our results showed the barrier function was improved after BoNT-A treatment, but the urothelial apoptosis and mast cell activation expression did not improve after repeated BoNT-A injections. The cause why the discrepancy occurs after BoTN-A injections remained further study. We speculated that the bladder biopsy was taken at six months after the latest BoNT-A injection, which might lower the therapeutic efficacy of BoNT-A on neurogenic inflammation due to SCI. In addition, the presence of asymptomatic UTI in one third of patients during the BoNT-A treatment course might also have affect on this result. Put together, although BoNT-A injection can improve barrier function in SCI bladders, the increased suburothelial inflammation and urothelial apoptosis did not show significant improvement after three BoNT-A injections. Nevertheless, the persistent effects of BoNT-A on increase of bladder capacity and decrease of detrusor pressure are beneficial to the SCI patients with refractory urinary incontinence.

A limitation of the present study is the small case number and short term follow-up. Secondly, around one-third of patients had asymptomatic UTI during follow-up might affect the results of anti-inflammatory effects of BoNT-A. Another limitation is that we did not analyze the patients smoking history, which might affect the urothelial function. Finally, there is no histologic assessment, which may provide compatible information to support our results. In addition, the therapeutic effects of sensory protein improvements of TRPV1, P2X receptors, connexin, and endothelial nitric oxide synthase have not yet been thoroughly investigated and require further study. Despite of these limitations, this preliminary study has demonstrated the therapeutic effect of BoNT-A treatment on improvement of urothelial dysfunction in the chronic SCI bladders.

4. Conclusions

Urothelial dysfunction and adhesive and junction protein concentrations in SCI bladders recovered after repeated 300 U BoNT-A injections. The therapeutic effects sustained up to six months after the third BoNT-A injection and reach the normal level. However, neurogenic inflammation and urothelial apoptosis after SCI was not significantly improved after repeated BoNT-A injections.

5. Materials and Methods

In this prospective study, 20 patients with chronic SCI and NDO refractory to anti-muscarinic treatment were consecutively enrolled. All patients received four sets of 300 U of BoNT-A (Allergan, Irvine, CA, USA) detrusor injection every six months. VUDS was routinely performed prior to enrolment to confirm the presence of DO with or without DSD. Patients were excluded if they had an active UTI or urinary tract cancer at enrolment, history of lower urinary tract surgery, or chronic systemic diseases such as congestive heart failure and chronic renal failure. Additionally, repeated BoNT-A injection would be hold when patients were found to have active UTI before treatment. All patients had been educated to perform intermittent catheterization (IC) due to possible urinary retention after BoNT-A injection. IC is the standard management in European Association of Urology (EAU) guideline for NLUTD patients who are unable to empty their bladder adequately [30].

All subjects gave their informed consent for inclusion before they participated in the study. The study was conducted in accordance with the Institutional Review Board, and the protocol was approved by the Ethics Committee of Buddhist Tzu Chi General Hospital (IRB: TCGH 101-61, 30 October 2016). Each patient was informed about the study rationale and procedures, and written informed consent to participate in the study was obtained before any bladder procedure. The patients received BoNT-A injection under intravenous general anesthesia in the operating room. Each vial of BoNT-A (100 U) was diluted with 10 mL of normal saline and 30 injections evenly distributed into the detrusor were given using a 23-gauge needle (Richard Wolf, Knittlingen, Germany) and a rigid cystoscopic injection instrument (22 French Richard Wolf, Knittlingen, Germany). Four bladder cold cup biopsies were taken randomly at the posterior wall above the interureteric ridge, and only the bladder mucosa and submucosa were taken to prevent bladder perforation. One bladder biopsy specimen was sent to the pathology department for hematoxylin and eosin staining to exclude the possibility of carcinoma *in situ*. The remaining three specimens were stored in optimum cutting temperature (OCT) and liquid nitrogen for further immunohistochemistry studies.

At six months after the previous BoNT-A treatment, patients underwent repeat VUDS and bladder biopsy and then received the next BoNT-A injection at that time. We also invited 10 female patients with stress urinary incontinence but without urgency frequency symptoms to serve as controls for comparison. All control patients had been proven free of bladder outlet obstruction by VUDS. The bladder tissue was obtained during anti-incontinence surgery and processed as the SCI patients. Male patient was not selected to serve as the controls, because the prostate might cause bladder outlet obstruction and affect the urothelial function [31].

Immunofluorescence staining and quantification of protein expression in the bladder tissues of SCI patients and controls were investigated for urothelial adhesive and junction proteins by measuring E-cadherin expression and ZO-1 expression, respectively. Mast cell activation was assessed by measuring tryptase levels. Urothelial cell apoptosis was evaluated using the terminal deoxynucleotidyl transferase dUTP nick end labelling (TUNEL) assay as described previously [21,32].

The urinary bladder specimens were immersed and fixed for 1 h in an ice-cold solution of 4% formaldehyde in phosphate buffered saline (PBS) (pH 7.4) (SIGMA, Saint Louis, MO, USA). They were then rinsed with ice-cold PBS containing 15% sucrose (SIGMA, Saint Louis, USA) for 12 h. Biopsy specimens were embedded in OCT medium and stored at −80 °C. Four sections per specimen were cut using a cryostat HM550 OP (Microm International GmbH, Walldorf, Germany) at a thickness of 8 μm and collected on new silane III-coated glass slides (Muto Pure Chemicals Co. Ltd., Tokyo, Japan). Sections were post-fixed in acetone (SIGMA, Saint Louis, MO, USA) at −20 °C and blocked with Power Blocking reagent 10× (ten multiplication) (BioGenex, Fremont, CA, USA). The sections were incubated overnight at 4 °C with primary antibodies to anti-human E-cadherin (BD Biosciences, San Jose, CA, USA) or anti-human tryptase (Chemicon, Temecula, CA, USA). After rinsing the sections with 0.1% Tween-20 in BPS, rabbit anti-mouse conjugated fluorescein isothiocyanate secondary antibodies (DakoCytomation Denmark A/S, Glostrup, Denmark) were applied to the sections and incubated for 1 h. Finally, the sections were counterstained with 4',6-diamidino-2-phenylindole (DAPI; Sigma Chemical Co., Saint Louis, MO, USA). Negative controls included the isotype of the primary antibody. We obtained the mean, maximum, range and standard deviation (SD) values of the staining intensity and the percent positive area measurements using three random hot spots within each specimen. The expression of E-cadherin and ZO-1 in the urothelium was quantified using ImageJ software, developed by the National Institutes of Health (Bethesda, MD, USA) [33]. Immunofluorescence (tryptase and TUNEL assays) was quantified by counting the number of positively stained cells/total cells per unit area (4 μm^2). The results were shown as the percentage of positive cells per 100 total cells. Differences in the expressions of proteins in the urothelium at baseline and 6 months after each BoNT-A injection were analyzed using the paired t-test. All calculations were performed using SPSS for Windows, version 16.0 (SPSS, Chicago, IL, USA). $p < 0.05$ was considered to indicate statistical significance.

Acknowledgments: We thanks support from the Tzu Chi fundation.

Author Contributions: Sheng-Fu Chen analyzed data and was the primary author of the manuscript. Chia-Hwei Chang collected the clinical and laboratory data. Hann-Chorng Kuo designed, oversaw, and performed the experiment and supervised the manuscript.

References

1. Van den Berg, M.E.; Castellote, J.M.; Mahillo-Fernandez, I.; de Pedro-Cuesta, J. Incidence of spinal cord injury worldwide: A systematic review. *Neuroepidemiology* **2010**, *34*, 184–192. [CrossRef] [PubMed]
2. Kuo, H.C. Quality of life after active urological management of chronic spinal cord injury in eastern Taiwan. *Eur. Urol.* **1998**, *34*, 37–46. [CrossRef] [PubMed]
3. Patki, P.S.; Hamid, R.; Arumugam, K.; Shah, P.J.; Craggs, M. Botulinum toxin-type A in the treatment of drug-resistant neurogenic detrusor overactivity secondary to traumatic spinal cord injury. *BJU Int.* **2006**, *98*, 77–82. [CrossRef] [PubMed]
4. Apodaca, G.; Kiss, S.; Ruiz, W.; Meyers, S.; Zeidel, M.; Birder, L. Disruption of bladder epithelium barrier function after spinal cord injury. *Am. J. Physiol. Ren. Physiol.* **2003**, *284*, F966–F976. [CrossRef] [PubMed]
5. Jiang, Y.H.; Liu, H.T.; Kuo, H.C. Urothelial dysfunction and chronic inflammation in patients with spinal cord injuries at different levels and correlation with urodynamic findings. *Neurourol. Urodyn.* **2015**, *34*, 757–762. [CrossRef] [PubMed]
6. Ginsberg, D.; Gousse, A.; Keppenne, V.; Sievert, K.D.; Thompson, C.; Lam, W.; Brin, M.F.; Jenkins, B.; Haag-Molkenteller, C. Phase 3 efficacy and tolerability study of onabotulinumtoxinA for urinary incontinence from neurogenic detrusor overactivity. *J. Urol.* **2012**, *187*, 2131–2139. [CrossRef] [PubMed]
7. Khera, M.; Somogyi, G.T.; Kiss, S.; Boone, T.B.; Smith, C.P. Botulinum toxin A inhibits ATP release from bladder urothelium after chronic spinal cord injury. *Neurochem. Int.* **2004**, *45*, 987–993. [CrossRef] [PubMed]
8. Liu, H.T.; Kuo, H.C. Intravesical botulinum toxin A injections plus hydrodistension can reduce nerve growth factor production and control bladder pain in interstitial cystitis. *Urology* **2007**, *70*, 463–468. [CrossRef] [PubMed]
9. Chen, S.F.; Chang, C.H.; Kuo, H.C. Effect of detrusor botulinum toxin a injection on urothelial dysfunction in patients with chronic spinal cord injury: A clinical and immunohistochemistry study before and after treatment. *Spinal Cord* **2016**. [CrossRef] [PubMed]

10. Giannantoni, A.; Mearini, E.; del Zingaro, M.; Porena, M. Six-year follow-up of botulinum toxin A intradetrusorial injections in patients with refractory neurogenic detrusor overactivity: Clinical and urodynamic results. *Eur. Urol.* **2009**, *55*, 705–711. [CrossRef] [PubMed]
11. Kuo, H.C.; Liu, S.H. Effect of repeated detrusor onabotulinumtoxinA injections on bladder and renal function in patients with chronic spinal cord injuries. *Neurourol. Urodyn.* **2011**, *30*, 1541–1545. [CrossRef] [PubMed]
12. Birder, L.; Andersson, K.E. Urothelial signaling. *Physiol. Rev.* **2013**, *93*, 653–680. [CrossRef] [PubMed]
13. Chuang, F.C.; Kuo, H.C. Increased urothelial cell apoptosis and chronic inflammation are associated with recurrent urinary tract infection in women. *PLoS ONE* **2013**, *8*. [CrossRef] [PubMed]
14. Cruz, C.D.; Cruz, F. Spinal cord injury and bladder dysfunction: New ideas about an old problem. *Sci. World J.* **2011**, *11*, 214–234. [CrossRef] [PubMed]
15. Schurch, B.; Stohrer, M.; Kramer, G.; Schmid, D.M.; Gaul, G.; Hauri, D. Botulinum-A toxin for treating detrusor hyperreflexia in spinal cord injured patients: A new alternative to anticholinergic drugs? Preliminary results. *J. Urol.* **2000**, *164*(3 Pt 1), 692–697. [CrossRef]
16. Karsenty, G.; Denys, P.; Amarenco, G.; de Seze, M.; Game, X.; Haab, F.; Kerdraon, J.; Perrouin-Verbe, B.; Ruffion, A.; Saussine, C.; *et al.* Botulinum toxin A (Botox) intradetrusor injections in adults with neurogenic detrusor overactivity/neurogenic overactive bladder: A systematic literature review. *Eur. Urol.* **2008**, *53*, 275–287. [CrossRef] [PubMed]
17. Mangera, A.; Andersson, K.E.; Apostolidis, A.; Chapple, C.; Dasgupta, P.; Giannantoni, A.; Gravas, S.; Madersbacher, S. Contemporary management of lower urinary tract disease with botulinum toxin A: A systematic review of botox (onabotulinumtoxinA) and dysport (abobotulinumtoxinA). *Eur. Urol.* **2011**, *60*, 784–795. [CrossRef] [PubMed]
18. Reitz, A.; Stohrer, M.; Kramer, G.; del Popolo, G.; Chartier-Kastler, E.; Pannek, J.; Burgdörfer, H.; Göcking, K.; Madersbacher, H.; Schumacher, S.; *et al.* European experience of 200 cases treated with botulinum-A toxin injections into the detrusor muscle for urinary incontinence due to neurogenic detrusor overactivity. *Eur. Urol.* **2004**, *45*, 510–515. [CrossRef] [PubMed]
19. Stoehrer, M.; Wolff, A.; Kramer, G.; Steiner, R.; Lmochner-Ernst, D.; Leuth, D.; Steude, U.; Ruebben, H. Treatment of neurogenic detrusor overactivity with botulinum toxin A: The first seven years. *Urol. Int.* **2009**, *83*, 379–385. [CrossRef] [PubMed]
20. Kuo, H.C. Urodynamic evidence of effectiveness of botulinum A toxin injection in treatment of detrusor overactivity refractory to anticholinergic agents. *Urology* **2004**, *63*, 868–872. [CrossRef] [PubMed]
21. Shie, J.H.; Kuo, H.C. Higher levels of cell apoptosis and abnormal E-cadherin expression in the urothelium are associated with inflammation in patients with interstitial cystitis/painful bladder syndrome. *BJU Int.* **2011**, *108*(2 Pt 2), E136–E141. [CrossRef] [PubMed]
22. Rovner, E.; Dmochowski, R.; Chapple, C.; Thompson, C.; Lam, W.; Haag-Molkenteller, C. OnabotulinumtoxinA improves urodynamic outcomes in patients with neurogenic detrusor overactivity. *Neurourol. Urodyn.* **2013**, *32*, 1109–1115. [CrossRef] [PubMed]
23. Giannantoni, A.; Conte, A.; Farfariello, V.; Proietti, S.; Vianello, A.; Nardicchi, V.; Santoni, G.; Amantini, C. Onabotulinumtoxin-A intradetrusorial injections modulate bladder expression of NGF, TrkA, p75 and TRPV1 in patients with detrusor overactivity. *Pharmacol. Res.* **2013**, *68*, 118–124. [CrossRef] [PubMed]
24. Collins, V.M.; Daly, D.M.; Liaskos, M.; McKay, N.G.; Sellers, D.; Chapple, C.; Grundy, D. OnabotulinumtoxinA significantly attenuates bladder afferent nerve firing and inhibits ATP release from the urothelium. *BJU Int.* **2013**, *112*, 1018–1026. [CrossRef] [PubMed]
25. Acharya, P.; Beckel, J.; Ruiz, W.G.; Wang, E.; Rojas, R.; Birder, L.; Apodaca, G. Distribution of the tight junction proteins ZO-1, occludin, and claudin-4, -8, and -12 in bladder epithelium. *Am. J. Physiol. Ren. Physiol.* **2004**, *287*, F305–F318. [CrossRef] [PubMed]
26. Janssen, D.A.; Hoenderop, J.G.; Jansen, K.C.; Kemp, A.W.; Heesakkers, J.P.; Schalken, J.A. The mechanoreceptor TRPV4 is localized in adherence junctions of the human bladder urothelium: A morphological study. *J. Urol.* **2011**, *186*, 1121–1127. [CrossRef] [PubMed]
27. Sant, G.R.; Kempuraj, D.; Marchand, J.E.; Theoharides, T.C. The mast cell in interstitial cystitis: Role in pathophysiology and pathogenesis. *Urology* **2007**, *69* (Suppl. 4), 34–40. [CrossRef] [PubMed]
28. Shie, J.H.; Liu, H.T.; Kuo, H.C. Increased cell apoptosis of urothelium mediated by inflammation in interstitial cystitis/painful bladder syndrome. *Urology* **2012**, *79*, 484.e7–484.e13. [CrossRef] [PubMed]

29. Kalsi, V.; Apostolidis, A.; Popat, R.; Gonzales, G.; Fowler, C.J.; Dasgupta, P. Quality of life changes in patients with neurogenic *vs.* idiopathic detrusor overactivity after intradetrusor injections of botulinum neurotoxin type A and correlations with lower urinary tract symptoms and urodynamic changes. *Eur. Urol.* **2006**, *49*, 528–535. [CrossRef] [PubMed]
30. Groen, J.; Pannek, J.; Castro Diaz, D.; del Popolo, G.; Gross, T.; Hamid, R.; Karsenty, G.; Kessler, T.M.; Schneider, M.; 't Hoen, L.; *et al.* Summary of European Association of Urology (EAU) Guidelines on Neuro-Urology. *Eur. Urol.* **2016**, *69*, 324–333. [CrossRef] [PubMed]
31. Yuk, S.M.; Shin, J.H.; Song, K.H.; Na, Y.G.; Lim, J.S.; Sul, C.K. Expression of brain derived-neurotrophic factor and granulocyte-colony stimulating factor in the urothelium: Relation with voiding function. *BMC Urol.* **2015**, *15*, 37. [CrossRef] [PubMed]
32. Shie, J.H.; Liu, H.T.; Wang, Y.S.; Kuo, H.C. Immunohistochemical evidence suggests repeated intravesical application of botulinum toxin A injections may improve treatment efficacy of interstitial cystitis/bladder pain syndrome. *BJU Int.* **2013**, *111*, 638–646. [CrossRef] [PubMed]
33. Kaczmarek, E.; Gorna, A.; Majewski, P. Techniques of image analysis for quantitative immunohistochemistry. *Rocz. Akad. Med. Bialymst.* **2004**, *49* (Suppl. 1), 155–158. [PubMed]

6

Botulinum Toxin A for Bladder Pain Syndrome/Interstitial Cystitis

Bin Chiu [1,†], Huai-Ching Tai [2], Shiu-Dong Chung [1,2,*,†] and Lori A. Birder [3,4]

1 Division of Urology, Department of Surgery, Far Eastern Memorial Hospital, Ban Ciao, New Taipei City 220, Taiwan; femhuro@gmail.com
2 Department of Urology, National Taiwan University Hospital, Taipei 100, Taiwan; taihuai48@hotmail.com
3 Department of Medicine-Renal Electrolyte Division, University of Pittsburgh School of Medicine, Pittsburgh, PA 15261, USA; lbirder@pitt.edu
4 Pharmacology & Chemical Biology, University of Pittsburgh School of Medicine, Pittsburgh, PA 15261, USA
* Correspondence: chungshiudong@gmail.com
† Present address: Graduate Program in Biomedical Informatics, College of Informatics, Yuan-Ze University, Chung-Li 320, Taiwan.

Academic Editor: Hann-Chorng Kuo

Abstract: Botulinum neurotoxin A (BoNT-A), derived from Clostridium botulinum, has been used clinically for several diseases or syndrome including chronic migraine, spasticity, focal dystonia and other neuropathic pain. Chronic pelvic or bladder pain is the one of the core symptoms of bladder pain syndrome/interstitial cystitis (BPS/IC). However, in the field of urology, chronic bladder or pelvic pain is often difficult to eradicate by oral medications or bladder instillation therapy. We are looking for new treatment modality to improve bladder pain or associated urinary symptoms such as frequency and urgency for patients with BPS/IC. Recent studies investigating the mechanism of the antinociceptive effects of BoNT A suggest that it can inhibit the release of peripheral neurotransmitters and inflammatory mediators from sensory nerves. In this review, we will examine the evidence supporting the use of BoNTs in bladder pain from basic science models and review the clinical studies on therapeutic applications of BoNT for BPS/IC.

Keywords: cystitis; botulinum toxin A; interstitial cystitis; intravesical injection

---

1. Introduction

Bladder pain syndrome/interstitial cystitis (BPS/IC) is a disease with clinical presentations of chronic pelvic/bladder pain, urinary frequency, and nocturia [1,2]. In the United States, it is estimated that about 6.5% or eight million women aged ⩾18 years could be diagnosed as BPS/IC [3]. The possible mechanism of BPS/IC remains unclear, although several pathogeneses including neurogenic inflammation, autoimmune disorder, mast-cell activation and urothelial dysfunction [4–8] have been reported. Cystoscopy with hydrodistention under anesthesia and biopsy if indicated is the first choice for diagnosis, classification and treatment [1,2,9]. Among patients with BPS/IC, mucosal fissure with bleeding and Hunner's ulcer are common findings after hydrodistension. According to guidelines of European Association of Urology, the available treatment options for patients with BPS/IC included the oral pentosan polysulfate sodium and intravesical Dimethyl sulfoxide (DMSO) which are both FDA-approved drugs [1,2]. Botulinum neurotoxins (BoNTs), which are produced by the bacterium Clostridium botulinum, have been widely applied medically since the first report of BoNTs for ocular strabismus in 1980 [10,11]. BoNT serotype A (BoNT-A) is the most widely used clinically, it can inhibit the release of neurotransmitters from nerve fibers and the urothelium [12–14]. Dykstra et al. firstly reported their experience of injections of BoNT-A into the external urethral sphincter to successfully treat detrusor sphincter dyssynergia of spinal cord injury patients [15]. Intravesical BoNT-A injection has been used in patients with BPS/IC since 2004. The pilot study reported that nine (69%) of 13 patients had subjective improvement after BoNT-A treatment [16]. However, recently, Gottsch et al. [16] investigated the efficacy of periurethral injection of 50 IU BoNTA in BPS/IC, and reported non-significant results on the main outcomes when compared with placebo. In the past decade, many studies have shown the efficacy of intravesical BoNT-A in BPS/IC though it has some side effects including urinary tract infection and urinary difficulty, and it seems to be a promising alternative treatment. In this review, we discuss the available mechanism and current medical evidence of BoNT-A for treating BPS/IC.

2. Mechanisms of BoNT-A

Internalization of BoNT/A begins with binding its ~100 kDa heavy chain to a specific receptor on the membrane of presynaptic neurons in the cholinergic nerve terminal. BoNT/A is then sequestered within a vesicle by endocytosis and undergoes a pH-dependent conformational change, leading to the translocation of its ~50 kDa light chain into the cytosol. After entering the cytosol, the light chain cleaves the SNAP-25 (synaptosome associated protein of molecular weight of 25 kDa), a subset of SNARE (soluble *N*-ethylmaleimide-sensitive fusion attachment protein receptor) proteins which mediate the fusion of the acetylcholine-containing vesicle with the presynaptic membrane. This interaction ultimately disrupts the release of neurotransmitter into the synapse, resulting in flaccid paralysis of the muscle [17]. There have been also several studies showing that BoNT/A inhibits the release of neurotransmitters that regulate pain and inflammation [18–20]. In an animal formalin-induced inflammatory pain model, the authors demonstrated the antinociceptive effects of BoNT-A [21]. Substance P and CGRP are neurotransmitters released by mainly C fibers, a primary nociceptive afferents of urinary bladder, Welch et al. found that BoNT can inhibit the release of substance P from cultured embryonic dorsal root ganglia neurons [22]. On the other hand, BoNT/A can diminish the amount of calcitonin gene-related peptide (CGRP) in rat trigeminal ganglia cells [23]. BoNT/A has been found to be able to reduce neurogenic inflammation, which is suggested to be associated with BPS/IC. In a capsaicin-induced prostatitis rat model, BoNT inhibited cyclooxygenase-2 expression [24]. Liu et al. demonstrated that BoNT-A injection to bladder can reduce the urine level of nerve growth factor, which is associated with neurogenic inflammation, by inhibiting the action of interleulkin-1, a proinflammatory cytokine [25]. In addition, BoNT can inhibit the delivery of the transient receptor potential vanilloid 1 (TRPV1) to neuron cell membranes [26].

TRPV1 has been identified to play an important role in the symptoms of urinary urgency, frequency and inflammatory pain in BPS/IC [27]. Liu et al. [27] showed that increased severity of bladder inflammation correlated with a higher expression of TRPV1-immunoreactive nerve fibers in BPS/IC patients' bladders and correlated with clinical symptoms. The number of suburothelial afferents expressing TRPV1 was significantly reduced after BoNT-A treatment. The decreased levels of these sensory receptors are associated with a decreased sensation of urgency [27]. In addition, inhibition of purinergic P2X3 receptors on afferent terminals, which resulted in less ATP release from the urothelium can improve the painful sensations in BPS/IC. Apostolidis et al. analyzed the expression of P2X3 receptors in the bladder biopsy specimen of patients with detrusor overactivity after intradetrusor injection of BoNT-A demonstrated that P2X3-immunoreactive fibers were decreased significantly and the reduction of P2X3 expression significantly correlated with reduction of urgency episodes and urodynamic parameters [28]. Taken together, BoNT-A might improve the underlying neuroregulatory disorders of the urinary bladder in BPS/IC patients.

3. Clinical Evidence of Intravesical BoNT-A for BPS/IC

Several studies have supported the efficacy of BoNT-A in BPS/IC.

Smith et al. [16] first demonstrated the results of 200 IU BoNT-A trigonal and bladder base injection in treating BPS/IC in 13 patients and they showed a significant overall reduction in pain scores. Based on the previous study [29], which found most nociceptive bladder afferents are located in the trigone, Pinto et al. [29] performed trigonal injection with 100 IU BoNT-A in 26 women with refractory BPS/IC. The results demonstrated that pelvic pain, daytime and night-time voiding frequency, O'Leary-Sant Interstitial Cystitis Symptom Index (ICSI) and quality of life of all patients improved significantly. The maximal cystometric capacity increased and the efficacy remained in >50% of the patients for 9 months [30]. Giannantoni et al. [31] analyzed the efficacy of 200 IU suburothelial OnabotulinumtoxinA injection to trigone and bladder floor in 14 patients and they found that 12 patients (85.7%) had improvements in terms of daytime frequency, nocturia, visual analogue scale (VAS) score and increased cystometric capacity. Chung et al. reported their experience of 100 IU suburothelial BoNT-A injection immediately followed by cystoscopic hydrodistention in 67 refractory BPS/IC patients and the ICSI and Interstitial Cystitis Problem Index (ICPI), VAS score for pain, functional bladder capacity, and global response assessment (GRA) were all significantly improved compared to baseline data [32]. In another long term follow-up study in 15 patients, Onabotulinumtoxin-A at 200 IU submucosally injected to the bladder trigone and lateral walls, 13 patients (86.6%) reported subjective improvement regarding the mean VAS score, and daytime and nighttime urinary frequency [33]. However, at one year after treatment, pain recurred in all patients and nine patients suffered from dysuria 1 month after BoNT-A injection. A prospective, randomized study evaluated the responses of 15 patients and 29 received suburothelial injection with 200 IU or 100 IU of BoNT-A followed by cystoscopic hydrodistension 2 weeks later and 23 patients received the cystoscopic hydrodistension without BoNT-A injection [34]. All patients remained on baseline medications of pentosan polysulphate throughout the study and the results showed that intravesical injections of BoNT-A followed by hydrodistension can provide significantly better clinical results than hydrodistension alone with the BPS/IC symptom and VAS score decreased functional bladder capacity and cystometric bladder capacity increased. Among the total 44 patients in the BoNT-A group, 31 (71%) had clinically improvements at 6 months [34]. There was no efficacy difference between different BoNT-A doses treatment groups however the adverse events were more common in the group of 200 IU compared to 100 IU group. In a recent prospective, open labeled, randomized comparative study, patients with refractory BPS/IC received immediate injection or 1-month delayed injection of botulinum toxin type A, the results showed that the response rate was 73.5% at 1 month, 58.8% at 3 months, 38.2% at 6 months and 20.6% at 12 months [35]. Further multivariate analysis suggested that past exposure to hydrodistension more than three times is associated with a better outcome [35]. Another multicenter, randomized, double-blind, placebo-controlled trial in 60 patients with IC/BPS refractory to conventional treatment alsoindicated that hydrodistension plus suburothelial injections of BoNT-A 100 IU can significantly improve the VAS score and increase cystometric bladder capacity at week 8 after treatment. Bladder tissue obtained from 19 BPS/IC patients before BoNT-A injections and hydrodistension expressed significantly higher nerve growth factor (NGF) levels versus controls, and the level decreased after BoNT-A treatment especially in patients who responded clinically [36]. These findings implied that BoNT-A has an effect in reducing neuroplasticity of sensory fibers in the bladder, and supported the hypothesis of BPS/IC partly originated from neurogenic inflammation.

4. Conclusions

Intravesical BoNT-A injection is promising in the treatment of BPS/IC. BoNT-A can relieve pain, urgency and frequency for refractory BPS/IC though the success rates are variable. BoNT-A can also improve the functional bladder capacity and urodynamic parameters. However, there was no randomized placebo-control study to investigate the efficacy and improvement of quality of life of BoNT-A for BPS/IC patients. Further well-designed larger-scale randomized trials with placebo controls are warranted.

Author Contributions: B.C. wrote the paper, H.-C.T. and S.-D.C. collected information and references; S.-D.C. and L.A.B. supervised and revised the paper.

References

1. Van de Merwe, J.P.; Nordling, J.; Bouchelouche, P.; Bouchelouche, K.; Cervigni, M.; Daha, L.K.; Elneil, S.; Fall, M.; Hohlbrugger, G.; Irwin, P.; et al. Diagnostic criteria, classification, and nomenclature for painfulbladder syndrome/interstitial cystitis: An ESSIC proposal. *Eur. Urol.* **2008**, *53*, 60–67. [CrossRef] [PubMed]
2. Hanno, P.M.; Burks, D.A.; Clemens, J.Q.; Dmochowski, R.R.; Erickson, D.; Fitzgerald, M.P.; Forrest, J.B.; Gordon, B.; Gray, M.; Mayer, R.D.; et al. AUA guideline for the diagnosis and treatment of interstitial cystitis/bladder pain syndrome. *J. Urol.* **2011**, *185*, 2162–2170. [CrossRef] [PubMed]
3. Curhan, G.C.; Speizer, F.E.; Hunter, D.J.; Curhan, S.G.; Stampfer, M.J. Epidemiology of interstitial cystitis: A population based study. *J. Urol.* **1999**, *161*, 549–552. [CrossRef]
4. Mayer, R. Interstitial cystitis pathogenesis and treatment. *Curr. Opin. Infect. Dis.* **2007**, *20*, 77–82. [CrossRef] [PubMed]
5. Nazif, O.; Teichman, J.M.; Gebhart, G.F. Neural upregulation in interstitial cystitis. *Urology* **2007**, *69*, 24–33. [CrossRef] [PubMed]
6. Sant, G.R.; Kempuraj, D.; Marchand, J.E.; Theoharides, T.C. The mast cell in interstitial cystitis: Role in pathophysiology and pathogenesis. *Urology* **2007**, *69*, 34–40. [CrossRef] [PubMed]
7. Van de Merwe, J.P.; Yamada, T.; Sakamoto, Y. Systemic aspects of interstitial cystitis, immunology and linkage with autoimmune disorders. *Int. J. Urol.* **2003**, *10* (Suppl. 1), S35–S38. [CrossRef] [PubMed]
8. Liu, H.T.; Kuo, H.C. Biomarkers for patients with interstitial cystitis/bladder pain syndrome. *Urol. Sci.* **2015**, *26*, 225–229. [CrossRef]
9. Lee, C.L.; Peng, C.H.; Kuo, H.C. Therapeutic effects and predictive factors for successful intravesical hyaluronic acid instillation in patients with interstitial cystitis/bladder pain syndrome. *Urol. Sci.* **2015**, *26*, 125–130. [CrossRef]
10. Scott, A.B. Botulinum toxin injection into extraocular muscles as an alternative to strabismus surgery. *J. Pediatr. Ophthalmol. Strabismus* **1980**, *17*, 21–25. [CrossRef]
11. Oh, H.M.; Chung, M.E. Botulinum Toxin for Neuropathic Pain: A Review of the Literature. *Toxins (Basel.)* **2015**, *7*, 3127–3154. [CrossRef] [PubMed]
12. Chuang, Y.C.; Yoshimura, N.; Huang, C.C.; Chiang, P.H.; Chancellor, M.B. Intravesical botulinum toxin A administration produces analgesia against acetic acid induced bladder pain response in rats. *J. Urol.* **2004**, *172*, 1529–1532. [CrossRef] [PubMed]
13. Kuo, H.C.; Liu, H.T.; Chuang, Y.C.; Birder, L.A.; Chancellor, M.B. Pilot study of liposome-encapsulated onabotulinumtoxina for patients with overactive bladder: A single-center study. *Eur. Urol.* **2014**, *65*, 1117–1124. [CrossRef] [PubMed]
14. Hung, S.Y.; Chancellor, D.D.; Chancellor, M.B.; Chuang, Y.C. Role of liposome in treatment of overactive bladder and interstitial cystitis. *Urol. Sci.* **2015**, *26*, 3–6. [CrossRef]
15. Dykstra, D.D.; Sidi, A.A.; Scott, A.B.; Pagel, J.M.; Goldish, G.D. Effects of botulinum A toxin on detrusor-sphincter dyssynergia in spinal cord injury patients. *J. Urol.* **1988**, *39*, 919–922.
16. Smith, C.P.; Radziszewski, P.; Borkowski, A.; Somogyi, G.T.; Boone, T.B.; Chancellor, M.B. Botulinum toxin A has antinociceptive effects in treating interstitial cystitis. *Urology* **2004**, *64*, 871–875. [CrossRef] [PubMed]
17. Lam, K.H.; Yao, G.; Jin, R. Diverse binding modes, same goal: The receptor recognition mechanism of botulinum neurotoxin. *Prog. Biophys. Mol. Biol.* **2015**, *117*, 225–231. [CrossRef] [PubMed]
18. Lucioni, A.; Bales, G.T.; Lotan, T.L.; McGehee, D.S.; Cook, S.P.; Rapp, D.E. Botulinum toxin type A inhibits sensory neuropeptide release in rat bladder models of acute injury and chronic inflammation. *BJU Int.* **2008**, *101*, 366–370. [CrossRef] [PubMed]
19. Peng, C.H.; Jhang, J.F.; Shie, J.H.; Kuo, H.C. Down regulation of vascular endothelial growth factor is associated with decreased inflammation after intravesical OnabotulinumtoxinA injections combined with hydrodistention for patients with interstitial cystitis—Clinical results and immunohistochemistry analysis. *Urology* **2013**, *82*. [CrossRef]
20. Apostolidis, A.; Dasgupta, P.; Fowler, C.J. Proposed mechanism for the efficacy of injected botulinum toxin in the treatment of human detrusor overactivity. *Eur. Urol.* **2006**, *49*, 644–650. [CrossRef] [PubMed]

21. Cui, M.; Khanijou, S.; Rubino, J.; Aoki, K.R. Subcutaneous administration of botulinum toxin A reduces formalin-induced pain. *Pain* **2004**, *107*, 125–133. [CrossRef] [PubMed]
22. Welch, M.J.; Purkiss, J.R.; Foster, K.A. Sensitivity of embryonic rat dorsal root ganglia neurons to Clostridium botulinum neurotoxins. *Toxicon* **2000**, *38*, 245–258. [CrossRef]
23. Durham, P.L.; Cady, R. Regulation of calcitonin gene-related peptide secretion from trigeminal nerve cells by botulinum toxin type A: Implications for migraine therapy. *Headache* **2004**, *44*, 35–42. [CrossRef] [PubMed]
24. Chuang, Y.C.; Yoshimura, N.; Huang, C.C.; Wu, M.; Chiang, P.H.; Chancellor, M.B. Intraprostatic botulinum toxin A injection inhibits cyclooxygenase-2 expression and suppresses prostatic pain on capsaicin induced prostatitis model in rat. *J. Urol.* **2008**, *180*, 742–748. [CrossRef] [PubMed]
25. Liu, H.T.; Kuo, H.C. Intravesical botulinum toxin A injections plus hydrodistension can reduce nerve growth factor production and control bladder pain in interstitial cystitis. *Urology* **2007**, *70*, 463–468. [CrossRef] [PubMed]
26. Xiao, L.; Cheng, J.; Zhuang, Y.; Qu, W.; Muir, J.; Liang, H.; Zhang, D. Botulinum toxin type A reduces hyperalgesia and TRPV1 expression in rats with neuropathic pain. *Pain Med.* **2013**, *14*, 276–286. [CrossRef] [PubMed]
27. Liu, B.L.; Yang, F.; Zhan, H.L.; Feng, Z.Y.; Zhang, Z.G.; Li, W.B.; Zhou, X.F. Increased severity of inflammation correlates with elevated expression of TRPV1 nerve fibers and nerve growth factor on interstitial cystitis/bladder pain syndrome. *Urol. Int.* **2014**, *92*, 202–208. [CrossRef] [PubMed]
28. Apostolidis, A.; Popat, R.; Yiangou, Y.; Cockayne, D.; Ford, A.P.; Davis, J.B.; Dasgupta, P.; Fowler, C.J.; Anand, P. Decreased sensory receptors P2X3 and TRPV1 in suburothelial nerve fibers following intradetrusor injections of botulinum toxin for human detrusor overactivity. *J. Urol.* **2005**, *174*, 977–982. [CrossRef] [PubMed]
29. Avelino, A.; Cruz, C.; Nagy, I.; Cruz, F. Vanilloid receptor 1 expression in the rat urinary tract. *Neuroscience* **2002**, *109*, 787–798. [CrossRef]
30. Pinto, R.; Lopes, T.; Frias, B.; Silva, A.; Silva, J.A.; Silva, C.M.; Cruz, C.; Cruz, F.; Dinis, P. Trigonal injection of botulinum toxin A in patients with refractory bladder pain syndrome/interstitial cystitis. *Eur. Urol.* **2010**, *58*, 360–365. [CrossRef] [PubMed]
31. Giannantoni, A.; Costantini, E.; Di Stasi, S.M.; Tascini, M.C.; Bini, V.; Porena, M. Botulinum A toxin intravesical injections in the treatment of painful bladder syndrome: A pilot study. *Eur. Urol.* **2006**, *49*, 704–709. [CrossRef] [PubMed]
32. Chung, S.D.; Kuo, Y.C.; Kuo, H.C. Intravesical onabotulinumtoxinA injections for refractory painful bladder syndrome. *Pain Phys.* **2012**, *15*, 197–202.
33. Giannantoni, A.; Porena, M.; Costantini, E.; Zucchi, A.; Mearini, L.; Mearini, E. Botulinum A toxin intravesical injection in patients with painful bladder syndrome: 1-Year followup. *J. Urol.* **2008**, *179*, 1031–1034. [CrossRef] [PubMed]
34. Kuo, H.C.; Chancellor, M.B. Comparison of intravesical botulinum toxin type A injections plus hydrodistention with hydrodistention alone for the treatment of refractory interstitial cystitis/painful bladder syndrome. *BJU Int.* **2009**, *104*, 657–661. [CrossRef] [PubMed]
35. Akiyama, Y.; Nomiya, A.; Niimi, A.; Yamada, Y.; Fujimura, T.; Nakagawa, T.; Fukuhara, H.; Kume, H.; Igawa, Y.; Homma, Y. Botulinum toxin type A injection for refractory interstitial cystitis: A randomized comparative study and predictors of treatment response. *Int. J. Urol.* **2015**, *22*, 835–841. [CrossRef] [PubMed]
36. Kuo, H.C.; Jiang, Y.H.; Tsai, Y.C.; Kuo, Y.C. Intravesical botulinum toxin-A injections reduce bladder pain of interstitial cystitis/bladder pain syndrome refractory to conventional treatment—A prospective, multicenter, randomized, double-blind, placebo-controlled clinical trial. *Neurourol. Urodyn.* **2016**, *35*, 609–614. [CrossRef] [PubMed]

7

Novel Applications of OnabotulinumtoxinA in Lower Urinary Tract Dysfunction

Jia-Fong Jhang and Hann-Chorng Kuo *

Department of Urology, Buddhist Tzu Chi General Hospital, and Tzu Chi University, Hualien 970, Taiwan; alur1984@hotmail.com

* Correspondence: hck@tzuchi.com.tw

Abstract: OnabotulinumtoxinA (BoNT-A) was first used to treat neurogenic lower urinary tract dysfunction (LUTD) 30 years ago. Recently, application of BoNT-A in LUTD have become more common since the approval of intravesical BoNT-A injection for patients with both overactive bladders (OAB) and neurogenic detrusor overactivity (NDO) by regulatory agencies in many countries. Although unlicensed, BoNT-A has been recommended to treat patients with interstitial cystitis/bladder pain syndrome (IC/BPS) under different guidelines. BoNT-A delivery with liposome-encapsulation and gelation hydrogel intravesical instillation provided a potentially less invasive and more convenient form of application for patients with OAB or IC/BPS. BoNT-A injections into the urethral sphincter for spinal cord injury patients with detrusor-sphincter dyssynergia have been used for a long time. New evidence revealed that it could also be applied to patients with non-neurogenic dysfunctional voiding. Previous studies and meta-analyses suggest that BoNT-A injections for patients with benign prostate hyperplasia do not have a better therapeutic effect than placebo. However, new randomized and placebo-controlled trials revealed intraprostatic BoNT-A injection is superior to placebo in specific patients. A recent trial also showed intraprostatic BoNT-A injection could significantly reduce pain in patients with chronic prostatitis. Both careful selection of patients and prudent use of urodynamic evaluation results to confirm diagnoses are essential for successful outcomes of BoNT-A treatment for LUTD.

Keywords: botulinum toxin; clinical trial; human; urodynamics

Key Contribution: This article summarized recent novel applications of BoNT-A for LUTD, and suggested the possible further works to improve the therapeutic efficacy.

---

1. Introduction

Lower urinary tract dysfunction (LUTD) is a condition presented by patients suffering from LUTD linked to one or more structures and/or functions of the lower urinary tract [1]. LUTD is common in both men and women, and the incidence and prevalence increase as people age [2]. A recent large cross-sectional study in China revealed 61.1% of women and 61.2% of men reported LUTD [2]. In general, the pathophysiology of LUTD could be classified into bladder or bladder outlet dysfunction, and treatments of LUTD should focus on etiology. However, not all LUTDs could be treated effectively, even if the etiology is definite. Treatment of functional LUTD, such as interstitial cystitis/bladder pain syndrome (IC/BPS), overactive bladder (OAB), and dysfunctional voiding (DV), remains a challenge to the urologist.

Botulinum toxin (BoNT) is a potent poisonous neurotoxin, which is produced by the bacterium *Clostridium botulinum* and related species [3]. Ingestion of BoNT-poisoned food causes intoxication by inhibiting the release of the neurotransmitter acetylcholine from nerve fibers, thereby inhibiting muscle contractions, which was first described in the early 17th century [4]. BoNT was first isolated in 1895, and now could be classified antigenically and serologically into eight distinguishable exotoxins (A, B, C1, C2, D, E, F, and G) [5]. In 1981, Scott first used onabotulinumtoxinA (BoNT-A) by injecting it into human eye muscles to correct strabismus successfully [6]. Since then, BoNT-A has been widely used to treat many neuropathic pain syndromes and dystonic diseases. In LUTD, the first application of BoNT-A targeted the urethral sphincter. Dykstra used transperineal or cystoscopic injection of BoNT-A into the urethral sphincter in patients with spinal cord injury (SCI) and detrusor-sphincter dyssynergia (DSD) in 1988 [7]. Currently, BoNT-A has been widely used in different kinds of LUTDs, especially in diseases that could not be easily treated with oral medications. In the American Urology Association (AUA) guidelines, BoNT-A injection into the urinary bladder is now a standard treatment for patients with refractory OAB and IC/BPS [8,9]. Newly published clinical trials also revealed novel applications of BoNT-A in different LUTDs and exhibited promising results. The aim of the current article is to review important new applications of BoNT-A in LUTDs and the associated evidence supporting its use.

2. Mechanisms of BoNT-A in LUTDs

BoNT-A, a potent neurotoxic protein, is well known for its ability to inhibit the release of the neurotransmitter acetylcholine from presynaptic efferent nerves at neuromuscular junctions [5]. BoNT-A consists of a 50-kDa light chain and a 100-kDa heavy endocytosis [10]. Subsequently, the light chain and heavy chain separate in the endosomal vesicle [11,12]. The light chain is the biologically active moiety of BoNT-A. The light chain of BoNT-A cleaves synaptosome-associated protein 25 in the presynaptic nerve terminal, and inhibits the release of acetylcholine by disrupting the fusion of vesicles with the neuron's cell membrane, finally causing flaccid paralysis of muscles [13,14]. Traditionally, the effects of BoNT-A in treating LUTDs, such as OAB and DSD, were believed to be attributed to the inhibition of detrusor or urethral sphincter contractions. Recently, evidence also revealed BoNT-A injection into the bladder also could regulate sensory nerve function by blocking the release of various noxious neurotransmitters, including adenosine triphosphate, calcitonin gene-related peptide, calcitonin gene-related peptide, and substance P [15,16]. Modulation of sensory nerve function might be the mechanism of BoNT-A in some sensory problems predominantly LUTD, such as IC/BPS. In addition, studies showed an anti-inflammatory effect for BoNT-A. Immunohistochemical evidence revealed decreased tryptase expression in the bladder after BoNT-A injections, which suggests a reduction in active mast cells in bladders of IC/BPS patients [17].

3. Intravesical BoNT-A Injection in OAB and Neurogenic Detrusor Overactivity

OAB is a clinical syndrome, which is characterized by urinary urgency, usually accompanied by frequency and nocturia, with or without urgency, urinary incontinence, in the absence of urinary tract infection (UTI), or other obvious pathology [18]. According to a recent large cross-sectional study in Asia, the prevalence of OAB was 20.8% overall (men 19.5%, women 22.1%) and increased significantly with age [19]. Treatments of OAB are usually started with behavioral therapy and then oral medications such as antimuscarinics or beta-agonists [8]. Although oral medications might be effective, a large-scale study showed that 46.2% of OAB patients discontinued antimuscarinics and stated the reason for treatment discontinuation was "did not work as expected" [20]. In patients with neurogenic detrusor overactivity (NDO) due to SCI, oral antimuscarinics have been reported to increase bladder capacity and decrease intravesical pressure [21]. However, the effect of antimuscarinics is usually poor in NDO patients with severe urgency and incontinence symptoms. In a large series of NDO patients with urinary incontinence, only 32% of patients could become continent after using oxybutynin and trospium [22]. Thus, treatment for patients with OAB and NDO, who were refractory to oral medications, is a daily common challenging problem in the urology clinic.

Intravesical BoNT-A injection for treating patients with SCI and NDO have been reported since 2000 [23]. Schurch first injected 200 to 300 units (U) of BoNT-A into the detrusor muscle of NDO patients [23]. At six weeks of follow-up, complete continence was observed in 17 of 19 (89.4%) cases in which anticholinergic medication was markedly decreased or withdrawn. Evidence from basic and clinical researchers revealed BoNT-A injection could block acetylcholine release from efferent nerves ending by cleaving Synaptosomal-associated protein 25, thereby temporarily inhibiting detrusor muscle contraction and improve bladder storage symptoms [24]. Further investigation also revealed that BoNT-A injection could also inhibit both noradrenaline and adenosine triphosphate release, which have a powerful influence on bladder sensation [25,26]. After years of work by many researchers and clinicians, intravesical BoNT-A injection has provided evidence demonstrating its utility as standard therapy in patients with both OAB and NDO [8,27]. The application of BoNT-A in OAB and NDO has also been approved by regulatory agencies in most countries.

Patients with NDO and OAB who respond to BoNT-A usually need repeat injections every 6 to 12 months [28]. The long-term efficacy of repeat BoNT-A injections was doubtful before, but recent long-term follow-up studies (>5 years) revealed that BoNT-A could decrease urinary incontinence rate and improve quality of life in patients with both NDO and OAB [29,30]. However, treatment compliance might be not satisfactory. Rahnama'i reported that only 25% of patients continued treatment during the six years of follow-up [29]. Most of these patients could not tolerate voiding urinary tract symptoms, urine retention, or urethral catheterization [29].

4. Intravesical Liposome-Encapsulated BoNT-A Instillation in OAB

In our prospective pilot randomized controlled study, liposome-encapsulated BoNT-A (Lipotoxin) bladder installation was used to treat patients with OAB [31]. At one month after treatment, the change in urinary frequency and urgency significantly improved in the Lipotoxin group but not in the normal saline instillation group. More importantly, no adverse event such as post-voiding residual volume (PVR), urinary retention, or UTI significantly increased or was reported by patients during the follow-up period. Bladder instillation of Lipotoxin in patients with OAB seems to be an effective treatment without significant adverse effects, but the long-term efficacy still needs to be proved in the future. Although the use of Lipotoxin for treating OAB patients is promising, it has not been used in patients with NDO until now. The therapeutic effect of Lipotoxin in NDO might be not adequate in this case.

Management is usually difficult in some patients who are characterized by urinary urgency, incontinence with incomplete bladder emptying, and with a urodynamic diagnosis of detrusor hyperactivity with impaired contractile function (DHIC) [32]. Recently, we reported our experience with suburothelial injection of 100 U of BoNT-A in patients with DHIC [33]. At six months of follow-up, the subjective urgency symptom scores improved significantly, but urgency episodes did not significantly improve in 21 patients. Acute urinary retention developed in 7 (33.3%) and UTI was noted in eight patients with DHIC (38.1%). The incidence of adverse effects of BoNT-A injection in patients with DHIC was relatively higher than that in patients with OAB. We concluded that the efficacy of intravesical BoNT-A injection for DHIC patients was limited and short-term. Physicians should inform patients of both potential benefits and risks of BoNT-A injection for the treatment of DHIC. A comprehensive urodynamic study before decision-making is recommended to rule out the coexistence of LUTD such as bladder neck dysfunction.

5. Intravesical BoNT-A Injection in Interstitial Cystitis/Bladder Pain Syndrome

IC/BPS is a clinical syndrome and includes a large group of patients who are defined by the AUA as having "an unpleasant sensation (pain, pressure, discomfort) perceived to be related to the urinary bladder, associated with LUTD of more than six weeks duration, in the absence of infection or other identifiable causes" [9]. The estimated prevalence of IC/BPS among adult females in the US ranges from 2.7% to 6.53% [34]. Until now, the etiology of IC/BPS is still uncertain, and its management is both frustrating and difficult [35]. Smith et al. first treated female IC/BPS patients with intravesical 100 to 200 U BoNT-A injection plus cystoscopic hydrodistention at the same time [36]. We also conducted a prospective, randomized, double-blind clinical trial to investigate the clinical efficacy of BoNT-A intravesical injection in patients with IC/BPS [37]. Our results showed a significantly greater reduction in pain and increase in cystometric bladder capacity in the BoNT-A group compared with the normal saline injection group at eight weeks of follow-up. Experimental studies conducted in both animals and humans provided laboratory evidence to support BoNT-A injections in the IC/BPS. BoNT-A injections into the bladder have been shown to block the release of noxious neurotransmitters including calcitonin, calcitonin gene-related peptide, glutamate, adenosine triphosphate, and substance P from neurons [38]. Now, intravesical BoNT-A injection is the fourth-line standard treatment in the AUA treatment guideline of IC/BPS [9].

A recent network meta-analysis compared BoNT-A injection with different intravesical therapy for IC/BPS, including bacillus Calmette-Guerin, resiniferatoxin, lidocaine, chondroitin sulfate, oxybutynin, and pentosan polysulfate [39]. The results indicate that in patients with IC/BPS BoNT-A injection has the highest probability of being the best therapy according to the global response assessment, and significantly improves bladder capacity. Recently, we conducted a double-blind, randomized trial to investigate the efficacy of intravesical Lipotoxin instillation in patients with IC/BPS [40]. Patients who received Lipotoxin therapy demonstrated a statistically significant decrease in O'Leary-Sant symptom scores and on the visual analog scale for pain. However, there was no significant difference in improvement between the Lipotoxin and normal saline instillation group. Nevertheless, no significant adverse effect developed in either group, the efficacy of Lipotxoin instillation in IC/BPS might be masked by the placebo effect, and further study is necessary to validate the actual effect. Rappaport et al. recently used TC-3 gel, a novel reverse-thermal gelation hydrogel to deliver BoNT-A into IC/BPS bladders [41]. A single intravesical instillation of 200 U of BoNT-A mixed with 40 mL TC-3 gel could significantly reduce both pain and O'Leary-Sant symptom scores at 12 weeks of follow-up. Preliminary results of instillation of a TC-3 gel-BoNT-A mixture are promising, but further prospective and randomized trials are necessary to prove its efficacy.

6. Urethral Sphincter BoNT-A Injection in Detrusor-Sphincter Dyssynergia

DSD is characterized by involuntary contractions of the external urethral sphincter during a detrusor contraction, which is caused by central nervous system injury between the pontine micturition center and the sacral spinal cord [42]. Patients with SCI and DSD usually suffer from incomplete bladder emptying and DO. Application of BoNT-A in DSD started as early as 1988 [7]. At that time, it was believed that the effect of BoNT-A could block acetylcholine release from presynaptic vesicles at the neuromuscular junction into the urethral sphincter [43]. However, clinical evidence to support its efficacy remains limited and randomized placebo-controlled trial data was limited until now. Our prospective study showed that 100 U of BoNT-A injection into the urethral sphincter could significantly decrease voiding detrusor pressure and increase maximum flow rate [44]. However, some patients might complain of an increase in incontinence grade and were dissatisfied with the BoNT-A injection. A recent prospective trial enrolled 59 SCI patients with both NDO and DSD. All these patients received both 200 U intravesical and 100 U urethral sphincter injections of BoNT-A at the same time [45]. Patients could experience a significant reduction of detrusor voiding pressure, urinary incontinence episode, and increased voiding volume at 12 weeks of follow-up. Twenty-five patients (42.4%) even reported complete dryness at follow-up. Patients with DSD may become incontinent after urethral sphincter BoNT-A injection, and it might adversely affect the quality of life in these patients. Simultaneously, BoNT-A injections in the detrusor and urethral sphincters are a reasonable treatment for SCI patients with both NDO and DSD. Using urodynamic study results to evaluate both urethral and bladder function in these patients and presenting a thorough explanation of all possible adverse effects as well as expectations is key to increase patient satisfaction.

7. Urethral Sphincter BoNT-A Injection in Dysfunctional Voiding

As urethral BoNT-A injection had been successfully used in the treatment of DSD in SCI patients, this treatment was further applied to adults with non-neurogenic voiding dysfunction due to bladder outlet obstruction and urethral sphincter overactivity. Fowler's syndrome consists of difficulty in passing urine or urinary retention due to failure to relax the urethral sphincter in patients without neurological or anatomical abnormality [46]. Treatment of Fowler's syndrome is complicated and patients usually need intermittent self-catheterization [46]. In 2016, an open-label, prospective study enrolled 10 women with difficult urination due to Fowler's syndrome and treated these patients with urethral injection of 100 U of BoNT-A [47]. At 10 weeks of follow-up, the maximal urinary flow rate was significantly increased and the residual volume was decreased. Even four of the five women, who initially had complete retention, could void spontaneously after the treatment. Recently, we also conducted a randomized, double-blind, and placebo-controlled study using BoNT-A injection into the urethral sphincter to treat patients with refractory DV (open bladder neck but a poorly relaxed urethral sphincter, and a normal-to-high voiding pressure with a low urinary flow) [48]. Our results revealed that patients who received BoNT-A injection had a significantly improved international prostate symptom score (IPSS), quality-of-life index, maximum flow rate, voided volume, and decreased detrusor voiding pressure at one month of follow-up. When compared with the normal saline injection group, however, only the total IPSS and voided volume improvement were significantly greater in the BoNT-A injection group. Improvement in other clinical parameters was not significantly different between the BoNT-A and normal saline injection groups. We concluded that urethral sphincter injection with either BoNT-A or placebo could safely and effectively ameliorate clinical symptoms and improve quality of life in patients with DV. Although the exact pathogenetic mechanism remains unknown, local injection itself might have a therapeutic effect on the relaxation of the urethral sphincter, regardless of pharmacologic effects of BoNT-A. Additional studies enrolling more patients with DV are necessary to elucidate the efficacy of BoNT-A urethral injection.

8. Intraprostatic BoNT-A Injection in Benign Prostate Hyperplasia

Benign prostate hyperplasia (BPH) resulting in bladder outlet obstruction is one of the most common conditions presented in the urology clinic. An epidemiological meta-analysis revealed the occurrence of BPH in age groups 40–49 years, 50–59 years, 60–69 years, 70–79 years, and 80 years and older was 2.9%, 29.0%, 44.7%, 58.1%, and 69.2%, respectively [49]. Mainstream treatment of BPH is usually started with oral medication including an α-adrenergic blocker and a 5-α-reductase inhibitor [50]. Surgical intervention such as transurethral prostate resection is indicated if BPH patients are refractory to treatment with oral medication [51]. The prostate is an organ composed of glandular tissue and fibromuscular stroma. The prostate may cause bladder outlet obstruction not only because of glandular hyperplasia, but also because it may be associated with the dysregulation of smooth muscle contractility in the stroma [52]. Relaxation of smooth muscle in the prostate stroma has been considered a potential target to treat patients with BPH in many pharmacological studies [52]. Given its inhibitory effect on neurotransmitter release from the neuromuscular junction, studies using 100 to 200 U intraprostatic injection of BoNT-A to treat patients with BPH started as early as 2003, and initial results showed promising therapeutic effects [53,54]. BPH patients who received intraprostatic BoNT-A injection experienced significant improvement in both symptom score and quality-of-life index at short-term follow-up (one month) [53,54]. In addition, evidence from both human and animal studies showed prostate apoptosis activity increased after BoNT-A injection [53,55]. However, two large, randomized, double-blind, placebo-controlled trials showed no significant difference between patients who received intraprostatic BoNT-A injection and placebo [56,57]. A meta-analysis including randomized, placebo-controlled trials also suggested that BoNT-A injection for patients with BPH does not have a significantly better therapeutic effect than does placebo [58]. On the other hand, a recent randomized placebo-controlled study, which enrolled only BPH patients with moderate to severe symptoms (IPSS $\geq$ 19) and pressure-flow study, indicated bladder outlet obstruction showed different results [59]. Patients received BoNT-A injection reported significantly greater improvement of IPSS, maximum flow rate, and PVR when compared with the placebo group at three months of follow-up. The follow-up urodynamic study in the BoNT-A injection group also showed a significant reduction in bladder outlet obstruction index (54%), which was not significantly changed in the placebo group. This study enrolled only BPH patients with evidence of bladder outlet obstruction and might be the reason why these results are different from previous studies. We suggested intraprostatic BoNT-A should be a reasonable treatment option for moderate to severe BPH patients who are refractory to oral medications and not willing to undergo surgical intervention. Careful selection of patients according to symptom severity and urodynamic study evaluation before treatment might be essential for successful outcome of this treatment.

9. Intraprostatic BoNT-A Injection in Chronic Prostatitis

Prostatitis is another common problem among many young and middle-aged male patients in the urology clinic. Male patients with chronic prostatitis usually present with pelvic pain/discomfort (perineal, testicular, penis, or pubic area) and voiding symptoms [60]. Treatments of chronic prostatitis should be treated first with oral antibiotics and an α-adrenergic blocker [61]. If there is no obvious symptomatic benefit, medications targeting neuropathic pain or neuromodulation procedures should be considered in these patients [61]. Giorgio et al. first used BoNT-A injection to treat voiding dysfunction in male patients with chronic prostatitis [62]. An animal study revealed the anti-inflammatory and analgesic effects of BoNT-A in prostatitis [63]. In rats with capsaicin-induced prostatitis, Chuang et al. showed that intraprostatic BoNT-A injection could both reduce pain and decrease infiltration of inflammatory cells in the prostate. Falahatkar et al. conducted a prospective, randomized, double-blind, placebo-controlled study to evaluate transurethral intraprostatic injection of 100 U of BoNT-A for patients with chronic prostatitis [64]. Significant improvement in pain score, National Institutes of Health chronic prostatitis symptom index, and quality of life were observed in the BoNT-A injection group at six months of follow-up. When compared with the placebo group, symptom improvements were significantly greater in the BoNT-A group. Another study compared the efficacy of transurethral and transrectal intraprostatic BoNT-A for chronic prostatitis [65]. Both groups demonstrated significant improvement in pain at six months of follow-up, but only patients in the transrectal injection group had significant improvement in the chronic prostatitis symptom index. Both anti-inflammatory and anti-nociceptive effects should be key factors for treating chronic prostatitis with BoNT-A. Although these pilot studies showed promising results of BoNT-A injection for treating chronic prostatitis, additional randomized placebo-controlled trials that enroll more patients are necessary to prove its efficacy.

In summary, both researchers and clinicians are determined to develop novel BoNT-A applications for treating LUTDs, improve the convenience of drug delivery, and decrease adverse effects. However, some patients continued to be dissatisfied with the outcome and opted to discontinue injections. For example, in a prospective study, only 68% of refractory OAB patients would like to continue to receive BoNT-A treatment after the first injection [66]. A study also detected neutralizing antibodies to BoNT-A in patients who had received bladder or urethral BoNT-A injections and suggested a possible cause of therapy failure [67]. Physicians should comprehensively evaluate voiding problems in patients and make diagnoses precisely before using BoNT-A to treat LUTDs. Further research that focuses on ways to improve BoNT-A with stronger effects and long-lasting formulations are necessary. Adjustment of BoNT-A dose according to urodynamics, study findings, or in combination with oral medications might improve the efficacy or prolong the duration of the therapeutic effect. A summary of novel applications of BoNT-A in LUTDs is provided in Table 1.

Table 1. Summary of novel applications of BoNT-A in Lower urinary tract dysfunctions (LUTDs).

LUTDs	Condition	BoNT-A Delivery Route	Study Design	Efficacy	Comment
LUTDs originated from bladder	IC/BPS	Intravesical injection	Randomized, placebo-controlled	Significantly greater reduction in pain and increase in bladder capacity in BoNT-A group compared with placebo group	First randomized, placebo-controlled trial for IC/BPS
		Instillation Lipotoxin	Randomized, placebo-controlled	No significant difference between Lipotoxin and placebo group	-
		Instillation gelation hydrogel	Prospective, non-controlled study	BoNT-A mixed with hydrogel significantly reduced the pain score at 12 weeks of follow up	-
	OAB	Instillation Lipotoxin	Randomized, placebo-controlled	Significantly improved frequency and urgency in Lipotoxin group but not in placebo group	-
	DHIC	Intravesical injection	Retrospective study	Subjective urgency symptom score significantly improved, but not incontinence episode	33% of patients experienced retention
LUTDs originated from bladder outlet	DV	Intrasphincter injection	Randomized, placebo-controlled	Significantly improved QoL, Qmax, IPSS, and VV in the study group. Only IPSS and VV improved greater than placebo group	-
	BPH	Intraprostatic injection	Randomized, placebo-controlled	Significantly greater improvement in IPSS, Qmax, and PVR compared with placebo group	Select patients with BPH urodynamic study
	Chronic prostatitis		Randomized, placebo-controlled	Significant improvement in pain score and QoL compared with placebo group	-

QoL: quality of life; Qmax: maximal urinary flow rate; IPSS: international prostate symptom score; VV: voided volume; PVR: post-voiding residual volume. IC/BPS: interstitial cystitis/bladder pain syndrome; OAB: overactive bladder; DHIC: detrusor hyperactivity with impaired contractile function; DV: dysfunctional voiding; BPH: benign prostate hyperplasia.

10. Conclusions

Since BoNT-A was first used to treat LUTD 30 years ago, applications have become increasingly prevalent and popular. Intravesical BoNT-A injection for patients with OAB or NDO has been widely used in daily urologic practice and proved by DHIC in the United States and many countries. For IC/BPS patients who have an inadequate response to initial treatment, intravesical BoNT-A injections also have been considered as standard treatment according to different clinical guidelines. BoNT-A delivery with liposome-encapsulation and gelation hydrogel intravesical installation provided a new class of less invasive and convenient application for patients with OAB or IC/BPS. Clinical trials revealed promising therapeutic results of novel BoNT-A applications, including DV, BPH, and chronic prostatitis. However, further randomized and placebo-controlled studies that enroll patients with accurate diagnoses are necessary to prove the efficacy of BoNT-A treatment. Both careful patient selection and prudent use of urodynamic study evaluation to confirm diagnoses are essential to achieve successful treatment outcomes.

References

1. Yang, C.C.; Weinfurt, K.P.; Merion, R.M.; Kirkali, Z.; Group, L.S. Symptoms of lower urinary tract dysfunction research network. *J. Urol.* **2016**, *196*, 146–152. [CrossRef] [PubMed]
2. Wang, Y.; Hu, H.; Xu, K.; Wang, X.; Na, Y.; Kang, X. Prevalence, risk factors and the bother of lower urinary tract symptoms in China: A population-based survey. *Int. Urogynecol. J.* **2015**, *26*, 911–919. [CrossRef] [PubMed]
3. Montecucco, C.; Molgo, J. Botulinal neurotoxins: Revival of an old killer. *Curr. Opin. Pharmacol.* **2005**, *5*, 274–279. [CrossRef] [PubMed]
4. Erbguth, F.J.; Naumann, M. Historical aspects of botulinum toxin: Justinus Kerner (1786–1862) and the "sausage poison". *Neurology* **1999**, *53*, 1850–1853. [CrossRef] [PubMed]
5. Nigam, P.K.; Nigam, A. Botulinum toxin. *Indian J. Dermatol.* **2010**, *55*, 8–14. [CrossRef] [PubMed]
6. Scott, A.B. Botulinum toxin injection of eye muscles to correct strabismus. *Trans. Am. Ophthalmol. Soc.* **1981**, *79*, 734–770. [PubMed]
7. Dykstra, D.D.; Sidi, A.A.; Scott, A.B.; Pagel, J.M.; Goldish, G.D. Effects of botulinum A toxin on detrusor-sphincter dyssynergia in spinal cord injury patients. *J. Urol.* **1988**, *139*, 919–922. [CrossRef]
8. Gormley, E.A.; Lightner, D.J.; Faraday, M.; Vasavada, S.P.; American Urological Association; Society of Urodynamics, Female Pelvic Medicine. Diagnosis and treatment of overactive bladder (non-neurogenic) in adults: AUA/SUFU guideline amendment. *J. Urol.* **2015**, *193*, 1572–1580. [CrossRef] [PubMed]
9. Hanno, P.M.; Erickson, D.; Moldwin, R.; Faraday, M.M.; American Urological Association. Diagnosis and treatment of interstitial cystitis/bladder pain syndrome: AUA guideline amendment. *J. Urol.* **2015**, *193*, 1545–1553. [CrossRef] [PubMed]
10. Franciosa, G.; Floridi, F.; Maugliani, A.; Aureli, P. Differentiation of the gene clusters encoding botulinum neurotoxin type a complexes in clostridium botulinum type a, ab, and a(b) strains. *Appl. Environ. Microbiol.* **2004**, *70*, 7192–7199. [CrossRef] [PubMed]
11. Dolly, J.O.; O'Connell, M.A. Neurotherapeutics to inhibit exocytosis from sensory neurons for the control of chronic pain. *Curr. Opin. Pharmacol.* **2012**, *12*, 100–108. [CrossRef] [PubMed]
12. Rummel, A. The long journey of botulinum neurotoxins into the synapse. *Toxicon* **2015**, *107*, 9–24. [CrossRef] [PubMed]
13. Dong, M.; Yeh, F.; Tepp, W.H.; Dean, C.; Johnson, E.A.; Janz, R.; Chapman, E.R. SV2 is the protein receptor for botulinum neurotoxin A. *Science* **2006**, *312*, 592–596. [CrossRef] [PubMed]
14. Fdez, E.; Jowitt, T.A.; Wang, M.C.; Rajebhosale, M.; Foster, K.; Bella, J.; Baldock, C.; Woodman, P.G.; Hilfiker, S. A role for soluble N-ethylmaleimide-sensitive factor attachment protein receptor complex dimerization during neurosecretion. *Mol. Biol. Cell* **2008**, *19*, 3379–3389. [CrossRef] [PubMed]
15. Aoki, K.R. Evidence for antinociceptive activity of botulinum toxin type A in pain management. *Headache* **2003**, *43* (Suppl. S1), S9–S15. [CrossRef] [PubMed]

16. Kaya, S.; Hermans, L.; Willems, T.; Roussel, N.; Meeus, M. Central sensitization in urogynecological chronic pelvic pain: A systematic literature review. *Pain Phys.* **2013**, *16*, 291–308.
17. Shie, J.H.; Liu, H.T.; Wang, Y.S.; Kuo, H.C. Immunohistochemical evidence suggests repeated intravesical application of botulinum toxin A injections may improve treatment efficacy of interstitial cystitis/bladder pain syndrome. *BJU Int.* **2013**, *111*, 638–646. [CrossRef] [PubMed]
18. Haylen, B.T.; de Ridder, D.; Freeman, R.M.; Swift, S.E.; Berghmans, B.; Lee, J.; Monga, A.; Petri, E.; Rizk, D.E.; Sand, P.K.; et al. An International Urogynecological Association (IUGA)/International Continence Society (ICS) joint report on the terminology for female pelvic floor dysfunction. *Int. Urogynecol. J.* **2010**, *21*, 5–26. [CrossRef] [PubMed]
19. Chuang, Y.C.; Liu, S.P.; Lee, K.S.; Liao, L.; Wang, J.; Yoo, T.K.; Chu, R.; Sumarsono, B. Prevalence of overactive bladder in China, Taiwan and South Korea: Results from a cross-sectional, population-based study. *Low Urin. Tract Symptoms* **2017**. [CrossRef] [PubMed]
20. Benner, J.S.; Nichol, M.B.; Rovner, E.S.; Jumadilova, Z.; Alvir, J.; Hussein, M.; Fanning, K.; Trocio, J.N.; Brubaker, L. Patient-reported reasons for discontinuing overactive bladder medication. *BJU Int.* **2010**, *105*, 1276–1282. [CrossRef] [PubMed]
21. Madersbacher, H.; Murtz, G.; Stohrer, M. Neurogenic detrusor overactivity in adults: A review on efficacy, tolerability and safety of oral antimuscarinics. *Spinal Cord* **2013**, *51*, 432–441. [CrossRef] [PubMed]
22. Hadiji, N.; Previnaire, J.G.; Benbouzid, R.; Robain, G.; Leblond, C.; Mieusset, R.; Enjalbert, M.; Soler, J.M. Are oxybutynin and trospium efficacious in the treatment of detrusor overactivity in spinal cord injury patients? *Spinal Cord* **2014**, *52*, 701–705. [CrossRef] [PubMed]
23. Schurch, B.; Stohrer, M.; Kramer, G.; Schmid, D.M.; Gaul, G.; Hauri, D. Botulinum-A toxin for treating detrusor hyperreflexia in spinal cord injured patients: A new alternative to anticholinergic drugs? Preliminary results. *J. Urol.* **2000**, *164*, 692–697. [CrossRef]
24. Cruz, F. Targets for botulinum toxin in the lower urinary tract. *Neurourol. Urodyn.* **2014**, *33*, 31–38. [CrossRef] [PubMed]
25. Schulte-Baukloh, H.; Priefert, J.; Knispel, H.H.; Lawrence, G.W.; Miller, K.; Neuhaus, J. Botulinum toxin A detrusor injections reduce postsynaptic muscular M2, M3, P2X2, and P2X3 receptors in children and adolescents who have neurogenic detrusor overactivity: A single-blind study. *Urology* **2013**, *81*, 1052–1057. [CrossRef] [PubMed]
26. Andersson, K.E.; Arner, A. Urinary bladder contraction and relaxation: Physiology and pathophysiology. *Physiol. Rev.* **2004**, *84*, 935–986. [CrossRef] [PubMed]
27. Groen, J.; Pannek, J.; Castro Diaz, D.; Del Popolo, G.; Gross, T.; Hamid, R.; Karsenty, G.; Kessler, T.M.; Schneider, M.; t' Hoen, L.; et al. Summary of European Association of Urology (EAU) guidelines on neuro-urology. *Eur. Urol.* **2016**, *69*, 324–333. [CrossRef] [PubMed]
28. Tyagi, P.; Kashyap, M.; Yoshimura, N.; Chancellor, M.; Chermansky, C.J. Past, Present and future of chemodenervation with botulinum toxin in the treatment of overactive bladder. *J. Urol.* **2017**, *197*, 982–990. [CrossRef] [PubMed]
29. Rahnamai, M.S.; Marcelissen, T.A.T.; Brierley, B.; Schurch, B.; de Vries, P. Long-term compliance and results of intravesical botulinum toxin A injections in male patients. *Neurourol. Urodyn.* **2017**, *36*, 1855–1859. [CrossRef] [PubMed]
30. Ginsberg, D.A.; Drake, M.J.; Kaufmann, A.; Radomski, S.; Gousse, A.E.; Chermansky, C.J.; Magyar, A.; Nicandro, J.P.; Nitti, V.W.; 191622-096 Investigators. Long-Term treatment with onabotulinumtoxina results in consistent, durable improvements in health related quality of life in patients with overactive bladder. *J. Urol.* **2017**, *198*, 897–904. [CrossRef] [PubMed]
31. Kuo, H.C.; Liu, H.T.; Chuang, Y.C.; Birder, L.A.; Chancellor, M.B. Pilot study of liposome-encapsulated onabotulinumtoxina for patients with overactive bladder: A single-center study. *Eur. Urol.* **2014**, *65*, 1117–1124. [CrossRef] [PubMed]
32. Hoag, N.; Gani, J. Underactive bladder: Clinical features, urodynamic parameters, and treatment. *Int. Neurourol. J.* **2015**, *19*, 185–189. [CrossRef] [PubMed]
33. Wang, C.C.; Lee, C.L.; Kuo, H.C. Efficacy and safety of intravesical onabotulinumtoxina injection in patients with detrusor hyperactivity and impaired contractility. *Toxins* **2016**, *8*. [CrossRef] [PubMed]

34. Berry, S.H.; Elliott, M.N.; Suttorp, M.; Bogart, L.M.; Stoto, M.A.; Eggers, P.; Nyberg, L.; Clemens, J.Q. Prevalence of symptoms of bladder pain syndrome/interstitial cystitis among adult females in the United States. *J. Urol.* **2011**, *186*, 540–544. [CrossRef] [PubMed]
35. Bosch, P.C.; Bosch, D.C. Treating interstitial cystitis/bladder pain syndrome as a chronic disease. *Rev. Urol.* **2014**, *16*, 83–87. [PubMed]
36. Smith, C.P.; Radziszewski, P.; Borkowski, A.; Somogyi, G.T.; Boone, T.B.; Chancellor, M.B. Botulinum toxin a has antinociceptive effects in treating interstitial cystitis. *Urology* **2004**, *64*, 871–875. [CrossRef] [PubMed]
37. Kuo, H.C.; Jiang, Y.H.; Tsai, Y.C.; Kuo, Y.C. Intravesical botulinum toxin-A injections reduce bladder pain of interstitial cystitis/bladder pain syndrome refractory to conventional treatment—A prospective, multicenter, randomized, double-blind, placebo-controlled clinical trial. *Neurourol. Urodyn.* **2016**, *35*, 609–614. [CrossRef] [PubMed]
38. Jhang, J.F.; Kuo, H.C. Novel treatment of chronic bladder pain syndrome and other pelvic pain disorders by onabotulinumtoxina injection. *Toxins* **2015**, *7*, 2232–2250. [CrossRef] [PubMed]
39. Zhang, W.; Deng, X.; Liu, C.; Wang, X. Intravesical treatment for interstitial cystitis/painful bladder syndrome: A network meta-analysis. *Int. Urogynecol. J.* **2017**, *28*, 515–525. [CrossRef] [PubMed]
40. Chuang, Y.C.; Kuo, H.C. A prospective, multicenter, double-blind, randomized trial of bladder instillation of liposome formulation onabotulinumtoxina for interstitial cystitis/bladder pain syndrome. *J. Urol.* **2017**, *198*, 376–382. [CrossRef] [PubMed]
41. Rappaport, Y.H.; Zisman, A.; Jeshurun-Gutshtat, M.; Gerassi, T.; Hakim, G.; Vinshtok, Y.; Stav, K. Safety and feasibility of intravesical instillation of botulinum toxin-a in hydrogel-based slow-release delivery system in patients with interstitial cystitis-bladder pain syndrome: A pilot study. *Urology* **2018**, *114*, 60–65. [CrossRef] [PubMed]
42. Chancellor, M.B.; Kaplan, S.A.; Blaivas, J.G. Detrusor-external sphincter dyssynergia. *Ciba Found. Symp.* **1990**, *151*, 195–206. [PubMed]
43. Jhang, J.F.; Kuo, H.C. Botulinum toxin a and lower urinary tract dysfunction: Pathophysiology and mechanisms of action. *Toxins* **2016**, *8*, 120. [CrossRef] [PubMed]
44. Kuo, H.C. Satisfaction with urethral injection of botulinum toxin A for detrusor sphincter dyssynergia in patients with spinal cord lesion. *Neurourol. Urodyn.* **2008**, *27*, 793–796. [CrossRef] [PubMed]
45. Huang, M.; Chen, H.; Jiang, C.; Xie, K.; Tang, P.; Ou, R.; Zeng, J.; Liu, Q.; Li, Q.; Huang, J.; et al. Effects of botulinum toxin A injections in spinal cord injury patients with detrusor overactivity and detrusor sphincter dyssynergia. *J. Rehabil. Med.* **2016**, *48*, 683–687. [CrossRef] [PubMed]
46. Osman, N.I.; Chapple, C.R. Fowler's syndrome—A cause of unexplained urinary retention in young women? *Nat. Rev. Urol.* **2014**, *11*, 87–98. [CrossRef] [PubMed]
47. Panicker, J.N.; Seth, J.H.; Khan, S.; Gonzales, G.; Haslam, C.; Kessler, T.M.; Fowler, C.J. Open-label study evaluating outpatient urethral sphincter injections of onabotulinumtoxinA to treat women with urinary retention due to a primary disorder of sphincter relaxation (Fowler's syndrome). *BJU Int.* **2016**, *117*, 809–813. [CrossRef] [PubMed]
48. Jiang, Y.H.; Wang, C.C.; Kuo, H.C. OnabotulinumtoxinA urethral sphincter injection as treatment for non-neurogenic voiding dysfunction—A randomized, double-blind, placebo-controlled study. *Sci. Rep.* **2016**, *6*. [CrossRef] [PubMed]
49. Wang, W.; Guo, Y.; Zhang, D.; Tian, Y.; Zhang, X. The prevalence of benign prostatic hyperplasia in mainland China: Evidence from epidemiological surveys. *Sci. Rep.* **2015**, *5*. [CrossRef] [PubMed]
50. Nitti, V.W. Pressure flow urodynamic studies: The gold standard for diagnosing bladder outlet obstruction. *Rev. Urol.* **2005**, *7* (Suppl. S6), S14–S21. [PubMed]
51. McVary, K.T.; Roehrborn, C.G.; Avins, A.L.; Barry, M.J.; Bruskewitz, R.C.; Donnell, R.F.; Foster, H.E., Jr.; Gonzalez, C.M.; Kaplan, S.A.; Penson, D.F.; et al. Update on AUA guideline on the management of benign prostatic hyperplasia. *J. Urol.* **2011**, *185*, 1793–1803. [CrossRef] [PubMed]
52. Drescher, P.; Eckert, R.E.; Madsen, P.O. Smooth muscle contractility in prostatic hyperplasia: Role of cyclic adenosine monophosphate. *Prostate* **1994**, *25*, 76–80. [CrossRef] [PubMed]
53. Chuang, Y.C.; Chiang, P.H.; Huang, C.C.; Yoshimura, N.; Chancellor, M.B. Botulinum toxin type A improves benign prostatic hyperplasia symptoms in patients with small prostates. *Urology* **2005**, *66*, 775–779. [CrossRef] [PubMed]

54. Maria, G.; Brisinda, G.; Civello, I.M.; Bentivoglio, A.R.; Sganga, G.; Albanese, A. Relief by botulinum toxin of voiding dysfunction due to benign prostatic hyperplasia: Results of a randomized, placebo-controlled study. *Urology* **2003**, *62*, 259–264. [CrossRef]
55. Chuang, Y.C.; Huang, C.C.; Kang, H.Y.; Chiang, P.H.; Demiguel, F.; Yoshimura, N.; Chancellor, M.B. Novel action of botulinum toxin on the stromal and epithelial components of the prostate gland. *J. Urol.* **2006**, *175*, 1158–1163. [CrossRef]
56. McVary, K.T.; Roehrborn, C.G.; Chartier-Kastler, E.; Efros, M.; Bugarin, D.; Chen, R.; Patel, A.; Haag-Molkenteller, C. A multicenter, randomized, double-blind, placebo controlled study of onabotulinumtoxinA 200 U to treat lower urinary tract symptoms in men with benign prostatic hyperplasia. *J. Urol.* **2014**, *192*, 150–156. [CrossRef] [PubMed]
57. Marberger, M.; Chartier-Kastler, E.; Egerdie, B.; Lee, K.S.; Grosse, J.; Bugarin, D.; Zhou, J.; Patel, A.; Haag-Molkenteller, C. A randomized double-blind placebo-controlled phase 2 dose-ranging study of onabotulinumtoxinA in men with benign prostatic hyperplasia. *Eur. Urol.* **2013**, *63*, 496–503. [CrossRef] [PubMed]
58. Shim, S.R.; Cho, Y.J.; Shin, I.S.; Kim, J.H. Efficacy and safety of botulinum toxin injection for benign prostatic hyperplasia: A systematic review and meta-analysis. *Int. Urol. Nephrol.* **2016**, *48*, 19–30. [CrossRef] [PubMed]
59. Totaro, A.; Pinto, F.; Pugliese, D.; Vittori, M.; Racioppi, M.; Foschi, N.; Bassi, P.F.; Sacco, E. Intraprostatic botulinum toxin type "A" injection in patients with benign prostatic hyperplasia and unsatisfactory response to medical therapy: A randomized, double-blind, controlled trial using urodynamic evaluation. *Neurourol. Urodyn.* **2018**, *37*, 1031–1038. [CrossRef] [PubMed]
60. Wagenlehner, F.M.; van Till, J.W.; Magri, V.; Perletti, G.; Houbiers, J.G.; Weidner, W.; Nickel, J.C. National Institutes of Health Chronic Prostatitis Symptom Index (NIH-CPSI) symptom evaluation in multinational cohorts of patients with chronic prostatitis/chronic pelvic pain syndrome. *Eur. Urol.* **2013**, *63*, 953–959. [CrossRef] [PubMed]
61. Rees, J.; Abrahams, M.; Doble, A.; Cooper, A.; Prostatitis Expert Reference Group. Diagnosis and treatment of chronic bacterial prostatitis and chronic prostatitis/chronic pelvic pain syndrome: A consensus guideline. *BJU Int.* **2015**, *116*, 509–525. [CrossRef] [PubMed]
62. Maria, G.; Destito, A.; Lacquaniti, S.; Bentivoglio, A.R.; Brisinda, G.; Albanese, A. Relief by botulinum toxin of voiding dysfunction due to prostatitis. *Lancet* **1998**, *352*, 625. [CrossRef]
63. Chuang, Y.C.; Yoshimura, N.; Wu, M.; Huang, C.C.; Chiang, P.H.; Tyagi, P.; Chancellor, M.B. Intraprostatic capsaicin injection as a novel model for nonbacterial prostatitis and effects of botulinum toxin A. *Eur. Urol.* **2007**, *51*, 1119–1127. [CrossRef] [PubMed]
64. Falahatkar, S.; Shahab, E.; Gholamjani Moghaddam, K.; Kazemnezhad, E. Transurethral intraprostatic injection of botulinum neurotoxin type A for the treatment of chronic prostatitis/chronic pelvic pain syndrome: Results of a prospective pilot double-blind and randomized placebo-controlled study. *BJU Int.* **2015**, *116*, 641–649. [CrossRef] [PubMed]
65. El-Enen, M.A.; Abou-Farha, M.; El-Abd, A.; El-Tatawy, H.; Tawfik, A.; El-Abd, S.; Rashed, M.; El-Sharaby, M. Intraprostatic injection of botulinum toxin-A in patients with refractory chronic pelvic pain syndrome: The transurethral vs. transrectal approach. *Arab J. Urol.* **2015**, *13*, 94–99. [CrossRef] [PubMed]
66. Malde, S.; Dowson, C.; Fraser, O.; Watkins, J.; Khan, M.S.; Dasgupta, P.; Sahai, A. Patient experience and satisfaction with Onabotulinumtoxin A for refractory overactive bladder. *BJU Int.* **2015**, *116*, 443–449. [CrossRef] [PubMed]
67. Schulte-Baukloh, H.; Bigalke, H.; Miller, K.; Heine, G.; Pape, D.; Lehmann, J.; Knispel, H.H. Botulinum neurotoxin type A in urology: Antibodies as a cause of therapy failure. *Int. J. Urol.* **2008**, *15*, 407–415. [CrossRef] [PubMed]

8

Comparing the Efficacy of OnabotulinumtoxinA, Sacral Neuromodulation and Peripheral Tibial Nerve Stimulation as Third Line Treatment for the Management of Overactive Bladder Symptoms in Adults

Chi-Wen Lo [1,2,3], Mei-Yi Wu [4], Stephen Shei-Dei Yang [2,3], Fu-Shan Jaw [1] and Shang-Jen Chang [2,3,*]

[1] Institute of Biomedical Engineering, National Taiwan University, Taipei 10617, Taiwan; chiwenlo0216@gmail.com (C.-W.L.); jaw@ntu.edu.tw (F.-S.J.)
[2] Division of Urology, Department of Surgery, Taipei Tzu Chi Hospital, The Buddhist Tzu Chi Medical Foundation, New Taipei 23142, Taiwan; urolyang@tzuchi.com.tw
[3] School of Medicine, Buddhist Tzu Chi University, Hualien 97071, Taiwan
[4] Department of Nephrology, Taipei Medical University-Shuang Ho Hospital, Taipei 23561, Taiwan; e220121@gmail.com
* Correspondence: krissygnet@gmail.com

Abstract: The American Urological Association guidelines for the management of non-neurogenic overactive bladder (OAB) recommend the use of OnabotulinumtoxinA, sacral neuromodulation (SNM), and peripheral tibial nerve stimulation (PTNS) as third line treatment options with no treatment hierarchy. The current study used network meta-analysis to compare the efficacy of these three modalities for managing adult OAB syndrome. We performed systematic literature searches of several databases from January 1995 to September 2019 with language restricted to English. All randomized control trials that compared any dose of OnabotulinumtoxinA, SNM, and PTNS with each other or a placebo for the management of adult OAB were included in the study. Overall, 17 randomized control trials, with a follow up of 3–6 months in the predominance of trials (range 1.5–24 months), were included for analysis. For each trial outcome, the results were reported as an average number of episodes of the outcome at baseline. Compared with the placebo, all three treatments were more efficacious for the selected outcome parameters. OnabotulinumtoxinA resulted in a higher number of complications, including urinary tract infection and urine retention. Compared with OnabotulinumtoxinA and PTNS, SNM resulted in the greatest reduction in urinary incontinence episodes and voiding frequency. However, comparison of their long-term efficacy was lacking. Further studies on the long-term effectiveness of the three treatment options, with standardized questionnaires and parameters are warranted.

Keywords: network meta-analysis; OnabotulinumtoxinA; overactive bladder; peripheral tibial nerve stimulation; sacral neuromodulation

Key Contribution: Updated systematic review to compare the efficacy of three existing third line treatments for the management of adult overactive bladder using network meta-analysis.

---

1. Introduction

Overactive bladder (OAB) syndrome is defined as "the presence of urinary urgency, usually accompanied by frequency and nocturia, with or without urgency urinary incontinence, in the absence of urinary tract infection (UTI) or other obvious pathology" [1]. The prevalence of OAB syndrome increases with age and there is no significant gender difference [2]. Non-neurogenic OAB impairs the patient's quality of life (QoL) and behavioral therapy is recommended as the first line treatment. If behavioral therapy fails, oral medications, including antimuscarinics and β3 agonists, are recommended as the second line therapy [3]. When there is inadequate symptom control or intolerable side effects due to second line management, the American Urological Association (AUA) guidelines recommend either OnabotulinumtoxinA, sacral neuromodulation (SNM), or peripheral tibial nerve stimulation (PTNS) as third line therapy options for OAB symptoms. Third line therapy is undertaken if the patient desires further treatment and is willing to engage in treatment, and/or further treatment is determined by clinicians to be in the patient's best interests. At present, the decision on which third line therapy to perform is based on the clinicians' and patient's preference, and there is not an evidence-based hierarchy available for guidance [3].

There have been several previously published randomized control studies, which compared pairwise treatments with a placebo [4,5]. However, there has not been a direct comparison of the three available treatments, and there has also been a lack of efficiency and safety comparisons between the three treatment options. When multiple treatment modalities are considered, a network meta-analysis could help compare their efficacies. Therefore, we conducted a systemic review to compare the efficacy of OnabotulinumtoxinA, SNM, and PTNS for the treatment of OAB symptoms, using a network meta-analysis.

2. Results

2.1. Included Studies

A Preferred reporting items for systematic reviews and meta-analyses (PRISMA) flow diagram flowchart summarizing the literature search is shown in Figure 1 [6]. The initial search identified 1940 and 5722 potential studies from PubMed and EMBASE, respectively. After the removal of duplicates the total number of articles was 7662. After screening, a total of 5738 articles were excluded based on their title and/or abstract, while another 185 articles were removed after a full-text assessment. A total of 20 articles met the qualitative inclusion criteria, while 17 trials, including 3038 participants, met the criteria for systematic review and network meta-analysis.

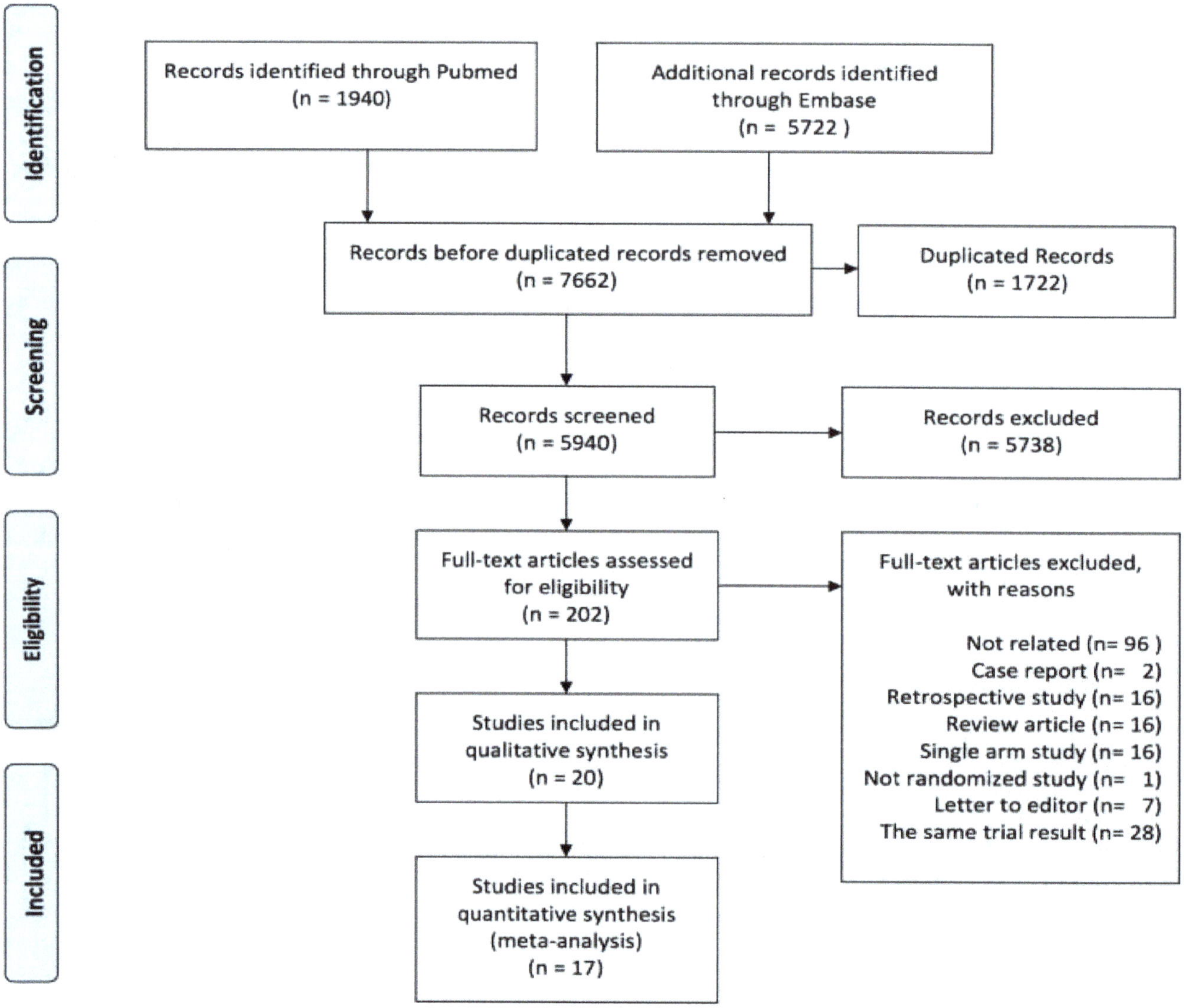

Figure 1. Preferred reporting items for systematic reviews and meta-analyses (PRISMA) flow diagram of the study selection process for network meta-analysis. The figure was generated using the PRISMA 2009 Flow Diagram.

2.2. Study and Participant Characteristics

The number of patients, the study design, and the inclusion and exclusion criteria for each of the included studies are listed in Table 1. As the three investigated treatment modalities are used for third line OAB syndromes management, most of the included patients were refractory or intolerant to the first and second line treatments.

Table 1. Characteristics of the included randomized controlled trials.

Author, Year [ref.]	Trial Registration	Study Design	Participants	Exclusion Criteria	Group Sample	Follow-up (month)	Outcomes
OnabotulinumtoxinA vs. placebo							
2007 Sahai [7]	ISRCTN 16995641	Randomized, Double blinded	OAB symptoms > 6 months, refractory or intolerant to medication	Neurological disease, BOO, anticoagulant therapy, pregnancy, IC, indwelling catheter, PVR >200 mL, previous bladder surgery, UC, UTI, neuromuscular transmission disease	Cystoscopy injection OnabotulinumtoxinA 200U (n = 16) vs. Cystoscopy Injection with Placebo (n = 18)	6	Change in MMC, Urgency, UUI, urinary frequency/day, IIQ-7, UDI-6, MBC, PVR, UTI, CIC
2009 Flynn [8]	N/A	Randomized, Double blinded	OAB symptoms with UUI, refractory to medication, multiple daily incontinence and pad weight/day > 100 gm	Neurological condition, fecal incontinence or absent detrusor contraction	Cystoscopy injection OnabotulinumtoxinA 200 U/ 300 U n = 15) vs. Cystoscopy injection with Placebo (n = 7)	1.5	Incontinence, urinary frequency/ day, nocturia/ IIQ7, UDI6, pads/day, pads weight/ day, MBC, PVR, UTI, CIC
2010 Dmochowski [9]	N/A	Randomized, Double blinded	OAB symptoms with UUI > 6 months, refractory or intolerant to medication	CIC, pelvic/urological abnormalities, disease related bladder dysfunction	OnabotulinumtoxinA 50 U/100 U/150 U/200 U/300 U (n = 268) vs. Cystoscopy injection with Placebo (n = 43)	9	UUI, KHQ, UTI, CIC, PVR >200 mL, urine retention
2011 Rovner [10]	N/A	Randomized, Double blinded	OAB symptoms with UUI, refractory or intolerant to medication	Predominant SUI, pelvic or urologic abnormality or disease affect bladder function, frequent UTI, PVR >200, or VV >3000	OnabotulinumtoxinA 50 U/100 U/150 U/200 U/300 U (n = 268) vs. Placebo (n = 43)	9	UUI, urinary frequency/day, Voided volume, MBC, CIC, PVR >200 mL
2012 Denys [11]	NCT 00231491	Randomized, Double blinded	OAB syndrome and Detrusor overactivity (≥3 urgency/ 3 days, frequency), refractory or intolerant to medication	UTI, predominant SUI, PVR >150, Qmax <15, anticoagulation/ antineoplastic or exposed to OnabotulinumtoxinA	OnabotulinumtoxinA 50 U/100 U/150 U (n = 70) vs. placebo (n = 29)	6	Urgency, UUI, urinary frequency, pads/day, MBC, PVR > 50% reduction, > 75% reduction UIE, EQ-5D, IQoL, UTI, CIC

Table 1. *Cont.*

Author, Year [ref.]	Trial Registration	Study Design	Participants	Exclusion Criteria	Group Sample	Follow-up (month)	Outcomes
2012 Tincello [12]	ISRCTN 26091555	Randomized, Double blinded	OAB symptoms and Detrusor overactivity (frequency, ≥2 urgency /day), refractory or intolerant to medication	SUI, neurologic disease, voiding dysfunction or contraindicated to OnabotulinumtoxinA	OnabotulinumtoxinA 200 U (n = 122) vs. placebo (n = 118)	3	Incontinence, urgency, urinary frequency/day, IQoL, UTI, CIC
2013 Chapple [13]	NCT 00910520	Randomized, Double blinded	OAB syndrome with UUI, refractory or intolerant to medication in the past 12 months	Previous OnabotulinumtoxinA treatment, with neurologic reason, predominance of SUI and pelvic/ urologic abnormalities, bladder surgery or disease affect bladder function	OnabotulinumtoxinA 100 U (n = 277) vs. placebo (n = 271)	6	Incontinence, urgency, UUI, urinary frequency/day, nocturia, continent, PVR, > 50% reduction UIE, ICIQ-SF, IUSS, IQoL, UTI, CIC,
2011 Dowson [14]	ISRCTN 57577615	Randomized, Double blinded	Bladder oversensitivity, refractory or intolerant to medication	Pregnancy, breast feeding, IC, neurological condition, BOO, indwelling catheter, previous bladder surgery, previous OnabotulinumtoxinA treatment, anticoagulation agent use	OnabotulinumtoxinA 100 U (n = 10) vs. placebo (n = 11)	3	Urinary frequency/day, Urgency, UUI, IIQ-7, UDI-6, PPBC, MBC, UTI, CIC
2013 Nitti [15]	NCT 00910845	Randomized, Double blinded	OAB syndrome, refractory or intolerant to medication	Predominance of SUI	OnabotulinumtoxinA 100 U (n = 278) vs. placebo (n = 272)	3	Incontinence, urgency, urinary frequency/day, nocturia, PVR, UUI, I-QoL, KHQ, UTI, CIC
OnabotulinumtoxinA vs. PTNS							
2017 Sherif [16]	N/A	Randomized	OAB symptoms, refractory or intolerant to medication	Nerve damage, pregnant, pacemaker, defibrillator, UTI, coagulopathy, BOO, neurogenic bladder, previous RT or bladder cancer, s/p incontinence surgery	OnabotulinumtoxinA 100 U (n = 30) vs. PTNS (n = 30)	9	Incontinence, urgency, urinary frequency/day, nocturia, OABSS, QoL, frequency, nocturia, PVR, Urgency scale, MBC, UTI, CIC

Table 1. *Cont.*

Author, Year [ref.]	Trial Registration	Study Design	Participants	Exclusion Criteria	Group Sample	Follow-up (month)	Outcomes
				PTNS vs. placebo			
2010 Finazzi-Agro [17]	N/A	Randomized, Double blinded	female, UI with detrusor overactivity incontinence, refractory or intolerant to medication	Pregnancy or plan / UTI, fistula, stone, Interstitial cystitis, DM, pacemaker/ defibrillator	PTNS (n = 17) vs. placebo (n = 15)	3	Incontinence, urinary frequency/day, nocturia, >50% reduction UIE
2010 Peters [18]	N/A	Randomized, Double blinded	OAB syndrome (OAB-q ≥4, voiding ≥10/day), refractory or intolerant to medication	Pregnant or plan/ neurogenic bladder/ previous use of OnabotulinumtoxinA / pacemaker/ defibrillator/ UTI/ use of TENS	PTNS (n = 103) vs. placebo (n = 105)	3	urinary frequency/day, nocturia, OAB-qSF, SF-36, GRA, voiding volume, UUI
2016 Scaldazza [19]	N/A	Randomized	Female with OAB syndrome	SUI, UTI, neurological disease, bladder stone, POP, pregnancy, DM, anti-incontinence surgery, pelvic tumor, radiation	PTNS (n = 30) vs. placebo (n = 30)	3	urinary frequency/day, voiding volume, nocturia, OAB-qSF, PPIUS, PGI-I >50% reduction UIE
				SNM vs. Placebo			
1999 Schmidt [20]	N/A	Randomized	UUI, poor response to anti-cholinergic agents	Neurological condition, SUI, pelvic pain symptoms	SNM (n = 34) vs. delay SNM (n = 42)	6	Incontinence, pads/day, >50% reduction UIE, SF-36, implant revision
2000 Hassouna [21]	N/A	Randomized	Urgency/ frequency symptoms, refractory to medication	Neurological condition, SUI, pelvic pain symptoms	SNM (n = 25) vs. no SNM (n = 26)	6	Urinary frequency/day, MBC, >50% reduction UIE, implant revision, SF-36
2000 Weil [22]	N/A	Randomized	Refractory urinary urge incontinence	SUI, SCI, CVA within 6 months, DD, bleeding complication, VUR or hydronephrosis, UTI, pelvic pain	SNM (n = 22) vs. conservative treatment (n = 20)	6	Incontinence, pad use, implant revision rate, >50% reduction UIE

Table 1. *Cont.*

Author, Year [ref.]	Trial Registration	Study Design	Participants	Exclusion Criteria	Group Sample	Follow-up (month)	Outcomes
SNM vs. OnabotulinumtoxinA							
2016 Amundsen [23,24]	NCT 01502956	Randomized	UUI, refractory or intolerant to 1st and 2nd line therapy	Neurological disease, PVR >150	SNM (n = 174) vs. OnabotulinumtoxinA 200U (n = 190)	24	UUI, urinary incontinence, pads, nocturia urinary frequency/day, CIC, UTI, > 50% reduction UIE, Questionnaire SF, Satisfaction Questionnaire, PGI-I, Sandvik

CIC: clean intermittent catheterization; OABSS: overactive bladder symptom score; UTI: urinary tract infection; I-QoL: Incontinence Quality of Life Questionnaire; IIQ-7: Incontinence Impact Questionnaire, short form; MBC: maximal bladder capacity; SUI: Stress urinary incontinence; UDI-6: Urogenital Distress Inventory, Short Form; UUI: urge urinary incontinence; >50% reduction UIE: >50% reduction in urinary incontinence episodes; KHQ: King's Health Questionnaire score; Questionnaire SF: Questionnaire short form; PGI-I: Patient Global Impression of Improvement; SF-36: Short Form 36 Health survey; PPIUS: Patient Perception of Intensity of Urgency Scale; OAB-qSF: Overactive bladder questionnaire short form; GRA: Global response assessment.

2.3. Networks

There was sufficient evidence available for analysis of the following efficacy and safety endpoints: urinary frequency per day, incontinence episodes per day, ≥50% reduction of symptoms, patients with urinary tract infections (UTIs), and post-treatment urine retention needing clean intermittent catheterization (CIC). There was a lack of sufficient data to make comparisons between the three treatment modalities with regard to the QoL, urgency, urge incontinence episodes/day, maximal bladder capacity, and nocturia. Results of the pair-wise comparison meta-analyses are shown in Table 2.

Table 2. Pairwise meta-analyses result for different endpoints.

Endpoint	Comparison	N	I^2 (%)	p Value	Standard Mean Difference (95% CI)
Urinary frequency/ day	OnabotulinumtoxinA vs. Placebo	4	92	< 0.001	−0.65 (-0.24−−1.06)
	PTNS vs. OnabotulinumtoxinA	1			−1.02 (−1.55−−0.48)
	PTNS vs. Placebo	3	37.1	0.204	−0.37 (-0.03−−0.70)
	SNM vs. Placebo	1			−1.12 (-0.53−−1.71)
Urge urine incontinence	OnabotulinumtoxinA vs. Placebo	2	70.7	0.065	−0.37 (−0.05—0.79)
Urgency Episode	OnabotulinumtoxinA vs. Placebo	4	97.6	<0.001	−0.84 (-0.08—1.60)
Maximal	PTNS vs. Placebo	1			1.35 (0.79–1.92)
	SNM vs. Placebo	1			0.91 (0.33–1.48)
I-QoL	OnabotulinumtoxinA vs. Placebo	2	99.1	<0.001	0.98 (−0.89–2.86)
	PTNS vs. Placebo	1			0.86 (0.13–1.59)
Incontinence	OnabotulinumtoxinA vs. Placebo	3	97.8	<0.001	-0.84 (-1.62—0.06)
	PTNS vs. OnabotulinumtoxinA	1			0.54 (0.02–1.06)
	PTNS vs. Placebo	1			-1.49 (-2.28—0.70)
	SNM vs. Placebo	2	74.6	0.047	-2.10 (-3.07—1.12)
≥50% Improvement	Placebo vs. OnabotulinumtoxinA	2	0.0	0.410	0.53 (0.40–0.70)
	PTNS vs. OnabotulinumtoxinA	2	0.0	0.371	0.50 (0.32–0.76)
	Placebo vs. PTNS	3	52.5	0.122	0.21 (0.07–0.61)
	SNM vs. Placebo	1			1.27 (0.87–1.87)
Urinary tract infection	OnabotulinumtoxinA vs. Placebo	8	0	0.486	2.55 (1.89–3.43)
	PTNS vs. OnabotulinumtoxinA	1			0.20 (0.01–4.34)
	SNM vs. OnabotulinumtoxinA	1			0.33 (0.19–0.56)
Clean intermittent catherization	OnabotulinumtoxinA vs. Placebo	9	0	0.786	5.95 (3.08–11.46)
	PTNS vs. OnabotulinumtoxinA	1			0.20 (0.01–4.34)
	SNM vs. OnabotulinumtoxinA	1			0.01 (0.00–0.23)

2.4. Risk of Bias Assessment

A summary of the included studies and a risk of bias graph are shown in Figure 2. The four studies that compared SNM with delayed SNM were rated as having a high risk of bias in the 'measurement of outcome' category because the self-reporting results could have been influenced by the placebo effect. As these papers did not describe the randomization method or specify whether the assessors were blinded, we had some concerns regarding the randomization process when the risk of bias was evaluated. All of the studies, except the four that compared the efficacy of SNM with the delayed SNM group, were judged as having a 'low risk' of bias or as having 'some concerns'.

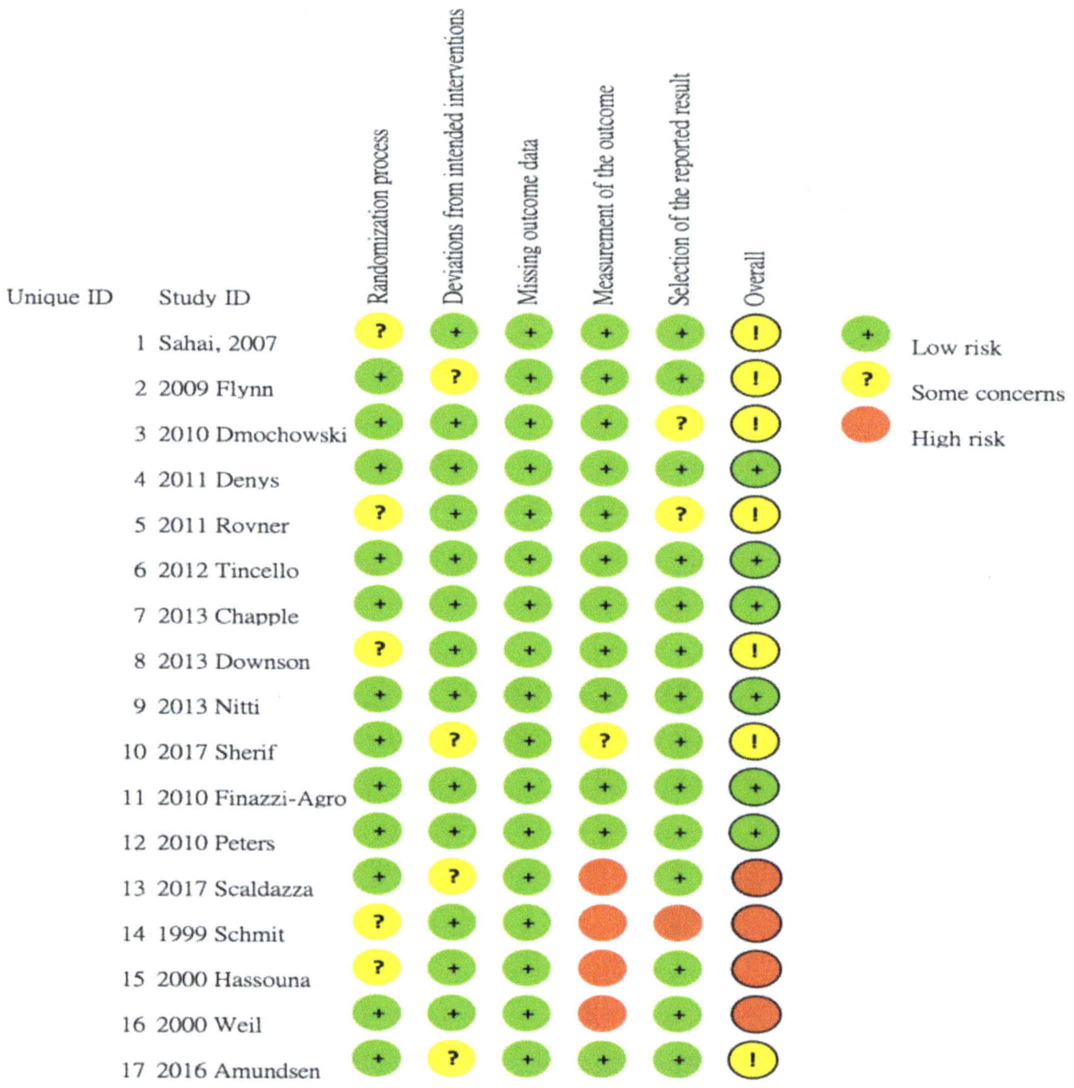

Figure 2. Risk of bias graph and summary of the included studies: Reviewers' judgments regarding each risk of bias item for the included studies. The figure was generated using RoB 2 tool (the 22 August 2019 version)

2.5. Network Meta-Analysis on the Outcomes of Interests

2.5.1. Efficacy

Urinary Frequency per Day

A total of nine studies contributed to the comparison of urine frequency per day [6–14]. Pair-wise comparisons with a random effects (RE) model revealed that all three modalities were more efficacious than the placebo (Table 2). The NMA (Network Meta-analysis) identified a greater reduction in the total number of micturition per day for SNM compared with the placebo, PTNS, and OnabotulinumtoxinA. There were no significant differences observed between OnabotulinumtoxinA and SNM (Table 3). The ranking probability results are shown in Figure 3. The ranking results for urinary frequency reduction was as follows: SNM ranked first, OnabotulinumtoxinA ranked second, PTNS ranked third, and placebo ranked fourth (Figure 3A).

Table 3. Summary of results from NMA (on the lower triangle) and traditional pairwise meta-analysis (on the upper triangle).

	Placebo	OnabotulinumtoxinA	PTNS	SNM
Urinary frequency/ Day (SMD, 95% CI)				
Placebo	0	−0.65 (-0.24—1.06)	−0.37 (-0.03—0.70)	−1.12 (-0.53—1.71)
OnabotulinumtoxinA	−1.72 (-1.23—2.21)	0	−1.02 (−1.55-−0.48)	
PTNS	−0.80 (-0.15—1.14)	−0.92 (−1.59-−0.26)	0	
SNM	−8.10 (-4.04—12.16)	−6.38 (-2.29—10.47)	−7.30 (−3.19—11.41)	0
Incontinence/ Day (SMD, 95% CI)				
Placebo	0	−0.84 (−0.06–1.62)	−1.49 (−0.70–2.28)	−2.10 (-1.12–3.07)
OnabotulinumtoxinA	−1.96 (-0.92—3.00)	0	−0.54 (-0.03—1.06)	
PTNS	−2.05 (-0.56—3.53)	-0.08 (−1.37–1.53)	0	
SNM	-10.96 (-8.60—13.31)	−8.99 (−6.42—11.57)	−8.91 (-6.12—11.70)	0
Urinary tract infection (OR, 95% CI)				
Placebo	1	2.54 (1.89–3.44)		
OnabotulinumtoxinA	3.06 (2.26–4.15)	1	0.20 (0.01–4.35)	0.33 (0.19–0.56)
PTNS	0.57 (0.03–12.62)	0.19 (0.01–4.06)	1	
SNM	10.73 (0.39–1.38)	0.24 (0.14–0.42)	1.28 (0.06–29.29)	1
Clean intermittent catheterization (OR, 95% CI)				
Placebo	1	5.95 (3.08–11.46)		
OnabotulinumtoxinA	6.92 (3.18–15.06)	1	0.20 (0.01–4.34)	0.01 (0.00–0.23)
PTNS	1.29 (0.05–31.93)	0.19 (0.01–4.19)	1	
SNM	0.08 (0.00–1.46)	0.01 (0.00–0.19)	0.06 (0.00–4.01)	1

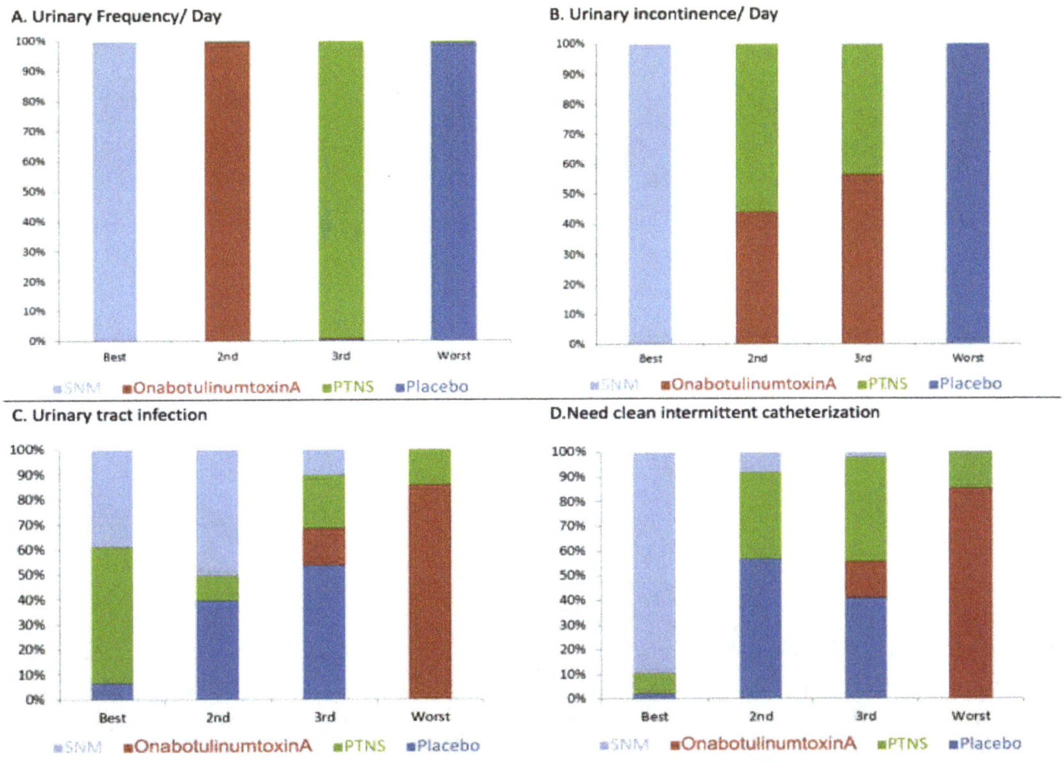

Figure 3. Treatment rankings for (**A**) urinary frequency/day, (**B**) incontinence, (**C**) urinary tract infection, and (**D**) urine retention needing clean intermittent catheterization.

Urinary Incontinence Episodes per Day

There were seven studies used to compare the efficacy of the three modalities on the number of incontinence episodes per day at 12 weeks follow-up [12,13,15–17,20,22]. Pair-wise comparisons with a RE model revealed that all three modalities were more efficacious than the placebo (Table 2). The NMA demonstrated that SNM was associated with a greater reduction in the total number of incontinence episodes per day compared with the placebo, PTNS, and OnabotulinumtoxinA. There was no significant difference between the efficacy of OnabotulinumtoxinA and PTNS (Table 3). The ranking results for incontinence episode reduction was as follows: SNM ranked first, PTNS ranked second, OnabotulinumtoxinA ranked third, and placebo ranked fourth (Figure 3B).

≥50% Symptom Improvement at 12 Weeks Follow-up

The network of eligible comparisons for >50% symptom improvement is shown in Figure 4D. There were eight studies that reported parameters including ≥50% improvement in symptoms at 12 weeks follow-up. Pair-wise comparisons with a RE model revealed all three modalities were more efficacious than the placebo. However, there was a significant inconsistency expected in ≥50% reduction of symptoms improvement. Therefore, network meta-analysis and ranking probability was not conducted with regard to this parameter.

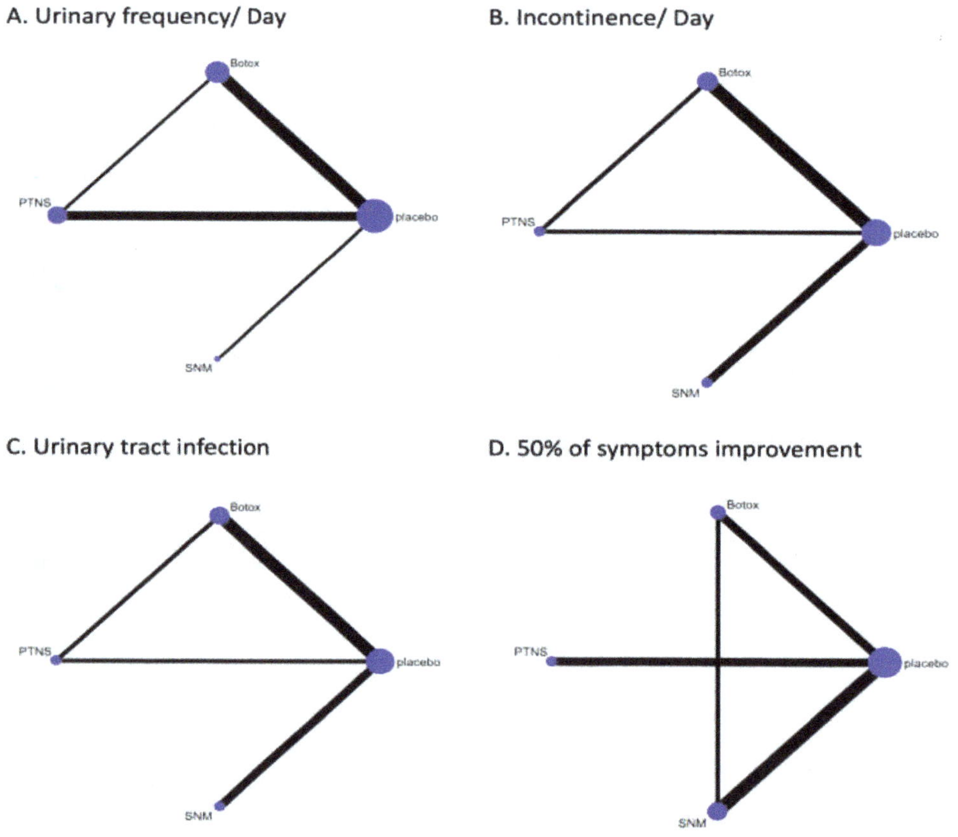

Figure 4. Network of treatment comparisons between OnabotulinumtoxinA (Botox), sacral neuromodulation (SNM), percutaneous tibial nerve stimulation (PTNS) in regard to **(A)** urinary frequency/day, **(B)** incontinence, **(C)** urinary tract infection, and **(D)** ≥50% of symptoms improvement. The figure was generated using R 3.3.2 software.

2.6. Complications

2.6.1. Urinary Tract Infection

Estimates of the treatment effectiveness on the occurrence of UTIs were informed by 10 studies [7–9,11–16,23,24]. The RE model revealed that OnabotulinumtoxinA was associated with a higher incidence of UTIs compared with the placebo, SNM, and PTNS (Table 3). The ranking results for the post-management risk of UTIs was as follows: PTNS ranked best, SNM ranked second, placebo ranked third, and OnabotulinumtoxinA ranked worst (Figure 3C).

2.6.2. Urine Retention Needing Clean Intermittent Catheterization

Estimates on the effect of treatments on post-management urine retention were reported in 11 studies [7–16,23,24]. The RE model demonstrated that OnabotulinumtoxinA was associated with a higher occurrence of post-treatment urine retention needing catherization compared with the placebo, SNM, and PTNS (Table 3). The ranking results for post-management risk of post-treatment urine retention was as follows: SNM ranked best, placebo ranked second, PTNS ranked third, and OnabotulinumtoxinA ranked worst (Figure 3D).

3. Discussion

The AUA guidelines suggest intra-detrusor injection with OnabotulinumtoxinA (evidence grade B), SNM (evidence grade C), or PTNS (evidence grade C) as the third-line treatment modalities for adult OAB [3]. In the absence of a direct head to head comparison of the three treatment modalities for adult OAB symptoms, the present detailed systemic review and network meta-analysis is the first review to combine all updated evidence and compares the efficacy of any dose of OnabotulinumtoxinA, sacral neuromodulation and PTNS. The compared outcomes included voiding frequency/day, urinary incontinence episodes/day, and ≥50% reduction in symptoms. Pairwise meta-analysis revealed that all three modalities were more efficacious than a placebo with regard to the outcomes of interests, including urinary frequency, incontinence, and achieving ≥50% of symptoms improvement. SNM achieved the greatest reduction in urinary incontinence episodes and voiding frequency/day. OnabotulinumtoxinA was associated with the highest risk of urine retention and UTI episodes in the follow-up period. As none of the included studies used a unified or standard questionnaire to evaluate the QoL, the results regarding QoL were not pooled for the meta-analysis. We suggested that International Continence Society or International Urogynecology Association should unify the QoL questionnaire based on evidence and experts' opinion for a better evaluation of post treatment result.

The cost of the treatment and the insurance payment system may influence the patient's preference for a specific therapy. A cost analysis was performed to assess the economic effectiveness of each treatment. Based on a literature review, SNM was considered to be the most expensive treatment compared with a OnabotulinumtoxinA injection and PTNS in the short term [25–27]. However, in a model of middle- and long-term treatment, the cost-effectiveness of SNM was comparable with OnabotulinumtoxinA [25,28]. There was no comparison between OnabotulinumtoxinA and PTNS. Martinson et al. constructed the Markov model to simulate the cost-effectiveness of PTNS and they concluded that PTNS was the least costly therapy compared with OnabotulinumtoxinA and SNM [26]. However, different regional health insurance and health care payment systems could affect the simulation result and lead to different outcomes. A local cost-effectiveness analysis is more valuable for urologists.

The current study primarily compared short-term efficacy at 12 weeks follow-up and data comparing long-term efficacy is lacking. Amundsen et al. conducted a randomized control trial with a 6 years follow-up, which confirmed the middle- to long-term efficacy, QoL and satisfaction with treatment for OnabotulinumtoxinA injection and SNM [24]. However, there has been no previous report on the long-term efficacy of PTNS. The present study did not compare long-term adherence between treatment modalities.

The major drawbacks for management with antimuscarinics lie in the low rates of adherence to the medication [29,30]. Adherence at 12 months was 39% for mirabegron vs. 14–35% for antimuscarinics [29]. The effects of OnabotulinumtoxinA persist for 6–9 months and the effect can be extended with repeated injections [31]. Long-term adherence to OnabotulinumtoxinA injections is less discussed. Patient preference is an important factor, especially when comprehensive data is not available to assist in the decision-making progress. No significant difference in patient satisfaction was reported between SNM and OnabotulinumtoxinA in the ROSETTA trials [23,24] or studies by Hoag et al. [32]. Since all three of the investigated third line treatments are effective, health care providers should carefully discuss the pros and cons of each treatment with the patient and determine the appropriate strategy based on each individual situation.

The adverse effects of an OnabotulinumtoxinA injection include hematuria, bacteriuria, UTIs, urine retention, and increased post-void residual urine [33]. The rate of post-therapeutic complications, including urine retention that needed clean intermittent catheterization and UTIs, were compared between treatments. Intravesical injection with OnabotulinumtoxinA lead to a significantly higher rate of CIC and UTIs. Nevertheless, the higher rate of CIC was not consistent among the included trials and the literature review, therefore this conclusion could be controversial. Side effects associated with SNM included pain at the stimulator and lead sites, lead migration, infection, and the requirement for surgical revision [21–24,32]. A screen test before implantation and two-stage implantation could increase the success rate [34]. The revision rate varied from 3–32% and the removal rate varied from 8.6–13% [24,35]. With improvements in battery longevity and better localization of lead placement, these revision and removal rates could be reduced. The only side effects of PTNS were local adverse events, including minor bleeding spots and temporary pain [4].

There were several limitations to the current network meta-analysis study. First, the variable qualities and publication biases of the included studies may compromise the results of the network meta-analysis. There was considerable heterogeneity across the study designs, including participants, scheduled follow-ups, questionnaires, evaluated parameters, OnabotulinumtoxinA dose, and SNM and PTNS protocols. The U.S Food and Drug Administration approved intra-detrusor injection of OnabotulinumtoxinA is 100 U [3], while the included ROSETTA trial used 200 U [23,24]. Different protocols were also used for PTNS. Second, the variable or ambiguous and potentially post-hoc definitions for the outcome parameters used in each study made it difficult to unify and compare the treatment results between the studies. However, because of the heterogeneity of enrolled patients, existing of high-risk bias and lacking long-term outcomes comparison, more high-quality studies are necessary to clarify this benefit and risk of the current available 3rd line therapy for overactive bladder symptoms. A strength of the current study was that it collected 17 randomized controlled trials published in English over three decades and used network meta-analysis to compare the three existing therapeutic options.

4. Conclusions

The results revealed that all three modalities were efficacious in managing adult OAB syndrome, and all were better than a placebo on the specific symptoms reported to be the outcome of the study. This review shows that at 12 weeks follow-up, SNM yielded the greatest reduction in urinary incontinence episodes and urinary frequency/day. OnabotulinumtoxinA resulted in a higher incidence of complications, including urinary tract infection and urinary retention.

As there is a lack of head to head comparison studies among SNM, PTNS, and OnabotulinumtoxinA for the treatment of adult OAB symptoms, the current network meta-analysis represents the best available evidence for the comparison of these three treatment modalities.

5. Material and Methods

5.1. Search Strategy and Eligibility Criteria

To identify appropriate studies for a network meta-analysis, two independent investigators (CWL and SJC) conducted a comprehensive electronic literature search of PubMed, EMBASE, Cochrane Central Register of Controlled Trials (CENTRAL), Wiley, and ClinicalTrial.gov for trials published between January 1995 and September 2019, with a language restriction of English. The present study followed PRISMA recommendations. The terms and related synonyms "overactive bladder", "bladder overactivity", "detrusor overactivity", "urinary incontinence", "urgency", "urgent incontinence", "detrusor overactivity" and "Botulinum A toxin" or "OnabotulinumtoxinA" or "Botox" or "botulinumtoxin A" or "sacral neuromodulation" or "sacral nerve stimulation" or "percutaneous tibial nerve stimulation" or "posterior tibial nerve stimulation" were combined in the search strategy. MeSH terms, key words and other free terms were used for searching and Boolean operators (OR and AND) were used to combine the searches. The reference lists of the included articles, as well as the guidelines for the AUA and European Association of Urology were manually reviewed, and external peer reviewers were asked to contribute any additional trials.

Studies were considered eligible if they were randomized controlled trials that compared any dose of OnabotulinumtoxinA, SNM, and PTNS therapy with each other or a placebo, in adults with OAB syndrome with reported efficacy at 12 weeks follow-up. It was required that the studies provided detailed data on the treatments and outcomes of the participants.

5.2. Data Extraction and Quality Asessment

Two investigators (CWL and SJC) independently reviewed the titles and abstracts to check their relevance and adherence to the eligibility criteria. The full text of articles was assessed if their eligibility was not clear from the abstract. A preliminary network was constructed based on the intervention and comparators in the included trials. The homogeneity of the included trials was also evaluated.

Two investigators (CWL and SJC) reviewed the quality of the included studies. The risk of bias was evaluated using the RoB 2 (Version 2 of the Cochrane risk-of-bias tool for randomized trials) tool to evaluate the quality of evidence [36]. The following domains were evaluated: random sequence generation, allocation concealment, blinding, incomplete data on outcomes, selective reporting, and other bias. The Grading of Recommendation, Assessment, Development, and Evaluation Working Group approach for rating the quality of treatment effect estimates was also followed. Urination frequency/day, incontinence, and ≥50% symptom improvement were selected because of their relevance to clinical symptom improvement. The quality of evidence was rated as very low, low, moderate or high.

When standard deviation data was missing or only 95% confidence intervals (CI) were listed, the standard deviation was calculated using the formula in the Cochrane handbook for systematic reviews of interventions, or it was calculated from the figure data in the article or supplemental data.

5.3. Network Development

If the data was available, theoretical networks were developed for each outcome based on the similarities between studies. The outcomes included QoL, lower urinary tract symptoms at 12 weeks follow-up, including urinary incontinence episodes, urgency episodes, urge urinary incontinence episodes/day and urinary frequency/day, achieving ≥50% of symptoms improvement, nocturia, and complications including post-treatment urine retention that needed intermittent catheterization and urinary tract infections.

5.4. Statistical Analysis

The network meta-analysis was performed using R 3.3.2 software (Bell Laboratories, Madison, WI, USA, 2016) and STATA version 15.0 (StataCorp. LP, College Station, TX, USA, 2017). All outcomes of interests were compared pairwise by calculating I^2 statistics. Study heterogeneity was assessed using the R package. Node splitting analysis was performed to evaluate inconsistencies by comparing differences between the direct and indirect evidence. Dichotomous variables and continuous variables were expressed as odds ratios (ORs) with 95% CIs and weighted mean differences with 95% CIs, respectively. A RE model was used to calculate evidence inconsistencies because of the existence of heterogeneity among the included trials and each intervention comparison. The ranking probabilities for the different OAB symptoms interventions were also calculated with regard to each outcome of interest. Additionally, publication bias was evaluated according to the symmetry characteristics of funnel plots, with a symmetrical and concentrated distribution of dots implying no significant deviation.

Author Contributions: Conceptualization, S.-J.C.; methodology, M.-Y.W.; software, M.-Y.W.; validation, C.-W.L. and S.-J.C.; formal analysis, M.-Y.W.; investigation, C.-W.L.; data curation, C.-W.L.; writing—original draft preparation, C.-W.L.; writing—review and editing, S.-J.C.; visualization, C.-W.L.; supervision, F.-S.J. and S.S.-D.Y. All authors have read and agree to the published version of the manuscript.

References

1. Abrams, P.; Cardozo, L.; Fall, M.; Griffiths, D.; Rosier, P.; Ulmsten, U.; Van Kerrebroeck, P.; Victor, A.; Wein, A.; Standardisation Sub-Committee of the International Continence Society. The standardisation of terminology of lower urinary tract function: Report from the standardisation sub-committee of the international continence society. *Neurourol. Urodyn.* **2002**, *21*, 167–178. [CrossRef] [PubMed]
2. Irwin, D.E.; Kopp, Z.S.; Agatep, B.; Milsom, I.; Abrams, P. Worldwide prevalence estimates of lower urinary tract symptoms, overactive bladder, urinary incontinence and bladder outlet obstruction. *BJU Int.* **2011**, *108*, 1132–1138. [CrossRef] [PubMed]
3. Lightner, D.J.; Gomelsky, A.; Souter, L.; Vasavada, S.P. Diagnosis and treatment of overactive bladder (Non-Neurogenic) in adults: AUA/SUFU guideline amendment 2019. *J. Urol.* **2019**, *202*, 558–563. [CrossRef] [PubMed]
4. Niu, H.L.; Ma, Y.H.; Zhang, C.J. Comparison of OnabotulinumtoxinA versus sacral neuromodulation for refractory urinary urge incontinence: A systematic review and meta-analysis of randomized controlled trials. *Int. J. Surg.* **2018**, *60*, 141–148. [CrossRef] [PubMed]
5. Arruda, R.M.; Takano, C.C.; Girão, M.J.B.C.; Haddad, J.M.; Aleixo, G.F.; Castro, R.A. Treatment of non-neurogenic overactive bladder with OnabotulinumtoxinA: Systematic review and meta-analysis of prospective, randomized, placebo-controlled clinical trials. *Rev. Bras. Ginecol. Obstet.* **2018**, *40*, 225–231. [CrossRef]
6. Moher, D.; Liberati, A.; Tetzlaff, J.; Altman, D.G.; The PRISMA Group. Preferred Reporting Items for Systematic Reviews and Meta-Analyses: The PRISMA Statement. *Ann. Intern. Med.* **2009**, *151*, 264–269. [CrossRef]
7. Sahai, A.; Khan, M.S.; Dasgupta, P. Efficacy of botulinum toxin-A for treating idiopathic detrusor overactivity: Results from a single center, randomized, double-blind, placebo controlled trial. *J. Urol.* **2007**, *177*, 2231–2236. [CrossRef]
8. Flynn, M.K.; Amundsen, C.L.; Perevich, M.; Liu, F.; Webster, G.D. Outcome of a randomized, double-blind, placebo controlled trial of botulinum A toxin for refractory overactive bladder. *J. Urol.* **2009**, *181*, 2608–2615. [CrossRef]
9. Dmochowski, R.; Chapple, C.; Nitti, V.W.; Chancellor, M.; Everaert, K.; Thompson, C.; Daniell, G.; Zhou, J.; Haag-Molkenteller, C. Efficacy and safety of onabotulinumtoxinA for idiopathic overactive bladder: A double-blind, placebo controlled, randomized, dose ranging trial. *J. Urol.* **2010**, *184*, 2416–2422. [CrossRef]
10. Rovner, E.; Kennelly, M.; Schulte-Baukloh, H.; Zhou, J.; Haag-Molkenteller, C.; Dasgupta, P. Urodynamic results and clinical outcomes with intradetrusor injections of onabotulinumtoxinA in a randomized, placebo-controlled dose-finding study in idiopathic overactive bladder. *Neurourol. Urodyn.* **2011**, *30*, 556–562. [CrossRef] [PubMed]

11. Denys, P.; Le Normand, L.; Ghout, I.; Costa, P.; Chartier-Kastler, E.; Grise, P.; Hermieu, J.F.; Amarenco, G.; Karsenty, G.; Saussine, C.; et al. Efficacy and safety of low doses of onabotulinumtoxinA for the treatment of refractory idiopathic overactive bladder: A multicentre, double-blind, randomised, placebo-controlled dose-ranging study. *Eur. Urol.* **2012**, *61*, 520–529. [CrossRef] [PubMed]
12. Tincello, D.G.; Kenyon, S.; Abrams, K.R.; Mayne, C.; Toozs-Hobson, P.; Taylor, D.; Slack, M. Botulinum toxin a versus placebo for refractory detrusor overactivity in women: A randomised blinded placebo-controlled trial of 240 women (the RELAX study). *Eur. Urol.* **2012**, *62*, 507–514. [CrossRef] [PubMed]
13. Chapple, C.; Sievert, K.D.; MacDiarmid, S.; Khullar, V.; Radziszewski, P.; Nardo, C.; Thompson, C.; Zhou, J.; Haag-Molkenteller, C. OnabotulinumtoxinA 100 U significantly improves all idiopathic overactive bladder symptoms and quality of life in patients with overactive bladder and urinary incontinence: A randomised, double-blind, placebo-controlled trial. *Eur. Urol.* **2013**, *64*, 249–256. [CrossRef] [PubMed]
14. Dowson, C.; Sahai, A.; Watkins, J.; Dasgupta, P.; Khan, M.S. The safety and efficacy of botulinum toxin-A in the management of bladder oversensitivity: A randomised double-blind placebo-controlled trial. *Int. J. Clin. Pract.* **2011**, *65*, 698–704. [CrossRef]
15. Nitti, V.W.; Dmochowski, R.; Herschorn, S.; Sand, P.; Thompson, C.; Nardo, C.; Yan, X.; Haag-Molkenteller, C.; EMBARK Study Group. OnabotulinumtoxinA for the treatment of patients with overactive bladder and urinary incontinence: Results of a phase 3, randomized, placebo controlled trial. *J. Urol.* **2013**, *189*, 2186–2193. [CrossRef]
16. Sherif, H.; Khalil, M.; Omar, R. Management of refractory idiopathic overactive bladder: Intradetrusor injection of botulinum toxin type A versus posterior tibial nerve stimulation. *Can. J. Urol.* **2017**, *24*, 8838–8846.
17. Finazzi-Agro, E.; Petta, F.; Sciobica, F.; Pasqualetti, P.; Musco, S.; Bove, P. Percutaneous tibial nerve stimulation effects on detrusor overactivity incontinence are not due to a placebo effect: A randomized, double-blind, placebo controlled trial. *J. Urol.* **2010**, *184*, 2001–2006. [CrossRef]
18. Peters, K.M.; Carrico, D.J.; Perez-Marrero, R.A.; Khan, A.U.; Wooldridge, L.S.; Davis, G.L.; Macdiarmid, S.A. Randomized trial of percutaneous tibial nerve stimulation versus Sham efficacy in the treatment of overactive bladder syndrome: Results from the SUmiT trial. *J. Urol.* **2010**, *183*, 1438–1443. [CrossRef]
19. Scaldazza, C.V.; Morosetti, C.; Giampieretti, R.; Lorenzetti, R.; Baroni, M. Percutaneous tibial nerve stimulation versus electrical stimulation with pelvic floor muscle training for overactive bladder syndrome in women: Results of a randomized controlled study. *Int. Braz. J. Urol.* **2017**, *43*, 121–126. [CrossRef]
20. Schmidt, R.A.; Jonas, U.; Oleson, K.A.; Janknegt, R.A.; Hassouna, M.M.; Siegel, S.W.; van Kerrebroeck, P.E. Sacral nerve stimulation for treatment of refractory urinary urge incontinence. Sacral Nerve Stimulation Study Group. *J. Urol.* **1999**, *162*, 352–357. [CrossRef]
21. Hassouna, M.M.; Siegel, S.W.; Nyeholt, A.A.; Elhilali, M.M.; van Kerrebroeck, P.E.; Das, A.K.; Gajewski, J.B.; Janknegt, R.A.; Rivas, D.A.; Dijkema, H.; et al. Sacral neuromodulation in the treatment of urgency-frequency symptoms: A multicenter study on efficacy and safety. *J. Urol.* **2000**, *163*, 1849–1854. [CrossRef]
22. Weil, E.H.; Ruiz-Cerda, J.L.; Eerdmans, P.H.; Janknegt, R.A.; Bemelmans, B.L.; van Kerrebroeck, P.E. Sacral root neuromodulation in the treatment of refractory urinary urge incontinence: A prospective randomized clinical trial. *Eur. Urol.* **2000**, *37*, 161–171. [CrossRef]
23. Amundsen, C.L.; Richter, H.E.; Menefee, S.A.; Komesu, Y.M.; Arya, L.A.; Gregory, W.T.; Myers, D.L.; Zyczynski, H.M.; Vasavada, S.; Nolen, T.L.; et al. OnabotulinumtoxinA vs Sacral Neuromodulation on Refractory Urgency Urinary Incontinence in Women: A Randomized Clinical Trial. *JAMA* **2016**, *316*, 1366–1374. [CrossRef] [PubMed]
24. Amundsen, C.L.; Komesu, Y.M.; Chermansky, C.; Gregory, W.T.; Myers, D.L.; Honeycutt, E.F.; Vasavada, S.P.; Nguyen, J.N.; Wilson, T.S.; Harvie, H.S.; et al. Two-year outcomes of sacral neuromodulation versus OnabotulinumtoxinA for refractory urgency urinary incontinence: A randomized trial. *Eur. Urol.* **2018**, *74*, 66–73. [CrossRef] [PubMed]
25. Arlandis, S.; Castro, D.; Errando, C.; Fernandez, E.; Jimenez, M.; Gonzalez, P.; Crespo, C.; Staeuble, F.; Rodriguez, J.M.; Brosa, M. Cost-effectiveness of sacral neuromodulation compared to botulinum neurotoxin a or continued medical management in refractory overactive bladder. *Value Health* **2011**, *14*, 219–228. [CrossRef]
26. Martinson, M.; MacDiarmid, S.; Black, E. Cost of neuromodulation therapies for overactive bladder: Percutaneous tibial nerve stimulation versus sacral nerve stimulation. *J. Urol.* **2013**, *189*, 210–216. [CrossRef] [PubMed]

27. Siddiqui, N.Y.; Amundsen, C.L.; Visco, A.G.; Myers, E.R.; Wu, J.M. Cost-effectiveness of sacral neuromodulation versus intravesical botulinum A toxin for treatment of refractory urge incontinence. *J. Urol.* **2009**, *182*, 2799–2804. [CrossRef] [PubMed]
28. Leong, R.K.; de Wachter, S.G.; Joore, M.A.; van Kerrebroeck, P.E. Cost-effectiveness analysis of sacral neuromodulation and botulinum toxin a treatment for patients with idiopathic overactive bladder. *BJU Int.* **2011**, *108*, 558–564. [CrossRef]
29. Wagg, A.; Franks, B.; Ramos, B.; Berner, T. Persistence and adherence with the new beta-3 receptor agonist, mirabegron, versus antimuscarinics in overactive bladder: Early experience in Canada. *Can. Urol. Assoc. J.* **2015**, *9*, 343–350. [CrossRef]
30. Yeaw, J.; Benner, J.S.; Walt, J.G.; Sian, S.; Smith, D.B. Comparing adherence and persistence across 6 chronic medication classes. *J. Manag. Care Pharm.* **2009**, *15*, 728–740. [CrossRef]
31. Carlson, K.; Civitarese, A.; Baverstock, R. OnabotulinumtoxinA for the treatment of idiopathic overactive bladder is effective and safe for repeated use. *Can. Urol. Assoc. J.* **2017**, *11*, e179–e183. [CrossRef] [PubMed]
32. Hoag, N.; Plagakis, S.; Pillay, S.; Edwards, A.W.; Gani, J. Sacral neuromodulation for refractory overactive bladder after prior intravesical onabotulinumtoxinA treatment. *Neurourol. Urodyn.* **2017**, *36*, 1377–1381. [CrossRef] [PubMed]
33. Martins-Silva, C.; Cruz, F. Efficacy and safety of OnabotulinumtoxinA in patients with urinary incontinence due to neurogenic detrusor overactivity: Update of the pivotal randomised, double-blind, placebo-controlled trials. *Eur. Urol. Focus* **2016**, *2*, 329–331. [CrossRef]
34. Banakhar, M.A.; Al-Shaiji, T.; Hassouna, M. Sacral neuromodulation and refractory overactive bladder: An emerging tool for an old problem. *Ther. Adv. Urol.* **2012**, *4*, 179–185. [CrossRef] [PubMed]
35. Siegel, S.W.; Catanzaro, F.; Dijkema, H.E.; Elhilali, M.M.; Fowler, C.J.; Gajewski, J.B.; Hassouna, M.M.; Janknegt, R.A.; Jonas, U.; van Kerrebroeck, P.E.; et al. Long-term results of a multicenter study on sacral nerve stimulation for treatment of urinary urge incontinence, urgency-frequency, and retention. *Urology* **2000**, *56*, 87–91. [CrossRef]
36. S Sterne, J.A.C.; Savovic, J.; Page, M.J.; Elbers, R.G.; Blencowe, N.S.; Boutron, I.; Cates, C.J.; Cheng, H.Y.; Corbett, M.S.; Eldridge, S.M.; et al. RoB 2: A revised tool for assessing risk of bias in randomised trials. *BMJ* **2019**, *366*, l4898. [CrossRef]

9

Can Botulinum Toxin A Still Have a Role in Treatment of Lower Urinary Tract Symptoms/Benign Prostatic Hyperplasia Through Inhibition of Chronic Prostatic Inflammation?

Bing-Juin Chiang [1,2,3], **Hann-Chorng Kuo** [4,5] **and Chun-Hou Liao** [1,2,*]

1 College of Medicine, Fu-Jen Catholic University, New Taipei City 24205, Taiwan; bingjuinchiang@gmail.com
2 Department of Urology, Cardinal Tien Hospital, New Taipei City 23148, Taiwan
3 Department of Life Science, College of Science, National Taiwan Normal University, Taipei 11677, Taiwan
4 Department of Urology, Buddhist Tzu Chi General Hospital, and Tzu Chi University, Hualien 97002, Taiwan; hck@tzuchi.com.tw
5 School of Medicine, Tzu Chi University, Hualien 97004, Taiwan
* Correspondence: liaoch22@gmail.com

Abstract: Patients with benign prostatic hyperplasia (BPH) can exhibit various lower urinary tract symptoms (LUTS) owing to bladder outlet obstruction (BOO), prostatic inflammation, and bladder response to BOO. The pathogenesis of BPH involves an imbalance of internal hormones and chronic prostatic inflammation, possibly triggered by prostatic infection, autoimmune responses, neurogenic inflammation, oxidative stress, and autonomic dysfunction. Botulinum toxin A (BoNT-A) is well recognized for its ability to block acetylcholine release at the neuromuscular junction by cleaving synaptosomal-associated proteins. Although current large clinical trials have shown no clinical benefits of BoNT-A for the management of LUTS due to BPH, BoNT-A has demonstrated beneficial effects in certain subsets of BPH patients with LUTS, especially in males with concomitant chronic prostatitis/chronic pelvic pain syndrome and smaller prostate. We conducted a review of published literature in Pubmed, using Botulinum toxin, BPH, BOO, inflammation, LUTS, and prostatitis as the key words. This article reviewed the mechanisms of BPH pathogenesis and anti-inflammatory effects of BoNT-A. The results suggested that to achieve effectiveness, the treatment of BPH with BoNT-A should be tailored according to more detailed clinical information and reliable biomarkers.

Keywords: lower urinary tract symptoms; botulinum toxin; benign prostatic hyperplasia; prostatitis; inflammation

Key Contribution: Botulinum Toxin A still have a role in treatment of lower urinary tract symptoms/benign prostatic hyperplasia through inhibition of chronic prostatic inflammation in selected patients.

---

1. Introduction

Benign prostatic hyperplasia (BPH) is a term exclusively used for describing benign histological patterns in the European Association of Urology (EAU) and the American Urological Association (AUA) guidelines [1,2]. BPH could lead to benign prostatic enlargement (BPE) or benign prostatic obstruction (BPO) resulting in male lower urinary tract symptoms (LUTS). LUTS are grouped into three categories: storage (increased daytime frequency, nocturia, urgency, and urinary incontinence), voiding (hesitancy, slow stream, intermittent stream, straining, and terminal dribble), and post-micturition (post-micturition dribble and feeling of incomplete emptying) symptoms [3]. In addition to BPH, other causes of male LUTS include structural or functional abnormalities of the bladder and its surrounding tissues, and some non-urological conditions [4]. Lower urinary tract dysfunction (LUTD) is defined as signs observed by the physician, including simple means, to verify and quantify symptoms [3]. From a clinical perspective, BPH usually refers to LUTD caused by BPE or BPO.

We conducted a review of published literature in Pubmed, using Botulinum toxin, BPH, bladder outlet obstruction (BOO), inflammation, LUTS, and prostatitis as the key words. We reviewed the mechanisms of BPH pathogenesis and anti-inflammatory effects of BoNT-A. We tried to determine the role of botulinum toxin A (BoNT-A) in treatment of LUTS/BPH.

2. Ambiguous Mechanisms of LUTS Related to BPH

Prevalence of LUTS generally increases with age. A large cross-sectional population-based study from the Asia-Pacific region reported LUTS prevalence to be higher in men than women [5]. More men had voiding symptoms (45.3%) than women (31.3%) [5], and the phenomenon could be attributed to BPH. Interestingly, the epidemiologic study showed more storage symptoms (49.9%) in men than voiding symptoms (45.3%). This could be attributed to BOO, which is capable of reducing bladder blood flow and subsequently causes chronic bladder ischemia, as reported by various epidemiologic and clinical studies [6–8]. BOO is also associated with repeated episodes of prolonged detrusor ischemia in pigs with an artificially implanted ring around urethra [9]. BOO causes a reduction in acetylcholine esterase staining nerves in detrusor muscle and expression of hypoxia-inducible factor 1 alpha, a cellular marker of hypoxia [10,11]. Moreover, experimentally, BOO has been shown to exhibit elevated cystometric voiding pressure, reduced urine flow rates, generated bladder hyperactivity, and increased bladder detrusor hypertrophy [12,13]. Further, BOO related bladder ischemia also causes denervation supersensitivity, leading to a fundamental reorganization of the detrusor's electrical activity and C-fiber mediated micturition reflexes [13–16]. BOO with high bladder pressure could also induces adaptive change of bladder wall, including detrusor muscle hypertrophy, bladder wall fibrosis and reduced bladder compliance [17]. Therefore, besides the preconceived voiding symptoms, BPH also causes varied storage symptoms related to bladder response to BOO. In addition, the prevalence of prostatitis-like symptoms in a community-based study was 11.5% and 8.5% in younger (<50 years) and older (≥50 years) men, respectively [18]. This study also measured irritative and obstructive voiding symptom severity (score, 0 to 10), where men with prostatitis-like symptoms showed significantly higher urinary symptom score. Prostatic inflammation is believed to play an important role in the BPH pathogenesis and progression [19,20]. In brief, most BPH related LUTS arises from BPE/BOO, prostatic inflammation, and bladder response to BPE/BOO. Therefore, it is difficult to distinguish the specific etiology of male LUTS through clinical practice. Although the exact mechanism underlying BPH related LUTS is unknown, its treatment should probably be tailored according to the cause of LUTS.

3. Mechanism of BPH Related to BOO

BPH causes obstruction by inducing functional and morphological changes in the prostate. Functionally, an increase in prostatic smooth muscle tone has been confirmed, which is influenced sympathetically [21]. Moreover, the presence of metabolic syndrome is associated with increased sympathetic nervous system activity and LUTS [22,23]. In such cases, alpha(α)-adrenergic antagonists can improve BPH-induced male LUTS [24]. Morphologically, BPH is characterized by unregulated proliferation of connective tissues, smooth muscles, and glandular epithelium [25]. Tissue proliferation leads to increased prostate volume (PV), subsequently compressing the prostatic urethra. McNeal found that BPH patients had an increase in BPH nodules in the periurethral zone and size of glandular nodules [26]. Further, either epithelium or fibro-muscular stroma proliferation could be found in the resected BPH tissues [27,28].

4. Mechanism of BPH-Imbalance of Internal Hormones

Abundant evidence showed that development of BPH requires testicular androgen [29]. Conversion of dihydrotestosterone (DHT), a metabolite of testosterone, in the prostate is considered as a major factor involved in the BPH pathogenesis. Elevated serum DHT level is associated with larger PV and higher prevalence of BPH [30]. Prostatic DHT and androgen receptor (AR) levels increase with age [31], whereas testosterone level declines with age. Increase in estrogen to testosterone ratio has been recognized as an important factor inducing the development of prostatic inflammation and cytokines [32]. In such cases, administration of 5α-reductase type II inhibitor resulted in increased plasma testosterone levels and further reduced the prostatic inflammation, suggesting the protective effect of testosterone against inflammation compared to that of DHT [33,34]. Imbalance in testosterone and estrogen levels also contributes to decreased activity of some suppressor cells, which maintain tolerance to prostatic antigen and prevent autoimmunity [35,36]. Moreover, the insulin-like growth factor (IGF) signaling pathway has been implicated in BPH development [37]. An IGF receptor antagonist, metformin, has an anti-proliferative effect, which attenuated testosterone-induced BPH in rats by decreasing the expression of estrogen receptor alpha [38]. Furthermore, neurotransmitter serotonin (5-HT) could possibly play a role in the pathogenesis of BPH. 5-HT can downregulate ARs and prevent prostate branching [39]. However, 5-HT depletion contributes to BPH development through modulation of ARs [39]. In summary, imbalance of internal hormones results in the development of BPH and prostatic inflammation.

5. Mechanism of BPH-Chronic Inflammation

A previous clinical study showed that men with prostatitis-like symptoms have significantly higher urinary symptom score [18]. Young-onset prostatitis was positively associated with LUTS [40]. Chronic inflammation along with BPH can coexist in human pathologic specimens [41]. Correlations were found between histopathology of chronic inflammation and severity of LUTS in a subgroup of patients from the randomized REDUCE (reduction in the use of corticosteroids in exacerbated COPD) trial [42]. Moreover, nonsteroidal anti-inflammatory drugs were inversely associated with the onset of LUTS [43]. These clinical results suggested the involvement of prostatic inflammation in the pathogenesis of BPH with LUTS.

The most important cytokine involved in the development of BPH is interleukin (IL)-8, which can directly promote epithelial and stromal proliferation [44]. Plasma IL-8 could serve as a reliable surrogate marker of prostatic inflammatory conditions, including chronic prostatitis and BPH [45]. Moreover, IL-8 can induce stromal cells for the emergence of a reactive myofibroblast phenotype [46]. Human BPH cells, including epithelial and stromal cells, act as antigen-presenting cells (APCs), which can secrete IL-8 and associated cytokines [47]. These cytokines promote prostatic immune cells upregulation for more specific cytokines, which in turn recruit more lymphomononuclear cells. These recruited lymphomononuclear cells express cognate receptors, CXCR1 and CXCR2, which induce proliferation of prostatic cells through autocrine/paracrine effect and generation of fibroblast grow factors [48]. Therefore, the cross-talk between the BPH and immune cells creates a positive feedback loop that can amplify inflammation, and the intraprostatic chronic inflammatory processes are induced and sustained.

6. Etiology of Prostatic Inflammation

The etiology of prostatic inflammatory process remains unclear. It is believed that several possible mechanisms are responsible for triggering a prostatic inflammatory response. Firstly, infection-induced inflammation hypothesis is evidenced by the presence of bacterial and viral strains in BPH tissue specimens [49]. Toll-like receptors (TLRs) expressed by BPH cells recognize structurally conserved molecules derived from pathogens. TLRs-mediated production of proinflammatory cytokines (IL-6) and chemokines (IL-8 and CXCL10) initiate and enhance the inflammatory process [50]. Secondly, autoimmune responses could be involved in prostatic inflammation. Epidemiologic studies showed that the prevalence of chronic prostatitis/chronic pelvic pain syndrome (CP/CPPS) is eight times more than bacterial prostatitis [51]. Prostate, as well as testes, are considered as immunologically privileged organs [52]; however, self-antigens release following a tissue injury results in autoimmunity [53]. Autoantibodies against prostate-specific antigen (PSA) or prostate acid phosphatase (PAP) were shown to be involved in the prostatic inflammatory process [54]. PSA has been demonstrated to be able to activate CD4+ T cells [55]. In addition, BPH cells, as well as other APCs, produce high levels of IL-12 and IL-23, promoting CD4+ T cell activation and differentiation [47], which in turn, differentiate into interferon gamma-secreting T-helper (Th) type 1 and IL-17-secreting Th17 cells [48]. These downstream pro-inflammatory cytokines manifest a positive feedback signal to inflammatory interaction between BPH and immune cells. Thirdly, neurogenic inflammation plays an important role in chronic prostatic inflammation. Neurotrophin, a nerve growth factor (NGF), is responsible for mediating prostatic neurogenic inflammation. The serum NGF level was found to be correlated with the severity of pain in CP/CPPS [56]. Moreover, damaged tissue has been found to contain higher NGF level [57], which can cause mast cells degranulation [58]. Infiltrating mast cells in BPH tissues can promote BPH development via activation of IL-6/Signal transducer and activator of transcription 3/Cyclin D1 signaling pathway [59]. NGF can also sensitize sensory nerve and induce production of neuropeptides, including substance P and calcitonin gene-related peptide (CGRP) [60]. Further, substance P can stimulate reactive oxygen species generation via its proinflammatory activity [61]. Prostatitis following intraprostatic formalin injection has been reported to induce prostate-to-bladder afferent cross-sensitization, increased urothelial NGF expression, and subsequent bladder overactivity [62]. Fourthly, oxidative stress can be one of the causes of inflammation. Interestingly, the ARR2PB-Nox4(ARR2PB-NADPH oxidase 4) transgenic mice showed increased prostate weight, increased epithelial proliferation, and histological changes, including epithelial proliferation, stromal thickening, and fibrosis through Nox4 promoting oxidative stress [63].

Furthermore, it is believed that chronic pelvic ischemia can generate oxidative stress [64]. Elderly patients with LUTS showed decreased prostate perfusion on transrectal color Doppler ultrasonography [7]. Serum glutathione peroxidase and superoxide dismutase levels, which have antioxidant effects, reportedly declined in dogs with BPH [65]. Oxidative stress also triggers prostate cells proliferation through the activation of cyclooxygenase (COX) pathways [66,67], whereas COX-2 inhibition can induce significant apoptosis in the prostate cell [67]. Fifthly, the autonomic nervous system (ANS) also contributes to prostatic inflammation and growth. Adrenergic innervation plays a role in prostate growth. ANS hyperactivity is significantly associated with LUTS, and serum norepinephrine level increased after tilt predicted prostate size [68]. Moreover, chronic administration of α1-adrenergic agonists induces proliferation of prostatic cells in a rat model [69]. Besides, norepinephrine can stimulate the proliferation of human non-epithelial prostatic cells [70]. α1-adrenoceptors have been linked with inflammatory pathways through activation of transforming growth factor β signaling cascade, regulating various events associated with the BPH development [69,71]. In summary, the major etiology of chronic prostatic inflammation includes prostatic infection, autoimmune responses, neurogenic inflammation, oxidative stress, and autonomic dysfunction.

7. Anti-Inflammatory Effects of Botulinum Toxin A (BoNT-A)

BoNT-A is well-recognized for its ability to block acetylcholine release at the neuromuscular junction by cleaving synaptosomal-associated proteins [72]. Intraprostatic injection of BoNT-A has been shown to induce relaxation of prostatic muscle through downregulation of α-adrenergic receptor expression and reducing smooth muscle contractility [73,74]. On the other hand, BoNT-A also causes morphological atrophy of the glands via chemodenervation and anti-inflammatory effects [75,76]. Clinically, BoNT-A has demonstrated therapeutic anti-inflammatory effects, including the reduction of pain, edema, erythema, and heat emission [77]. A study in a complete Freund's adjuvant-induced arthritic rat model revealed the anti-inflammatory effect of BoNT-A by attenuating anti-ionized calcium-binding adaptor molecule 1 and IL-1β immune-reactive cells [78]. Moreover, BoNT-A reduces rosacea-associated skin inflammation by directly inhibiting mast cell degranulation [79]. Intravesical BoNT-A injections plus hydrodistension reduce bladder pain and NGF levels in patients with interstitial cystitis [80], probably through blocking bladder pain responses and CGRP release from afferent nerve terminals, as depicted in a rat model [81]. BoNT-A may also inhibit peripheral and subsequent central sensitizations via suppressing substance P, glutamate, and adenosine triphosphate, showing reduction of somatic and visceral pain [82]. Interestingly, BoNT-A pretreatment could inhibit intraprostatic capsaicin injection-induced COX-2 expression in prostate and spinal cord [83]. Furthermore, BoNT-A also significantly prevented oxidative stress in vascular endothelial cells in cutaneous ischemia/reperfusion injured mouse model [84]. It has been shown that BoNT-A inhibits IL-8/CXCR1 signaling cascade in endothelial cells through inhibiting Rho signaling pathways [85]. In summary, BoNT-A exhibits anti-inflammatory effect by suppressing cytokine generation, mast cell activation, neurogenic inflammation, and oxidative stress in different organs. These reports from the basic research of BoNT-A potentially strengthened evidence for its therapeutic effects in patients with BPH; however, further studies are warranted for some of the proven anti-inflammatory effects on prostatic growth and inflammation.

8. Clinical Perspectives

Although previous single-arm studies showed promising results in improving international prostate symptom score (IPSS), maximal flow rate (Qmax), PV, and post-void residual urine volume (PVR) following intraprostatic injection of BoNT-A, two recent large scale randomized control trials failed to show significant efficacy of BoNT-A on all outcomes [76,86–92]. Moreover, a systematic review including three large randomized placebo-control studies (experimental group, $n = 260$; control group, $n = 262$) showed only marginal benefits to IPSS (−1.02; 95% confidence interval: −1.97, −0.07) for the BTX-A versus placebo groups. There were no significant differences in Qmax, PV, and PVR between the two groups, which was attributed to the placebo effect [93]. The EAU guidelines on the management of non-neurogenic male LUTS documented that "Results from clinical trials have shown no clinical benefits for BoNT-A compared to placebo for the management of LUTS due to BPO," and strongly recommended not to offer intraprostatic BoNT-A injection treatment to patients with male LUTS [1]. Intraprostatic BoNT-A injection is also not listed as one of the treatment choices in the AUA guidelines [2]. However, it is difficult to explain how intraprostatic BoNT-A injection significantly decrease PV, as reported by other meta-analyses [94–96].

Although limited reports are available for the therapeutic effects of BoNT-A on CP/CPPS, several beneficial effects on LUTS have been noted. In an uncontrolled randomized clinical trial conducted in men with refractory CP/CPPS, the patients were classified into two groups according to the route of BoNT-A injection, transurethral or transrectal. After intraprostatic injection of BoNT-A (100 U), Qmax, voiding score, and quality of life (QoL) were significantly improved in both groups during the follow-up period [97], with mean initial PV ranging from 36.4 to 37.9 ml among the groups. Another randomized, controlled study of transurethral intraprostatic injection of BTX-A (100 or 200 U depending on PV) showed significant improvement not only in pain score and QoL but also in the urinary domain of chronic prostatitis symptom index 1-month post-injection [98]. Other outcomes, including IPSS, frequency of diurnal, and nocturnal urination, showed significant reduction compared to baseline at 1, 3 and 6-month after BoNT-A injection. The mean initial PV in the experimental group was 22.27 mL. Chuang et al. reported that 16 men with symptomatic BPH and PV <30 mL were successfully treated with transperineal intraprostatic BoNT-A injection [89], with significant improvement in PV and IPSS following BoNT-A injection. However, the mean PV of men included in the two largest randomized trials failed to show beneficial effects on PV (range, 43.8–48.8 mL) [91,92]. Therefore, these results imply that intraprostatic injection of BoNT-A might be effective in relieving LUTS in patients with small prostate and refractory CP/CPPS. As mentioned above, patients suffering from BPH and CP/CPPS might show overlapping symptoms due to similar etiologies shared by BPH and prostatitis.

9. Conclusions

Based on the current basic and clinical studies, BoNT-A could still be effective in certain subsets of BPH with LUTS, especially in males with concomitant CP/CPPS and smaller prostate. However, this hypothesis requires further validation through randomized controlled clinical studies. In addition, it is imperative to consider exploring biomarkers of BPH, including NGF level, mast cells/distribution of activated subtypes of immune cells in biopsies, inflammatory-associated cytokines, or ANS dysfunction, as determining predictors of the treatment efficacy. Therefore, for effectiveness, the treatment of BPH with BoNT-A should be tailored according to more detailed clinical information and reliable biomarkers.

Author Contributions: Conceptualization, B.-J.C. and H.-C.K.; methodology, B.-J.C., H.-C.K. and C.-H.L.; writing—original draft preparation, B.-J.C.; writing—review and editing, B.-J.C., H.-C.K. and C.-H.L.; supervision, H.-C.K. and C.-H.L.; project administration, H.-C.K.

References

1. Gravas, S.; Cornu, J.N.; Drake, M.J.; Gacci, M.; Gratzke, C.; Herrmann, T.R.W.; Mamoulakis, C.; Rieken, M.; Speakman, M.J.; Tikkinen, K.A.O.; et al. Management of Non-Neurogenic Male LUTS. Available online: https://uroweb.org/guideline/treatment-of-non-neurogenic-male-luts/ (accessed on 1 January 2019).
2. Foster, H.E.; Barry, M.J.; Gandhi, M.C.; Kaplan, S.A.; Kohler, T.S.; Lerner, L.B.; Lightner, D.J.; Parsons, J.K.; Roehrborn, C.G.; Welliver, C.; et al. Benign Prostatic Hyperplasia: Surgical Management of Benign Prostatic Hyperplasia/Lower Urinary Tract Symptoms (2018, Amended 2019). Available online: https://www.auanet.org/guidelines/benign-prostatic-hyperplasia- (accessed on 1 January 2019).
3. Abrams, P.; Cardozo, L.; Fall, M.; Griffiths, D.; Rosier, P.; Ulmsten, U.; van Kerrebroeck, P.; Victor, A.; Wein, A. The standardisation of terminology of lower urinary tract function: Report from the Standardisation Sub-committee of the International Continence Society. *Am. J. Obstet. Gynecol.* **2002**, *187*, 116–126. [CrossRef] [PubMed]
4. Chapple, C.R.; Wein, A.J.; Abrams, P.; Dmochowski, R.R.; Giuliano, F.; Kaplan, S.A.; McVary, K.T.; Roehrborn, C.G. Lower urinary tract symptoms revisited: A broader clinical perspective. *Eur. Urol.* **2008**, *54*, 563–569. [CrossRef]
5. Chapple, C.; Castro-Diaz, D.; Chuang, Y.C.; Lee, K.S.; Liao, L.; Liu, S.P.; Wang, J.; Yoo, T.K.; Chu, R.; Sumarsono, B. Prevalence of lower urinary tract symptoms in China, Taiwan, and South Korea: Results from a cross-sectional, population-based study. *Adv. Ther.* **2017**, *34*, 1953–1965. [CrossRef] [PubMed]
6. Ponholzer, A.; Temml, C.; Wehrberger, C.; Marszalek, M.; Madersbacher, S. The association between vascular risk factors and lower urinary tract symptoms in both sexes. *Eur. Urol.* **2006**, *50*, 581–586. [CrossRef] [PubMed]
7. Pinggera, G.M.; Mitterberger, M.; Steiner, E.; Pallwein, L.; Frauscher, F.; Aigner, F.; Bartsch, G.; Strasser, H. Association of lower urinary tract symptoms and chronic ischaemia of the lower urinary tract in elderly women and men: Assessment using colour Doppler ultrasonography. *BJU Int.* **2008**, *102*, 470–474. [CrossRef] [PubMed]
8. Azadzoi, K.M.; Pontari, M.; Vlachiotis, J.; Siroky, M.B. Canine bladder blood flow and oxygenation: Changes induced by filling, contraction and outlet obstruction. *J. Urol.* **1996**, *155*, 1459–1465. [CrossRef]
9. Greenland, J.E.; Brading, A.F. The effect of bladder outflow obstruction on detrusor blood flow changes during the voiding cycle in conscious pigs. *J. Urol.* **2001**, *165*, 245–248. [CrossRef] [PubMed]
10. Gosling, J.A.; Gilpin, S.A.; Dixon, J.S.; Gilpin, C.J. Decrease in the autonomic innervation of human detrusor muscle in outflow obstruction. *J. Urol.* **1986**, *136*, 501–504. [CrossRef]
11. Koritsiadis, G.; Stravodimos, K.; Koutalellis, G.; Agrogiannis, G.; Koritsiadis, S.; Lazaris, A.; Constantinides, C. Immunohistochemical estimation of hypoxia in human obstructed bladder and correlation with clinical variables. *BJU Int.* **2008**, *102*, 328–332. [CrossRef]
12. Speakman, M.J.; Brading, A.F.; Gilpin, C.J.; Dixon, J.S.; Gilpin, S.A.; Gosling, J.A. Bladder outflow obstruction—A cause of denervation supersensitivity. *J. Urol.* **1987**, *138*, 1461–1466. [CrossRef]

13. Seki, N.; Karim, O.M.; Mostwin, J.L. The effect of experimental urethral obstruction and its reversal on changes in passive electrical properties of detrusor muscle. *J. Urol.* **1992**, *148*, 1957–1961. [CrossRef]
14. Greenland, J.E.; Hvistendahl, J.J.; Andersen, H.; Jorgensen, T.M.; McMurray, G.; Cortina-Borja, M.; Brading, A.F.; Frokiaer, J. The effect of bladder outlet obstruction on tissue oxygen tension and blood flow in the pig bladder. *BJU Int.* **2000**, *85*, 1109–1114. [CrossRef] [PubMed]
15. Steers, W.D.; Ciambotti, J.; Etzel, B.; Erdman, S.; de Groat, W.C. Alterations in afferent pathways from the urinary bladder of the rat in response to partial urethral obstruction. *J. Comp. Neurol.* **1991**, *310*, 401–410. [CrossRef] [PubMed]
16. Harrison, S.C.; Hunnam, G.R.; Farman, P.; Ferguson, D.R.; Doyle, P.T. Bladder instability and denervation in patients with bladder outflow obstruction. *Br. J. Urol.* **1987**, *60*, 519–522. [CrossRef] [PubMed]
17. Komninos, C.; Mitsogiannis, I. Obstruction-induced alterations within the urinary bladder and their role in the pathophysiology of lower urinary tract symptomatology. *Can. Urol. Assoc. J.* **2014**, *8*, E524–E530. [CrossRef]
18. Nickel, J.C.; Downey, J.; Hunter, D.; Clark, J. Prevalence of prostatitis-like symptoms in a population based study using the National Institutes of Health chronic prostatitis symptom index. *J. Urol.* **2001**, *165*, 842–845. [CrossRef]
19. Ficarra, V.; Rossanese, M.; Zazzara, M.; Giannarini, G.; Abbinante, M.; Bartoletti, R.; Mirone, V.; Scaglione, F. The role of inflammation in lower urinary tract symptoms (LUTS) due to benign prostatic hyperplasia (BPH) and its potential impact on medical therapy. *Curr. Urol. Rep.* **2014**, *15*, 463. [CrossRef]
20. He, Q.; Wang, Z.; Liu, G.; Daneshgari, F.; MacLennan, G.T.; Gupta, S. Metabolic syndrome, inflammation and lower urinary tract symptoms: Possible translational links. *Prostate Cancer Prostatic Dis.* **2016**, *19*, 7–13. [CrossRef]
21. Lepor, H. The pathophysiology of lower urinary tract symptoms in the ageing male population. *Br. J. Urol.* **1998**, *81* (Suppl. S1), 29–33. [CrossRef]
22. Tai, H.C.; Chung, S.D.; Ho, C.H.; Tai, T.Y.; Yang, W.S.; Tseng, C.H.; Wu, H.P.; Yu, H.J. Metabolic syndrome components worsen lower urinary tract symptoms in women with type 2 diabetes. *J. Clin. Endocrinol. Metab.* **2010**, *95*, 1143–1150. [CrossRef]
23. Soler, R.; Andersson, K.E.; Chancellor, M.B.; Chapple, C.R.; de Groat, W.C.; Drake, M.J.; Gratzke, C.; Lee, R.; Cruz, F. Future direction in pharmacotherapy for non-neurogenic male lower urinary tract symptoms. *Eur. Urol.* **2013**, *64*, 610–621. [CrossRef] [PubMed]
24. Kuei, C.H.; Liao, C.H.; Chiang, B.J. Significant intravesical prostatic protrusion and prostatic calcification predict unfavorable outcomes of medical treatment for male lower urinary tract symptoms. *Urol. Sci.* **2016**, *27*, 13–16. [CrossRef]
25. Auffenberg, G.B.; Helfand, B.T.; McVary, K.T. Established medical therapy for benign prostatic hyperplasia. *Urol. Clin. N. Am.* **2009**, *36*, 443–459. [CrossRef] [PubMed]
26. McNeal, J. Pathology of benign prostatic hyperplasia. Insight into etiology. *Urol. Clin. N. Am.* **1990**, *17*, 477–486.
27. Rohr, H.P.; Bartsch, G. Human benign prostatic hyperplasia: A stromal disease? New perspectives by quantitative morphology. *Urology* **1980**, *16*, 625–633. [CrossRef]
28. Franks, L.M. Benign nodular hyperplasia of the prostate; A review. *Ann. R. Coll. Surg. Engl.* **1953**, *14*, 92–106.
29. McConnell, J.D. Androgen ablation and blockade in the treatment of benign prostatic hyperplasia. *Urol. Clin. N. Am.* **1990**, *17*, 661–670.
30. Liao, C.H.; Li, H.Y.; Chung, S.D.; Chiang, H.S.; Yu, H.J. Significant association between serum dihydrotestosterone level and prostate volume among Taiwanese men aged 40–79 years. *Aging Male* **2012**, *15*, 28–33. [CrossRef]
31. McConnell, J.D. The pathophysiology of benign prostatic hyperplasia. *J. Androl.* **1991**, *12*, 356–363.
32. Harris, M.T.; Feldberg, R.S.; Lau, K.M.; Lazarus, N.H.; Cochrane, D.E. Expression of proinflammatory genes during estrogen-induced inflammation of the rat prostate. *Prostate* **2000**, *44*, 19–25. [CrossRef]
33. Zhu, Y.S.; Sun, G.H. 5α-reductase isozymes in the prostate. *J. Med Sci. (Taipei Taiwan)* **2005**, *25*, 1–12.
34. Nickel, J.C.; Downey, J.; Pontari, M.A.; Shoskes, D.A.; Zeitlin, S.I. A randomized placebo-controlled multicentre study to evaluate the safety and efficacy of finasteride for male chronic pelvic pain syndrome (category IIIA chronic nonbacterial prostatitis). *BJU Int.* **2004**, *93*, 991–995. [CrossRef] [PubMed]

35. Kramer, G.; Mitteregger, D.; Marberger, M. Is benign prostatic hyperplasia (BPH) an immune inflammatory disease? *Eur. Urol.* **2007**, *51*, 1202–1216. [CrossRef] [PubMed]
36. Nickel, J.C. Inflammation and benign prostatic hyperplasia. *Urol. Clin. N. Am.* **2008**, *35*, 109–115. [CrossRef] [PubMed]
37. Sreenivasulu, K.; Nandeesha, H.; Dorairajan, L.N.; Rajappa, M.; Vinayagam, V. Elevated insulin and reduced insulin like growth factor binding protein-3/prostate specific antigen ratio with increase in prostate size in Benign Prostatic Hyperplasia. *Clin. Chim. Acta* **2017**, *469*, 37–41. [CrossRef] [PubMed]
38. Mosli, H.H.; Esmat, A.; Atawia, R.T.; Shoieb, S.M.; Mosli, H.A.; Abdel-Naim, A.B. Metformin attenuates testosterone-induced prostatic hyperplasia in rats: A pharmacological perspective. *Sci. Rep.* **2015**, *5*, 15639. [CrossRef] [PubMed]
39. Carvalho-Dias, E.; Miranda, A.; Martinho, O.; Mota, P.; Costa, A.; Nogueira-Silva, C.; Moura, R.S.; Alenina, N. Serotonin regulates prostate growth through androgen receptor modulation. *Sci. Rep.* **2017**, *7*, 15428. [CrossRef] [PubMed]
40. Sutcliffe, S.; Giovannucci, E.; De Marzo, A.M.; Willett, W.C.; Platz, E.A. Sexually transmitted infections, prostatitis, ejaculation frequency, and the odds of lower urinary tract symptoms. *Am. J. Epidemiol.* **2005**, *162*, 898–906. [CrossRef] [PubMed]
41. Nickel, J.C. Prostatic inflammation in benign prostatic hyperplasia—The third component? *Can. J. Urol.* **1994**, *1*, 1–4. [PubMed]
42. Nickel, J.C.; Roehrborn, C.G.; O'Leary, M.P.; Bostwick, D.G.; Somerville, M.C.; Rittmaster, R.S. The relationship between prostate inflammation and lower urinary tract symptoms: Examination of baseline data from the REDUCE trial. *Eur. Urol.* **2008**, *54*, 1379–1384. [CrossRef] [PubMed]
43. St Sauver, J.L.; Jacobson, D.J.; McGree, M.E.; Lieber, M.M.; Jacobsen, S.J. Protective association between nonsteroidal antiinflammatory drug use and measures of benign prostatic hyperplasia. *Am. J. Epidemiol.* **2006**, *164*, 760–768. [CrossRef] [PubMed]
44. Castro, P.; Xia, C.; Gomez, L.; Lamb, D.J.; Ittmann, M. Interleukin-8 expression is increased in senescent prostatic epithelial cells and promotes the development of benign prostatic hyperplasia. *Prostate* **2004**, *60*, 153–159. [CrossRef] [PubMed]
45. Penna, G.; Mondaini, N.; Amuchastegui, S.; Degli Innocenti, S.; Carini, M.; Giubilei, G.; Fibbi, B.; Colli, E.; Maggi, M.; Adorini, L. Seminal plasma cytokines and chemokines in prostate inflammation: Interleukin 8 as a predictive biomarker in chronic prostatitis/chronic pelvic pain syndrome and benign prostatic hyperplasia. *Eur. Urol.* **2007**, *51*, 524–533. [CrossRef] [PubMed]
46. Schauer, I.G.; Ressler, S.J.; Tuxhorn, J.A.; Dang, T.D.; Rowley, D.R. Elevated epithelial expression of interleukin-8 correlates with myofibroblast reactive stroma in benign prostatic hyperplasia. *Urology* **2008**, *72*, 205–213. [CrossRef] [PubMed]
47. Penna, G.; Fibbi, B.; Amuchastegui, S.; Cossetti, C.; Aquilano, F.; Laverny, G.; Gacci, M.; Crescioli, C.; Maggi, M.; Adorini, L. Human benign prostatic hyperplasia stromal cells as inducers and targets of chronic immuno-mediated inflammation. *J. Immunol.* **2009**, *182*, 4056–4064. [CrossRef] [PubMed]
48. Fibbi, B.; Penna, G.; Morelli, A.; Adorini, L.; Maggi, M. Chronic inflammation in the pathogenesis of benign prostatic hyperplasia. *Int. J. Androl.* **2010**, *33*, 475–488. [CrossRef] [PubMed]
49. Sciarra, A.; Di Silverio, F.; Salciccia, S.; Autran Gomez, A.M.; Gentilucci, A.; Gentile, V. Inflammation and chronic prostatic diseases: Evidence for a link? *Eur. Urol.* **2007**, *52*, 964–972. [CrossRef] [PubMed]
50. Penna, G.; Fibbi, B.; Amuchastegui, S.; Corsiero, E.; Laverny, G.; Silvestrini, E.; Chavalmane, A.; Morelli, A.; Sarchielli, E.; Vannelli, G.B.; et al. The vitamin D receptor agonist elocalcitol inhibits IL-8-dependent benign prostatic hyperplasia stromal cell proliferation and inflammatory response by targeting the RhoA/Rho kinase and NF-kappaB pathways. *Prostate* **2009**, *69*, 480–493. [CrossRef] [PubMed]
51. Krieger, J.N.; Lee, S.W.; Jeon, J.; Cheah, P.Y.; Liong, M.L.; Riley, D.E. Epidemiology of prostatitis. *Int. J. Antimicrob. Agents* **2008**, *31* (Suppl. S1), S85–S90. [CrossRef] [PubMed]
52. Whitmore, W.F.; Gittes, R.F. Studies on the prostate and testis as immunologically privileged sites. *Cancer Treat. Rep.* **1977**, *61*, 217–222. [PubMed]
53. Zisman, A.; Zisman, E.; Lindner, A.; Velikanov, S.; Siegel, Y.I.; Mozes, E. Autoantibodies to prostate specific antigen in patients with benign prostatic hyperplasia. *J. Urol.* **1995**, *154*, 1052–1055. [CrossRef]

54. Motrich, R.D.; Maccioni, M.; Molina, R.; Tissera, A.; Olmedo, J.; Riera, C.M.; Rivero, V.E. Presence of INFγ-secreting lymphocytes specific to prostate antigens in a group of chronic prostatitis patients. *Clin. Immunol.* **2005**, *116*, 149–157. [CrossRef] [PubMed]
55. Ponniah, S.; Arah, I.; Alexander, R.B. PSA is a candidate self-antigen in autoimmune chronic prostatitis/chronic pelvic pain syndrome. *Prostate* **2000**, *44*, 49–54. [CrossRef]
56. Miller, L.J.; Fischer, K.A.; Goralnick, S.J.; Litt, M.; Burleson, J.A.; Albertsen, P.; Kreutzer, D.L. Nerve growth factor and chronic prostatitis/chronic pelvic pain syndrome. *Urology* **2002**, *59*, 603–608. [CrossRef]
57. Varilek, G.W.; Weinstock, J.V.; Pantazis, N.J. Isolated hepatic granulomas from mice infected with *Schistosoma mansoni* contain nerve growth factor. *Infect. Immun.* **1991**, *59*, 4443–4449. [PubMed]
58. Mazurek, N.; Weskamp, G.; Erne, P.; Otten, U. Nerve growth factor induces mast cell degranulation without changing intracellular calcium levels. *FEBS Lett.* **1986**, *198*, 315–320. [CrossRef]
59. Ou, Z.; He, Y.; Qi, L.; Zu, X.; Wu, L.; Cao, Z.; Li, Y.; Liu, L.; Dube, D.A.; Wang, Z.; et al. Infiltrating mast cells enhance benign prostatic hyperplasia through IL-6/STAT3/Cyclin D1 signals. *Oncotarget* **2017**, *8*, 59156–59164. [CrossRef] [PubMed]
60. Lindsay, R.M.; Harmar, A.J. Nerve growth factor regulates expression of neuropeptide genes in adult sensory neurons. *Nature* **1989**, *337*, 362–364. [CrossRef] [PubMed]
61. Chien, C.-T.; Yu, H.-J.; Lin, T.-B.; Lai, M.-K.; Hsu, S.-M. Substance P via NK_1 receptor facilitates hyperactive bladder afferent signaling via action of ROS. *Am. J. Physiol. Ren. Physiol.* **2003**, *284*, F840–F851. [CrossRef]
62. Funahashi, Y.; Takahashi, R.; Mizoguchi, S.; Suzuki, T.; Takaoka, E.; Ni, J.; Wang, Z.; DeFranco, D.B.; de Groat, W.C.; Tyagi, P. Bladder overactivity and afferent hyperexcitability induced by prostate-to-bladder cross-sensitization in rats with prostatic inflammation. *J. Physiol.* **2019**, *597*, 2063–2078. [CrossRef]
63. Vital, P.; Castro, P.; Ittmann, M. Oxidative stress promotes benign prostatic hyperplasia. *Prostate* **2016**, *76*, 58–67. [CrossRef] [PubMed]
64. Chiang, B.J.; Chen, T.W.; Chung, S.D.; Lee, W.Z.; Chien, C.T. Synthetic nickel-containing superoxide dismutase attenuates para-phenylenediamine-induced bladder dysfunction in rats. *Oncotarget* **2017**, *8*, 105735–105748. [CrossRef] [PubMed]
65. Dearakhshandeh, N.; Mogheiseh, A. Changes in the oxidative stress factors and inflammatory proteins following the treatment of BPH-induced dogs with an anti-proliferative agent called tadalafil. *J. Vet. Pharmacol. Ther.* **2019**. [CrossRef] [PubMed]
66. Sugar, L.M. Inflammation and prostate cancer. *Can. J. Urol.* **2006**, *13* (Suppl. S1), 46–47. [PubMed]
67. Di Silverio, F.; Gentile, V.; De Matteis, A.; Mariotti, G.; Giuseppe, V.; Luigi, P.A.; Sciarra, A. Distribution of inflammation, pre-malignant lesions, incidental carcinoma in histologically confirmed benign prostatic hyperplasia: A retrospective analysis. *Eur. Urol.* **2003**, *43*, 164–175. [CrossRef]
68. McVary, K.T.; Rademaker, A.; Lloyd, G.L.; Gann, P. Autonomic nervous system overactivity in men with lower urinary tract symptoms secondary to benign prostatic hyperplasia. *J. Urol.* **2005**, *174*, 1327–1433. [CrossRef] [PubMed]
69. Kim, J.; Yanagihara, Y.; Kikugawa, T.; Ji, M.; Tanji, N.; Masayoshi, Y.; Freeman, M.R. A signaling network in phenylephrine-induced benign prostatic hyperplasia. *Endocrinology* **2009**, *150*, 3576–3583. [CrossRef] [PubMed]
70. Kanagawa, K.; Sugimura, K.; Kuratsukuri, K.; Ikemoto, S.; Kishimoto, T.; Nakatani, T. Norepinephrine activates P44 and P42 MAPK in human prostate stromal and smooth muscle cells but not in epithelial cells. *Prostate* **2003**, *56*, 313–318. [CrossRef] [PubMed]
71. Huang, X.; Lee, C. Regulation of stromal proliferation, growth arrest, differentiation and apoptosis in benign prostatic hyperplasia by TGF-beta. *Front. Biosci.* **2003**, *8*, s740–s749.
72. Turton, K.; Chaddock, J.A.; Acharya, K.R. Botulinum and tetanus neurotoxins: Structure, function and therapeutic utility. *Trends Biochem. Sci.* **2002**, *27*, 552–558. [CrossRef]
73. Chuang, Y.C.; Huang, C.C.; Kang, H.Y.; Chiang, P.H.; Demiguel, F.; Yoshimura, N.; Chancellor, M.B. Novel action of botulinum toxin on the stromal and epithelial components of the prostate gland. *J. Urol.* **2006**, *175*, 1158–1163. [CrossRef]
74. Lin, A.T.; Yang, A.H.; Chen, K.K. Effects of botulinum toxin A on the contractile function of dog prostate. *Eur. Urol.* **2007**, *52*, 582–589. [CrossRef] [PubMed]

75. Chuang, Y.C.; Tu, C.H.; Huang, C.C.; Lin, H.J.; Chiang, P.H.; Yoshimura, N.; Chancellor, M.B. Intraprostatic injection of botulinum toxin type-A relieves bladder outlet obstruction in human and induces prostate apoptosis in dogs. *BMC Urol.* **2006**, *6*, 12. [CrossRef] [PubMed]
76. Chuang, Y.C.; Chiang, P.H.; Yoshimura, N.; De Miguel, F.; Chancellor, M.B. Sustained beneficial effects of intraprostatic botulinum toxin type A on lower urinary tract symptoms and quality of life in men with benign prostatic hyperplasia. *BJU Int.* **2006**, *98*, 1033–1037. [CrossRef] [PubMed]
77. Borodic, G.E.; Acquadro, M.; Johnson, E.A. Botulinum toxin therapy for pain and inflammatory disorders: Mechanisms and therapeutic effects. *Expert Opin. Investig. Drugs* **2001**, *10*, 1531–1544. [CrossRef] [PubMed]
78. Yoo, K.Y.; Lee, H.S.; Cho, Y.K.; Lim, Y.S.; Kim, Y.S.; Koo, J.H.; Yoon, S.J.; Lee, J.H.; Jang, K.H.; Song, S.H. Anti-inflammatory effects of botulinum toxin type A in a complete Freund's adjuvant-induced arthritic knee joint of hind leg on rat model. *Neurotox. Res.* **2014**, *26*, 32–39. [CrossRef] [PubMed]
79. Choi, J.E.; Werbel, T.; Wang, Z.; Wu, C.C.; Yaksh, T.L.; Di Nardo, A. Botulinum toxin blocks mast cells and prevents rosacea like inflammation. *J. Dermatol. Sci.* **2019**, *93*, 58–64. [CrossRef] [PubMed]
80. Liu, H.T.; Kuo, H.C. Intravesical botulinum toxin A injections plus hydrodistension can reduce nerve growth factor production and control bladder pain in interstitial cystitis. *Urology* **2007**, *70*, 463–468. [CrossRef]
81. Chuang, Y.C.; Yoshimura, N.; Huang, C.C.; Chiang, P.H.; Chancellor, M.B. Intravesical botulinum toxin A administration produces analgesia against acetic acid induced bladder pain responses in rats. *J. Urol.* **2004**, *172*, 1529–1532. [CrossRef]
82. Aoki, K.R. Review of a proposed mechanism for the antinociceptive action of botulinum toxin type A. *Neurotoxicology* **2005**, *26*, 785–793. [CrossRef]
83. Chuang, Y.C.; Yoshimura, N.; Huang, C.C.; Wu, M.; Chiang, P.H.; Chancellor, M.B. Intraprostatic botulinum toxin A injection inhibits cyclooxygenase-2 expression and suppresses prostatic pain on capsaicin induced prostatitis model in rat. *J. Urol.* **2008**, *180*, 742–748. [CrossRef]
84. Uchiyama, A.; Yamada, K.; Perera, B.; Ogino, S.; Yokoyama, Y.; Takeuchi, Y.; Ishikawa, O.; Motegi, S. Protective effect of botulinum toxin A after cutaneous ischemia-reperfusion injury. *Sci. Rep.* **2015**, *5*, 9072. [CrossRef]
85. Schraufstatter, I.U.; Chung, J.; Burger, M. IL-8 activates endothelial cell CXCR1 and CXCR2 through Rho and Rac signaling pathways. *Am. J. Physiol. Lung Cell. Mol. Physiol.* **2001**, *280*, L1094–L1103. [CrossRef]
86. Kuo, H.C. Prostate botulinum A toxin injection—An alternative treatment for benign prostatic obstruction in poor surgical candidates. *Urology* **2005**, *65*, 670–674. [CrossRef]
87. Silva, J.; Pinto, R.; Carvalho, T.; Botelho, F.; Silva, P.; Oliveira, R.; Silva, C.; Cruz, F.; Dinis, P. Intraprostatic botulinum toxin type A injection in patients with benign prostatic enlargement: Duration of the effect of a single treatment. *BMC Urol.* **2009**, *9*, 9. [CrossRef]
88. Maria, G.; Brisinda, G.; Civello, I.M.; Bentivoglio, A.R.; Sganga, G.; Albanese, A. Relief by botulinum toxin of voiding dysfunction due to benign prostatic hyperplasia: Results of a randomized, placebo-controlled study. *Urology* **2003**, *62*, 259–264. [CrossRef]
89. Chuang, Y.C.; Chiang, P.H.; Huang, C.C.; Yoshimura, N.; Chancellor, M.B. Botulinum toxin type A improves benign prostatic hyperplasia symptoms in patients with small prostates. *Urology* **2005**, *66*, 775–779. [CrossRef]
90. Brisinda, G.; Cadeddu, F.; Vanella, S.; Mazzeo, P.; Marniga, G.; Maria, G. Relief by botulinum toxin of lower urinary tract symptoms owing to benign prostatic hyperplasia: Early and long-term results. *Urology* **2009**, *73*, 90–94. [CrossRef]
91. McVary, K.T.; Roehrborn, C.G.; Chartier-Kastler, E.; Efros, M.; Bugarin, D.; Chen, R.; Patel, A.; Haag-Molkenteller, C. A multicenter, randomized, double-blind, placebo controlled study of onabotulinumtoxinA 200 U to treat lower urinary tract symptoms in men with benign prostatic hyperplasia. *J. Urol.* **2014**, *192*, 150–156. [CrossRef]
92. Marberger, M.; Chartier-Kastler, E.; Egerdie, B.; Lee, K.S.; Grosse, J.; Bugarin, D.; Zhou, J.; Patel, A.; Haag-Molkenteller, C. A randomized double-blind placebo-controlled phase 2 dose-ranging study of onabotulinumtoxinA in men with benign prostatic hyperplasia. *Eur. Urol.* **2013**, *63*, 496–503. [CrossRef]
93. Shim, S.R.; Cho, Y.J.; Shin, I.S.; Kim, J.H. Efficacy and safety of botulinum toxin injection for benign prostatic hyperplasia: A systematic review and meta-analysis. *Int. Urol. Nephrol.* **2016**, *48*, 19–30. [CrossRef]
94. Marchal, C.; Perez, J.E.; Herrera, B.; Machuca, F.J.; Redondo, M. The use of botulinum toxin in benign prostatic hyperplasia. *Neurourol. Urodyn.* **2012**, *31*, 86–92. [CrossRef]

95. Mangera, A.; Apostolidis, A.; Andersson, K.E.; Dasgupta, P.; Giannantoni, A.; Roehrborn, C.; Novara, G.; Chapple, C. An updated systematic review and statistical comparison of standardised mean outcomes for the use of botulinum toxin in the management of lower urinary tract disorders. *Eur. Urol.* **2014**, *65*, 981–990. [CrossRef]
96. Mangera, A.; Andersson, K.E.; Apostolidis, A.; Chapple, C.; Dasgupta, P.; Giannantoni, A.; Gravas, S.; Madersbacher, S. Contemporary management of lower urinary tract disease with botulinum toxin A: A systematic review of botox (onabotulinumtoxinA) and dysport (abobotulinumtoxinA). *Eur. Urol.* **2011**, *60*, 784–795. [CrossRef]
97. El-Enen, M.A.; Abou-Farha, M.; El-Abd, A.; El-Tatawy, H.; Tawfik, A.; El-Abd, S.; Rashed, M.; El-Sharaby, M. Intraprostatic injection of botulinum toxin-A in patients with refractory chronic pelvic pain syndrome: The transurethral vs. transrectal approach. *Arab J. Urol.* **2015**, *13*, 94–99. [CrossRef]
98. Falahatkar, S.; Shahab, E.; Gholamjani Moghaddam, K.; Kazemnezhad, E. Transurethral intraprostatic injection of botulinum neurotoxin type A for the treatment of chronic prostatitis/chronic pelvic pain syndrome: Results of a prospective pilot double-blind and randomized placebo-controlled study. *BJU Int.* **2015**, *116*, 641–649. [CrossRef]

10

Therapeutic Effects of Botulinum Toxin A, via Urethral Sphincter Injection on Voiding Dysfunction Due to Different Bladder and Urethral Sphincter Dysfunctions

Yu-Khun Lee and Hann-Chorng Kuo *

Department of Urology, Hualien Tzu Chi Hospital, Buddhist Tzu Chi Medical Foundation and Tzu Chi University, Hualien 970, Taiwan
* Correspondence: hck@tzuchi.com.tw

Abstract: Botulinum toxin A (BoNT-A) urethral sphincter injections have been applied in treating voiding dysfunction but the treatment outcome is not consistent. This study analyzed treatment outcomes between patients with different bladder and urethral sphincter dysfunctions. Patients with refractory voiding dysfunction due to neurogenic or non-neurogenic etiology were treated with urethral sphincter 100 U BoNT-A injections. The treatment outcomes were assessed by a global response assessment one month after treatment. The bladder neck opening and urodynamic parameters in preoperative videourodynamic study were compared between successful and failed treatment groups. A total of 80 non-neurogenic and 75 neurogenic patients were included. A successful outcome was noted in 92 (59.4%) patients and a failed outcome in 63 (40.6%). The treatment outcome was not affected by the gender, voiding dysfunction subtype, bladder dysfunction, or sphincter dysfunction subtypes. Except an open bladder neck and higher maximum flow rate, no significant difference was noted in the other variables between groups. Non-neurogenic patients with successful outcomes had a significantly higher detrusor pressure, and patients with neurogenic voiding dysfunction with successful results had higher maximum flow rates and smaller post-void residuals than those who failed the treatment. However, increased urinary incontinence was reported in 12 (13%) patients. BoNT-A urethral sphincter injection is effective in about 60% of either neurogenic or non-neurogenic patients with voiding dysfunction. An open bladder neck during voiding and a higher maximum flow rate indicate a successful treatment outcome.

Keywords: urethra; onabotulinumtoxinA; voiding; therapeutic outcome

Key Contribution: Urethral BoNT-A injection is effective for patients with voiding dysfunction especially in patients having an open bladder neck.

---

1. Introduction

Voiding dysfunction may result from detrusor underactivity (DU), bladder outlet obstruction (BOO), urethral sphincter hyperactivity, or poor relaxation of the external urethral sphincter (PRES) during micturition. A previous urodynamic study reported DU in 12.4% of men [1] and in 23.1% of women [2] with voiding lower urinary tract symptoms (LUTS). Urethral sphincter hyperactivity was noted in 17.0% of women [3], and PRES in 39.5% of men [1] and 17.6% of women [3] with voiding dysfunction. Voiding dysfunction may be neurogenic or non-neurogenic in origin, with symptoms of dysuria and large post-void residual (PVR) volume, and might result in upper urinary tract deterioration. Recently, botulinum toxin A (BoNT-A) has been applied as an injection into the urethral sphincter to treat voiding dysfunction refractory to medical treatment.

In the beginning, BoNT-A was used to treat patients with severe dysuria due to spinal cord injury (SCI) and detrusor sphincter dyssynergia (DSD) [4]. Reduction of the urethral sphincter hypertonicity through chemical denervation was noted after treatment. Patients usually can urinate more efficiently. BoNT-A has been safely used for treatment of neurogenic urethral sphincter spasticity in patients with DSD due to SCI, Parkinson's disease, cerebrovascular accidents (CVA), and multiple sclerosis (MS). The treatment outcome was initially reported satisfactorily, with adverse events of the increase of urinary incontinence and incomplete bladder emptying [5].

Because BoNT-A can improve voiding efficiency and detrusor contractility, this treatment has been further applied to treat patients with non-neurogenic voiding dysfunction (NNVD) due to urethral sphincter hyperactivity, PRES, and a non-relaxing urethral sphincter in patients with dysfunctional voiding (DV) or DU [6,7]. After BoNT-A injection, two thirds of patients voided smoothly and had significant decreases in PVR; the voiding derusor pressure was also decreased [7]. Even a dose of 50 U onabotulinumtoxinA could result in excellent and improved results overall in 39% of patients [8]. However, because the therapeutic outcome is not consistent and the therapeutic duration was short, urethral BoNT-A injection for voiding dysfunction remains an off-label treatment. In contrast, BoNT-A detrusor injection has already been licensed for use in patients with neurogenic detrusor overactivity (NDO) or non-neurogenic overactive bladder (OAB) to treat urinary incontinence [9]. Nevertheless, for patients with voiding dysfunction not due to BOO, urethral BoNT-A injections remain an attractive treatment modality for various types of adults with pediatric voiding dysfunctions [10,11].

Although BoNT-A has been used in treatment of voiding dysfunction for a long time, the success rate varies widely and patients might not be satisfied with the treatment outcome. Urethral BoNT-A injection had been shown to decrease voiding pressure in NNVD, but the success rate was not superior to normal saline injection [12]. For patients with Fowler's syndrome and urinary retention due to urethral sphincter hyperactivity, onabotulinumtoxinA injection could improve subjective and objective parameters [13]. In patients with DU and voiding dysfunction, a 60% success rate can be achieved after urethral BoNT-A injection [14]. Because voiding is a combination of detrusor contraction and relaxation of the bladder outlet structures, including the bladder neck, prostatic urethra (in men), urethral sphincter, pelvic floor muscles, and the urethra, voiding dysfunction might be caused by a different combination of bladder and bladder outlet dysfunctions during voiding. In patients with DU, a powerful abdominal pressure by straining is necessary, while in patients with DV or DSD, adequate relaxation of the urethral resistance is needed to achieve efficient voiding. BoNT-A urethral sphincter injection can reduce urethral sphincter resistance, but this therapeutic effect might not be adequate to restore voiding efficiency in all patients. This study retrospectively analyzed the results of our previously treated patients with voiding dysfunction and compared the therapeutic efficacy between patients with voiding dysfunction due to neurogenic versus non-neurogenic origin, and between different detrusor functions (DU versus non-DU) or urethral dysfunction (DV versus PRES).

2. Results

A total of 155 patients underwent their first-time urethral BoNT-A injection for their voiding dysfunction refractory to medical therapies. The patients included 80 with NNVD (22 men and 58 women, aged 66.6 ± 16.9 years) and 75 with neurogenic voiding dysfunction (NVD, 34 men and 41 women, aged 55.5 ± 19.7 years). Successful outcomes were reported in 92 (59.4%) patients, and a failed outcome was noted in 63 (40.6%). Table 1 lists the baseline patient demographics according to their voiding dysfunction subtypes, bladder dysfunction, and urethral sphincter dysfunctions between successful and failed subgroups. We found that the treatment outcome was not significantly different among different voiding dysfunction subtypes.

Table 1. Treatment outcome according to patient characteristics at baseline.

VD Characteristics		N	Successful Outcome	Failed Outcome	p Value
VD Subtype	Idiopathic VD	80	50 (62.5%)	30 (37.5%)	0.255
	Neurogenic VD	75	42 (56%)	33 (44%)	
Gender	Male	54	32 (59.3%)	22 (40.7%)	0.445
	Female	99	60 (60.6%)	39 (39.4%)	
Bladder Function	DO	57	36 (63.2%)	21 (36.8%)	0.819
	DU	59	34 (57.6%)	25 (42.4%)	
	DHIC	25	15 (60%)	10 (40%)	
	HSB	14	7 (50%)	7 (50%)	
Sphincter Function	DV	115	70 (60.9%)	45 (39.1%)	0.550
	DSD	237	14 (60.9%)	9 (39.1%)	
	PRES		8 (47.1%)	9 (52.9%)	

VD, voiding dysfunction; DO, detrusor overactivity; DU, detrusor underactivity; DHIC, detrusor hyperreflexia and inadequate contractility; HSB, hypersensitive bladder; DV, dysfunctional voiding; DSD, detrusor sphincter dyssynergia; PRES, poor relaxation of external sphincter.

When we compared the videourodynamic study (VUDS) characteristics between patients with successful and failed outcomes, only the baseline maximum flow rate (Qmax) and an open bladder neck during voiding showed a significant difference between groups (Table 2). In the 92 patients with a successful outcome, 89 (96.7%) had an open bladder neck, whereas of the 63 with failed outcomes, 54 (85.7%) had a tight bladder neck ($p < 0.001$). Patients with a successful outcome had a significantly higher Qmax than those with failed outcome ($p = 0.031$). However, this fact was only observed in patients without DU (7.82 ± 4.97 versus 2.0 ± 2.65 mL/s, $p = 0.004$), but not in patients with DU (5.05 ± 5.15 versus 6.0 ± 5.66 mL/s, $p = 0.804$).

Table 2. The video-urodynamic (VUDS) characteristics between patients with successful and failed treatment outcomes.

VUDS Findings		Successful Outcome	Failed Outcome	p Value
		($n = 92$)	($n = 63$)	
Age (years)		62 ± 18.8	64.7 ± 20.3	0.692
First sensation of filling (mL)		140.1 ± 73.0	132 ± 74.6	0.792
Cystometric bladder capacity		338 ± 142	267 ± 135	0.153
Detrusor pressure (cmH_2O)		25.2 ± 25.2	39.0 ± 40.7	0.344
Abdominal pressure (cmH_2O)		36.7 ± 36.3	34.3 ± 38.1	0.860
Maximum flow rate (mL/s)		6.76 ± 5.19	2.89 ± 3.52	0.031
Post-void residual volume (mL)		218 ± 5.19	202 ± 151	0.799
Open bladder neck		89 (96.7%)	9 (14.3%)	< 0.001
DU	Open BN	34 (94.4%)	2 (5.6%)	< 0.001
	Tight BN	2 (7.7%)	24 (92.3%)	
Non-DU	Open BN	55 (88.7%)	7 (11.3%)	< 0.001
	Tight BN	1 (3.2%)	30 (96.8%)	

DO, detrusor overactivity; DU, detrusor underactivity; BN, bladder neck.

The treatment outcome was also not related to the bladder dysfunction between NVD and NNVD patients (Table 3). Further analysis of the VUDS parameters revealed that in patients with NNVD and non-DU, patients with successful outcomes had significantly higher voiding detrusor pressure (Pdet) than those with failed outcomes ($p = 0.013$), but that was not found in patients with NNVD and DU ($p = 0.456$). In patients with NVD and non-DU, those with successful outcomes had significantly lower first sensation of filling (FSF, $p = 0.050$), smaller cystometric bladder capacity (CBC, $p = 0.010$), higher Qmax ($p = 0.044$), and smaller PVR ($p = 0.011$) than patients with failed outcomes. In patients with NVD and DV, those with successful outcomes ($n = 28$) had a significantly lower FSF and full sensation (FS) and smaller CBC ($p = 0.008$) than those with failed outcomes ($n = 24$). Patients of NVD and DSD and a successful outcome had a higher Qmax ($p = 0.042$) and smaller PVR ($p = 0.021$) than those who failed the treatment. Interestingly, significantly more patients with a successful outcome had an open bladder neck (BN) during VUDS than those with a failed outcome, in any subgroup of the bladder or urethral sphincter dysfunction. (Table 4)

Table 3. The video-urodynamic (VUDS) characteristics of voiding dysfunctions between patients with successful and failed treatment outcomes.

VUDS Findings		**Successful Outcome ($n = 92$)**	**Failed Outcome ($n = 63$)**	***p* Value**
Bladder Function				
Non-neurogenic	DU	19 (67.9%)	9 (32.1%)	0.316
	Non-DU	31 (59.6%)	21 (40.4%)	
Neurogenic	DU	16 (48.5%)	17 (51.5%)	0.177
	Non-DU	26 (61.9%)	16 (38.1%)	
Sphincter Function				
Non-neurogenic	DV	46 (62.2%)	28 (37.8%)	0.598
	PRES	4 (66.7%)	2 (33.3%)	
Neurogenic	DV	28 (53.8%)	24 (46.2%)	0.379
	DSD	14 (60.9%)	9 (39.1%)	

DU, detrusor underactivity; DV, dysfunctional voiding; DSD, detrusor sphincter dyssynergia; PRES, poor relaxation of external sphincter.

After urethral BoNT-A injection for treatment of voiding dysfunction, increased urinary incontinence was reported in 12 (13%) patients with successful outcomes, mostly occurring during sleep. De novo urinary tract infection was only observed in four (2.6%) patients overall.

Table 4. Comparison of the baseline video-urodynamic parameters between patients with successful and failed treatment outcomes in different bladder and urethral sphincter dysfunctions.

Voiding Dysfunction Subtypes		FSF/FS (mL)	CBC (mL)	Pdet (cmH_2O)	Pabd (cmH_2O)	Qmax (mL/s)	PVR (mL)	BN Condition	
								Tight	Open
NVD-non-DU (n = 42)	S	111 ± 52.3	262 ± 129	32.1 ± 26.7	18.9 ± 18.8	7.22 ± 6.03	162 ± 124	1 (8.3%)	26 (86.7%)
	F	157 ± 80.7	381 ± 149	26.0 ± 22.2	26.0 ± 26.1	3.60 ± 3.94	285 ± 174	11 (91.7%)	4 (13.3%)
	p	0.050	0.010	0.456	0.316	0.044	0.011	0.000	
NVD-DU (n = 33)	S	182 ± 104	384 ± 150	6.06 ± 8.65	71.3 ± 47.0	4.50 ± 4.26	253 ± 143	0 (0.0%)	16 (94.1%)
	F	230 ± 91.6	431 ± 124	2.53 ± 4.03	68.2 ± 35.9	3.76 ± 3.62	329 ± 161	16 (100%)	1 (5.9%)
	p	0.174	0.336	0.139	0.837	0.596	0.164	0.000	
NNVD-non-DU (n = 53)	S	132 ± 52.8	350 ± 140	39.6 ± 28.9	29.4 ± 32.6	8.00 ± 4.08	176 ± 137	1 (5.3%)	30 (88.2%)
	F	141 ± 57.0	343 ± 109	23.2 ± 17.5	39.1 ± 29.7	6.23 ± 4.57	228 ± 129	18 (94.7%)	4 (11.8%)
	p	0.576	0.836	0.013	0.272	0.144	0.168	0.000	
NNVD-DU (n = 27)	S	161 ± 72.4	373 ± 115	7.85 ± 8.20	40.0 ± 27.3	4.90 ± 5.57	275 ± 171	3 (33.3%)	17 (94.4%)
	F	180 ± 79.0	360 ± 171	7.86 ± 7.56	34.3 ± 40.7	3.57 ± 3.87	274 ± 182	6 (66.7%)	1 (5.6%)
	p	0.563	0.815	0.998	0.679	0.567	0.993	0.002	
NVD-DV (n = 52)	S	145 ± 66.4	323 ± 151	19.9 ± 25.3	38.5 ± 35.4	6.04 ± 6.33	202 ± 130	1 (5.9%)	25 (92.6%)
	F	215 ± 96.7	450 ± 149	9.89 ± 14.9	49.4 ± 37.5	3.50 ± 3.43	328 ± 177	16 (94.1)	2 (7.4%)
	p	0.013	0.008	0.139	0.329	0.129	0.016	0.000	
NVD-DSD (n = 23)	S	113 ± 102	261 ± 134	29.7 ± 24.8	31.4 ± 42.5	7.33 ± 3.74	157 ± 124	0 (0.0%)	15 (83.3%)
	F	168 ± 83.8	344 ± 102	21.8 ± 25.6	44.6 ± 43.9	3.91 ± 4.39	289 ± 148	8 (100%)	3 (16.7%)
	p	0.152	0.099	0.435	0.450	0.042	0.021	0.000	
NNVD-DV (n = 74)	S	144 ± 63.4	361 ± 132	28.1 ± 28.0	31.4 ± 29.1	6.92 ± 4.96	213 ± 160	4 (14.8%)	45 (93.8)
	F	149 ± 66.0	349 ± 127	20.9 ± 17.0	40.6 ± 32.7	5.77 ± 4.48	237 ± 135	23 (85.2%)	3 (6.3%)
	p	0.735	0.709	0.175	0.218	0.327	0.514	0.000	
NNVD-NR (n = 6)	S	138 ± 17.7	304 ± 65.1	5.00 ± 0.00	85.0 ± 35.4	3.50 ± 2.12	250 ± 70.7	0 (0.0%)	2 (66.7%)
	F	183 ± 38.9	305 ± 134	0.00 ± 0.00	12.5 ± 10.6	1.00 ± 1.41	350 ± 212	1 (100%)	1 (33.3%)
	p	0.275	0.993	0.218	0.109	0.300	0.592	1.000	

FSF, first sensation of filling; FS, full sensation; CBC, cystometric bladder capacity; Pdet, detrusor pressure; Pabd, abdominal pressure; Qmax, maximum flow rate; PVR, postvoid residual; BN, bladder neck; DO, detrusor overactivity; NVD, neurogenic voiding dysfunction; NNVD, non-neurogenic voiding dysfunction; DU, detrusor underactivity; DV, dysfunctional voiding; DSD, detrusor sphincter dyssynergia; NR, non-relaxing external sphincter; S, successful outcome; F, failed outcome.

3. Discussion

The results of this study revealed that BoNT-A urethral sphincter injection can improve voiding efficiency in about 60% of patients regardless of neurogenic or non-neurogenic etiology. Preoperative VUDS provides an important prognostic indicator for successful treatment. Patients with NNVD who had higher voiding detrusor pressure and smaller PVR might benefit more from urethral sphincter BoNT-A injection than those with lower voiding pressure. Patients who were found to have a tight bladder neck during VUDS and the DU patients with a very low Qmax might have less favorable therapeutic outcomes. In addition, patients with non-DU NVD and reduced bladder sensation might not benefit from urethral sphincter BoNT-A injection.

The application of BoNT-A in urology started from urethral sphincter injections for the treatment of DSD in patients with SCI and MS [4]. After that, the treatment was extended to treat DO and urinary incontinence in NVD and NNVD patients [8,15]. Double-blind placebo-controlled studies of therapeutic efficacy of BoNT-A urethral sphincter injection have also confirmed the validity and durability of this treatment in patients with SCI and DSD [4,16]. A 50% reduction of the occurrence of urinary tract infection after urethral sphincter BoNT-A injections for DSD has also been reported in a meta-analysis [17]. Previous studies have shown that urethral sphincter injections with 100 to 200 U of BoNT-A were effective in patients with voiding dysfunction due to MS, CVA, or SCI [8,18]. Patients with chronic CVA and chronic urinary retention might be able to get rid of clean intermittent catheterization (CIC) after the urethral injection of 100 U of BoNT-A [8,19].

Several small cohort studies also confirmed the successful therapeutic results in patients with NNVD and voiding dysfunction at doses of 100 U or 50 U of BoNT-A [7,20,21]. Some patients with NNVD and DU could also have recovery of detrusor contractility after urethral sphincter BoNT-A injections and long lasting therapeutic effects [22]. However, until now, urethral BoNT-A injection for voiding dysfunction remained an off-label treatment. Although urethral BoNT-A injection can result in relaxation of the striated urethral sphincter [12], patients with DU and a tight bladder outlet might not have a successful treatment outcome because the bladder neck cannot open on micturition [14]. The treatment results between patients with NVD and NNVD, or between patients with different bladder contractility and urethral sphincter tonicity have not been compared. In addition, although urethral sphincter BoNT-A injection is effective in improving voiding efficiency (VE) and decreasing PVR, incomplete emptying remains a problem to be solved, and postoperative urinary incontinence is still another de novo issue for women with SCI or MS [8,18,23,24]. Under these considerations, patients might not be completely satisfied with the treatment outcome of urethral sphincter BoNT-A injection [23,25]. Therefore, patient selection is important for a successful treatment.

Urination is a complex interaction with appropriate coordination among the central and peripheral neural controls, sustained detrusor contraction, adequate bladder neck relaxation, and complete relaxation of the external sphincter and pelvic floor muscles. With one or more defects of those micturition mechanisms, patients may develop NVD or NNVD. Patients with DSD or DV usually cannot achieve efficient voiding due to hypertonicity of the external sphincter. Patients with DU who use abdominal pressure to void might have voiding difficulty and incomplete bladder emptying due to a tight bladder neck or a non-relaxing urethral sphincter or pelvic floor. Patients with detrusor hyperreflexia (DHIC) might have significant PVR because of low detrusor contractility without any anatomical BOO. In the era of BoNT-A, although theoretically the urethral sphincter BoNT-A injection might produce benefits by reducing bladder outlet resistance in voiding dysfunction, the unrealistic expectations of BoNT-A urethral sphincter injections often results in failed treatment in patients not suitable for this treatment [23].

In this study, we found that an open bladder neck during VUDS is essential for successful BoNT-A injection in patients with NVD or NNVD. A tight bladder neck during voiding is an unfavorable prognostic factor for the successful outcome of BoNT-A treatment. If the bladder neck cannot be opened, urine output will be inhibited at this gate. On the contrary, after transurethral incision of the bladder neck, patients with DSD or DU usually can urinate by abdominal straining or detrusor contraction after the urethral BoNT-A injection. However, urinary incontinence might be a bothersome problem. Before urethral sphincter BoNT-A injection, patients should be informed about this potential adverse event. This adverse event is also the reason why many NVD patients finally select detrusor BoNT-A injections and periodic CIC for the solution of their voiding problem [23].

BoNT-A urethral sphincter injection results in decreased urethral pressure, increased Qmax, decreased PVR, and a reduction of autonomic dysreflexia in NVD patients with DSD due to SCI or MS [4,5,12,25]. The external sphincter hypertonicity might have different severity; therefore, injection of 100 U of BoNT-A might not be adequate for an efficient voiding in high grade DSD. In addition, because patients with NVD and DSD also have uninhibited DO, an increased urinary incontinence grade might develop after effective urethral sphincter BoNT-A injections [26].

NNVD due to DV is difficult to treat because the actual pathophysiology has not been elucidated and the only known LUTD is dysregulated urethral function with spastic or a non-relaxing external urethral sphincter during voiding [27]. DV results in voiding symptoms: Slow stream and large PVR. Therefore, attempts to reduce the hypertonicity or hyperactivity of the urethral sphincter by medication, and resume spontaneous voiding, always results in failure. It is also postulated that the psychologic voiding dysfunction due to anxiety or depression might be a cause of a low detrusor contractility and non-relaxing urethral sphincter through inhibiting detrusor contraction [28]. BoNT-A urethral sphincter injection can reduce urethral resistance but does not have an effect on the psychological insult; therefore, the successful outcome was only observed in 60% of patients with DV. If the bladder neck is not open during voiding, patients with DV might have more difficulty urinating.

DU may result from neurogenic, myogenic, obstructive, or idiopathic etiology. DU patients need to use abdominal pressure to void or depend on CIC. A sustained abdominal pressure is necessary to efficiently empty the bladder [29]. If the bladder outlet resistance is high at the level of bladder neck or urethral sphincter, patients need higher abdominal pressure to overcome the resistance, and therefore, they might not able to void efficiently. If the bladder neck is not open during voiding, urethral BoNT-A injections to the urethral sphincter might not be successful. Therefore, if VUDS shows a tight bladder neck, patients with DU and voiding dysfunction should undergo transurethral incision of the bladder neck first, otherwise, BoNT-A urethral sphincter injections might fail. In addition to an open BN, an adequate abdominal pressure is necessary for patients with DU who wish to void spontaneously after urethral BoNT-A injection.

Normal bladder sensation is another important factor for an efficient urination. The sensory afferents from the bladder urothelium and detrusor are essential parts of the voiding reflex circuit. Patients with DU might have reduced bladder sensations of filling and fullness [30]. The deficit of the bladder sensation will cause difficult initiation of voiding, as well as inefficient bladder emptying when the bladder has not been completely emptied [31]. Therefore, although the urethral resistance has been reduced after the BoNT-A injection, patients with DU and reduced bladder sensation might still have a poor outcome after treatment, especially in patients with NVD [32]. For these patients timed voiding and instruction of correct usage of abdominal pressure to void are mandatory after urethral sphincter BoNT-A injection in patients who have DU and reduced bladder sensation.

A limitation of this study is the mixed patient cohort. We aimed to find predictive factors for patients with different bladder and urethral sphincter dysfunctions. Interestingly, the success rates were similar between NVD and NNVD, and between different bladder or urethral sphincter dysfunctions. Treatment of voiding dysfunction is not an easy task. The possible causes of treatment failure have several different aspects [27]. Identification of the underlying causes of failure may improve the success rate after urethral sphincter BoNT-A injection. In this regard, VUDS before urethral BoNT-A treatment is mandatory to assess the vesicourethral dysfunction in patients with NVD and NNVD. Careful evaluation of the bladder neck opening and a higher Qmax at baseline may provide predictive value for a successful BoNT-A treatment outcome. However, urinary incontinence might be a de novo adverse event after urethral sphincter BoNT-A injection. Patients who are planning to undergo urethral sphincter BoNT-A injection for voiding dysfunction should be fully informed of the limited therapeutic efficacy and the possible adverse event of urinary incontinence before treatment.

4. Materials and Methods

This study retrospectively analyzed consecutive patients with voiding dysfunction who were refractory to medical treatment and received 100 U of BoNT-A (onabotulinumtoxinA, Allergan, Irvine, CA, USA) via urethral sphincter injection from 2011 to 2019. All patients underwent VUDS and cystoscopy to identify the underlying pathophysiology of lower urinary tract dysfunction before the BoNT-A injections. Patients with anatomical BOO, such as urethral stricture, bladder neck obstruction, or benign prostatic obstruction were excluded from the study. Only patients with DU who required spontaneous voiding by abdominal straining, had voiding dysfunction due to non-relaxing urethral sphincter, had spinal cord lesion(s) and DSD, and had DV were included in the final analysis. This study was approved by the ethics committee of the institution (IRB 105-151-B). Date of approval: 29 December 2016 to 14 December 2017. Informed consent was waived by the committee due to the retrospective nature of the study. All patients were informed of the potential adverse events after BoNT-A injection before treatment.

The treatment was performed in the operating room under light intravenous general anesthesia. A total of 100 U BoNT-A was given via transurethral sphincter injections [8]. One vial of 100 U onabotulinumtoxinA was reconstituted with normal saline to 4 mL, making the concentration equivalent to 25 U per mL. One mL of BoNT-A solution was injected into the urethral sphincter at the 3, 6, 9, and 12-o'clock positions transurethrally in men, and transcutaneous injection to the urethral sphincter along the urethral lumen at 1, 4, 7, and 10 o'clock positions of the sides of the urethral meatus in women.

A Foley catheter was indwelled overnight after BoNT-A injections and the voiding condition was requested to be reported at the out-patient clinic. The effect of BoNT-A on the urethral sphincter function appeared about 2–3 days after the treatment. The maximum therapeutic effect would reach about 2 weeks after BoNT-A injection [8]. Patients with DU and large PVR were instructed to void by Crede maneuver or abdominal straining, and CIC was recommended instead of an indwelling Foley catheter. The Qmax and PVR were measured and CIC was continued until PVR was reduced to less than 50% of the voided volume. Antibiotics were routinely given for 3 days to prevent urinary tract Infections and all medications for reduction of urethral resistance were discontinued after BoNT-A injections.

VUDS was performed in all patients at baseline. The VUDS parameters included the opening or closed bladder neck during voiding cystourethrography, the FSF, CBC, Qmax, Pdet, PVR, intra-abdominal pressure to void (in patients with DU), and VE were recorded. The terminology used in this study was based on the recommendations of the International Continence Society [33]. Patients with voiding dysfunction caused by SCI, CVA, MS, or peripheral neuropathy were categorized as having NVD, otherwise, patients were considered as NNVD. For analysis of the treatment outcome, the bladder dysfunctions were categorized into hypersensitive bladder, DO, DHIC, and DU groups. The urethral sphincter dysfunctions were caegorized as DV, DSD, and PRES, according to the electromyographic characteristics and images during the voiding phase.

The treatment outcome was assessed by self reported satisfaction and the change of the VE at 1 month after the BoNT-A injection. Patients were requested to report their global response assessment (GRA) after BoNT-A injection as: Excellent (+3), markedly improved (+2), mildly improved (+1), no change (0), or worsened (−1). Treatment success was defined as a report with GRA ≥ 1 and the VE $\geq 50\%$ after BoNT-A injection. If patients had VE of less than 50% and GRA equaled to 0 or −1, they were considered to have had failed treatment. Adverse events after BoNT-A injections were also recorded and appropriate treatments were given if needed.

Continuous variables were expressed as means ± standard deviations (SD). Categorical data were presented as numbers and percentages (%). We used chi-square test for categorical variables, and the Wilcoxon rank sum test for continuous variables to determine the p-values between successful and failed subgroups for statistical comparisons. All statistical assessments were two-sided and considered significant at a $p < 0.05$. All calculations were performed using SPSS for Windows, version 16.0 (SPSS, Chicago, IL, USA).

5. Conclusions

BoNT-A urethral sphincter injection is effective in approximately 60% of patients with voiding dysfunction due to NVD or NNVD, refractory to conventional medical treatment. Careful VUDS interpretation of bladder neck opening and measurements of a higher detrusor or abdominal pressure enabled us to select candidates suitable for urethral sphincter BoNT-A treatment.

Author Contributions: Y.-K.L.: Perform urodynamics and manuscript writing. H.-C.K.: Study design, data interpretation, and critical review.

Acknowledgments: This study was supported by the grant of Tzu Chi Medical Foundation TCMF-MP-107-02-01.

References

1. Jiang, Y.H.; Kuo, H.C. Video-urodynamic characteristics of non-neurogenic, idiopathic underactive bladder in men—A comparison of men with normal tracing and bladder outlet obstruction. *PLoS ONE* **2017**, *12*, e0174593. [CrossRef] [PubMed]
2. Yang, T.H.; Chuang, F.C.; Kuo, H.C. Urodynamic characteristics of detrusor underactivity in women with voiding dysfunction. *PLoS ONE* **2018**, *13*, e0198764. [CrossRef] [PubMed]
3. Hsiao, S.M.; Lin, H.H.; Kuo, H.C. Videourodynamic Studies of Women with Voiding Dysfunction. *Sci. Rep.* **2017**, *7*, 6845. [CrossRef] [PubMed]
4. Dykstra, D.D.; Sidi, A.A. Treatment of detrusor-sphincter dyssynergia with botulinum A toxin: A double-blind study. *Arch. Phys. Med. Rehabil.* **1990**, *71*, 24–26. [PubMed]
5. Schurch, B.; Hauri, D.; Rodic, B.; Curt, A.; Meyer, M.; Rossier, A.B. Botulinum-A toxin as a treatment of detrusor-sphincter dyssynergia: A prospective study in 24 spinal cord injury patients. *J. Urol.* **1996**, *155*, 1023–1029. [CrossRef]
6. Maria, G.; Destito, A.; Lacquaniti, S.; Bentivoglio, A.R.; Brisinda, G.; Albanese, A. Relief by botulinum toxin of voiding dysfunction due to prostatitis. *Lancet* **1998**, *352*, 625. [CrossRef]
7. Phelan, M.W.; Franks, M.; Somogyi, G.T.; Yokoyama, T.; Fraser, M.O.; Lavelle, J.P.; Yoshimura, N.; Chancellor, M.B. Botulinum toxin urethral sphincter injection to restore bladder emptying in men and women with voiding dysfunction. *J. Urol.* **2001**, *165*, 1107–1110. [CrossRef]
8. Kuo, H.C. Botulinum A toxin urethral injection for the treatment of lower urinary tract dysfunction. *J. Urol.* **2003**, *170*, 1908–1912. [CrossRef] [PubMed]
9. Mangera, A.; Apostolidis, A.; Andersson, K.E.; Dasgupta, P.; Giannantoni, A.; Roehrbom, C.; Novara, G.; Chapple, C. An updated systematic review and statistical comparison of standardised mean outcomes for the use of botulinum toxin in the management of lower urinary tract disorders. *Eur. Urol.* **2014**, *65*, 981–990. [CrossRef]
10. Mokhless, I.; Gaafar, S.; Fouda, K.; Shafik, M.; Assem, A. Botulinum A toxin urethral sphincter injection in children with nonneurogenic neurogenic bladder. *J. Urol.* **2006**, *176*, 1767–1770. [CrossRef] [PubMed]
11. Franco, I.; Landau-Dyer, L.; Isom-Batz, G.; Collett, T.; Reda, E.F. The use of botulinum toxin A injection for the management of external sphincter dyssynergia in neurologically normal children. *J. Urol.* **2007**, *178*, 1775–1779, discussion 1779–1780. [CrossRef] [PubMed]
12. Jiang, Y.H.; Wang, C.C.; Kuo, H.C. OnabotulinumtoxinA Urethral Sphincter Injection as Treatment for Non-neurogenic Voiding Dysfunction—A Randomized, Double-Blind, Placebo-Controlled Study. *Sci. Rep.* **2016**, *6*, 38905. [CrossRef] [PubMed]
13. Panicker, J.N.; Seth, J.H.; Khan, S.; Gonzales, G.; Haslam, C.; Kessler, T.M.; Fowler, C.J. Open-label study evaluating outpatient urethral sphincter injections of onabotulinumtoxinA to treat women with urinary retention due to a primary disorder of sphincter relaxation (Fowler's syndrome). *BJU Int.* **2016**, *117*, 809–813. [CrossRef] [PubMed]

14. Jiang, Y.H.; Jhang, J.F.; Chen, S.F.; Kuo, H.C. Videourodynamic factors predictive of successful onabotulinumtoxinA urethral sphincter injection for neurogenic or non-neurogenic detrusor underactivity. *Low Urin. Tract. Symptoms* **2019**, *11*, 66–71. [CrossRef] [PubMed]
15. Smith, C.P.; Chancellor, M.B. Emerging role of botulinum toxin in the treatment of voiding dysfunction. *J. Urol.* **2004**, *171*, 2128–2137. [CrossRef] [PubMed]
16. De Sèze, M.; Petit, H.; Gallien, P.; de Seze, M.P.; Joseph, P.A.; Mazaux, J.M.; Barat, M. Botulinum a toxin and detrusor sphincter dyssynergia: A double-blind lidocaine-controlled study in 13 patients with spinal cord disease. *Eur. Urol.* **2002**, *42*, 56–62.
17. Mehta, S.; Hill, D.; Foley, N.; Hsieh, J.; Ethans, K.; Potter, P.; Baverstock, R.; Teasell, R.W.; Wolfs, D. A meta-analysis of botulinum toxin sphincteric injections in the treatment of incomplete voiding after spinal cord injury. *Arch. Phys. Med. Rehabil.* **2012**, *93*, 597–603. [CrossRef] [PubMed]
18. Smith, C.P.; Nishiguchi, J.; O'Leary, M.; Yoshimura, N.; Chancellor, M.B. Single-institution experience in 110 patients with botulinum toxin A injection into bladder or urethra. *Urology* **2005**, *65*, 37–41. [CrossRef]
19. Chen, Y.H.; Kuo, H.C. Botulinum A toxin treatment of urethral sphincter pseudodyssynergia in patients with cerebrovascular accidents or intracranial lesions. *Urol. Int.* **2004**, *73*, 156–161. [CrossRef]
20. Leippold, T.; Reitz, A.; Schurch, B. Botulinum toxin as a new therapy option for voiding disorders: Current state of the art. *Eur. Urol.* **2003**, *44*, 165–174. [CrossRef]
21. Kuo, H.C. Effect of botulinum a toxin in the treatment of voiding dysfunction due to detrusor underactivity. *Urology* **2003**, *61*, 550–554. [CrossRef]
22. Kuo, H.C. Recovery of detrusor function after urethral botulinum A toxin injection in patients with idiopathic low detrusor contractility and voiding dysfunction. *Urology* **2007**, *69*, 57–61. [CrossRef] [PubMed]
23. Kuo, H.C. Satisfaction with urethral injection of botulinum toxin A for detrusor sphincter dyssynergia in patients with spinal cord lesion. *Neurourol. Urodyn.* **2008**, *27*, 793–796. [CrossRef] [PubMed]
24. Gallien, P.; Reymann, J.M.; Amarenco, G.; Nicolas, B.; de Seze, M.; Bellissant, E. Placebo-controlled, randomised, double-blind study of the effects of botulinum A toxin on detrusor sphincter dyssynergia in multiple sclerosis patients. *J. Neurol. Neurosurg Psychiatry* **2005**, *76*, 1670–1676. [CrossRef] [PubMed]
25. Mahfouz, W.; Karsenty, G.; Corcos, J. Injection of botulinum toxin type A in the urethral sphincter to treat lower urinary tract dysfunction: Review of indications, techniques and results: 2011 update. *Can J. Urol.* **2011**, *18*, 5787–5795. [PubMed]
26. Dykstra, D.D.; Sidi, A.A.; Scott, A.B.; Pagel, J.M.; Goldish, G.D. Effects of botulinum A toxin on detrusor-sphincter dyssynergia in spinal cord injury patients. *J. Urol.* **1988**, *139*, 919–922. [CrossRef]
27. Liao, Y.M.; Kuo, H.C. Causes of failed urethral botulinum toxin A treatment for emptying failure. *Urology* **2007**, *70*, 763–766. [CrossRef] [PubMed]
28. Chen, Y.C.; Kuo, H.C. Clinical and video urodynamic characteristics of adult women with dysfunctional voiding. *J. Formos. Med. Assoc.* **2014**, *113*, 161–165. [CrossRef] [PubMed]
29. Hoeritzauer, I.; Phé, V.; Panicker, J.N. Urologic symptoms and functional neurologic disorders. *Handb. Clin. Neurol.* **2016**, *139*, 469–481.
30. Jiang, Y.H.; Lee, C.L.; Jhang, J.F.; Kuo, H.C. Current pharmacological and surgical treatment of underactive bladder. *Investig. Clin. Urol.* **2017**, *29*, 187–191.
31. Jiang, Y.H.; Kuo, H.C. Urothelial Barrier Deficits, Suburothelial Inflammation and Altered Sensory Protein Expression in Detrusor Underactivity. *J. Urol.* **2017**, *197*, 197–203. [CrossRef] [PubMed]
32. Kuo, H.C. Therapeutic outcome and quality of life between urethral and detrusor botulinum toxin treatment for patients with spinal cord lesions and detrusor sphincter dyssynergia. *Int. J. Clin. Pract.* **2013**, *67*, 1044–1049. [CrossRef] [PubMed]
33. Abrams, P.; Cardozo, L.; Fall, M.; Griffiths, D.; Rosier, P.; Ulmsten, U.; van Kerrebroeck, P.; Victor, A.; Wein, A. The standardisation of terminology of lower urinary tract function: Report from the standardisation sub–committee of the international continence society. *Neurourol. Urodyn.* **2002**, *21*, 167–178. [CrossRef] [PubMed]

11

The Therapeutic Effects and Pathophysiology of Botulinum Toxin A on Voiding Dysfunction Due to Urethral Sphincter Dysfunction

Yao-Lin Kao [1], Kuan-Hsun Huang [2], Hann-Chorng Kuo [3] and Yin-Chien Ou [1,4,*]

1 Department of Urology, National Cheng Kung University Hospital, College of Medicine, National Cheng Kung University, Tainan 704, Taiwan; pleasewaitforg@hotmail.com
2 Department of Urology, Dalin Tzu Chi Hospital, Buddhist Tzu Chi Medical Foundation, Chiayi County 622, Taiwan; i5490108@hotmail.com
3 Department of Urology, Hualien Tzu Chi Hospital, Buddhist Tzu Chi Medical Foundation and Tzu Chi University, Hualien 970, Taiwan; hck@tzuchi.com.tw
4 College of Medicine, Institute of Clinical Medicine, National Cheng Kung University, Tainan 704, Taiwan
* Correspondence: i54921051@gmail.com

Abstract: Neurogenic and non-neurogenic urethral sphincter dysfunction are common causes of voiding dysfunction. Injections of botulinum toxin A (BoNT-A) into the urethral sphincter have been used to treat urethral sphincter dysfunction (USD) refractory to conventional treatment. Since its first use for patients with detrusor sphincter dyssynergia in 1988, BoNT-A has been applied to various causes of USD, including dysfunctional voiding, Fowler's syndrome, and poor relaxation of the external urethral sphincter. BoNT-A is believed to decrease urethral resistance via paralysis of the striated sphincter muscle through inhibition of acetylcholine release in the neuromuscular junction. Recovery of detrusor function in patients with detrusor underactivity combined with a hyperactive sphincter also suggested the potential neuromodulation effect of sphincteric BoNT-A injection. A large proportion of patients with different causes of USD report significant improvement in voiding after sphincteric BoNT-A injections. However, patient satisfaction might not increase with an improvement in the symptoms because of concomitant side effects including exacerbated incontinence, urinary urgency, and over-expectation. Nonetheless, in terms of efficacy and safety, BoNT-A is still a reasonable option for refractory voiding function. To date, studies focusing on urethral sphincter BoNT-A injections have been limited to the heterogeneous etiologies of USD. Further well-designed studies are thus needed.

Keywords: botulinum toxin; urethral sphincter; urethral sphincter dysfunction; lower urinary tract symptoms; urodynamics

Key Contribution: This article summarized the effects of sphincteric BoNT-A injections among various USDs in view of pathophysiology, urodynamic outcome, and subjective patient reports.

---

1. Introduction

Urethral sphincter dysfunction (USD) is one of the functional causes of voiding dysfunction (VD), which leads to slow or incomplete micturition in both males and females [1]. The condition can be either neurogenic or non-neurogenic. While detrusor sphincter dyssynergia (DSD) commonly stands for the well-known neurogenic cause [2], dysfunctional voiding (DV), Fowler's syndrome (FS), and poor relaxation of the external urethral sphincter (PRES) during voiding comprise the non-neurogenic causes [3,4]. Management of these functional disorders can be challenging if conventional treatment fails.

The introduction of a botulinum toxin A (BoNT-A) injection at the external urethral sphincter (EUS) was first performed in 1988 by Dykstra et al. [5]. Paralysis of the urethral sphincter and decreased urethral resistance were anticipated following the BoNT-A injection. The authors indeed found the signs of sphincter denervation and an improvement in voiding efficiency in patients with spinal cord injury (SCI) and DSD. Since then, extended use of BoNT-A in various urinary tract dysfunctions has been reported [6], however, the currently approved indications for BoNT-A for the lower urinary tract are neurogenic detrusor overactivity and overactive bladder [7]. To date, there have been only a handful of studies demonstrating the application of BoNT-A injections into the EUS, especially in the case of VDs other than DSD [8,9]. This review is an attempt to summarize the pathophysiology of BoNT-A and its therapeutic effects among different types of USD.

2. Biology and Mechanism of BoNT-A

Botulinum toxin is a neurotoxin produced by Clostridium botulinum [6]. It was first isolated as a crystalline product in 1946 [10] and was found to have a paralyzing effect on hyperactive muscles in the 1950s [11,12]. To date, eight immunologically antigenic distinct subtypes have been identified, i.e., subtypes A, B, C1, C2, D, E, F, and G [13]. Botulinum neurotoxin subtype A is potent, with the longest duration of action among these subtypes, and is commonly used in clinical practice [14]. Currently, several commercial forms of BoNT-A are available, where Botox® (Allergan, Irvine, CA, USA) and Dysport® (Ipsen, Slough, UK) are the two most widely used agents [15]. It should be noted that these products cannot be considered equivalent in terms of dose, efficacy, or safety owing to having different fragments of botulinum toxin and different manufacturing processes [6]. Although a few studies have suggested the efficacy of 1 unit of Botox to be similar to 3–5 units of Dysport [16,17], this simple linear exchange equation has been questioned in different BoNT-A applications [18].

The mechanism by which BoNT-A inhibits target muscle contractions is well-known as the blocking of acetylcholine release from presynaptic efferent nerves at the neuromuscular junctions via cleaving of synaptosome-associated protein 25 (SNAP-25) and preventing the docking of acetylcholine-containing vesicles to the neuronal cell membrane [19]. The toxin also blocks the release of other neurotransmitters, including adenosine triphosphate, substance P, calcitonin gene-related peptide, and downregulates sensory receptors such as vanilloid (TRPV1) and purinergic (P2 × 3) receptors [20,21] known as an afferent nerve desensitizer. The effect of BoNT-A on urethral striated muscle is thought to block the presynaptic release of acetylcholine in the neuromuscular junction and subsequently achieve a chemical sphincterotomy, which is believed to relieve the USD and improve VD [22,23]. An animal study has also shown a reduction in the release of norepinephrine in the urethra after BoNT-A injections at the EUS of rats, supporting its use in the treatment of EUS overactivity [24]. A decrease in maximum urethral pressure (MUP) of an average of 27 cm H_2O was noted after BoNT-A injection in DSD patients [5].

Besides the direct effect on the EUS, BoNT-A injections at the EUS may lead to recovery of bladder detrusor contractility in VD patients with detrusor underactivity (DU) and hyperactive EUS or PRES [25]. It has been proposed that the suppression of EUS contraction will deactivate the afferent signals inhibiting the bladder reflex [26,27], however, this neuromodulation effect still awaits further confirmation.

3. Urethral Sphincter BoNT-A Injections in Patients with Detrusor Sphincter Dyssynergia

DSD is defined as involuntary contractions of the EUS during detrusor contractions [28]. DSD is mainly caused by damage to the upper motor neurons lying between the pontine micturition center and the sacral spinal cord, such as in the morbidities associated with spinal cord injury (SCI), multiple sclerosis (MS), and transverse myelitis (TM) [29–33]. DSD usually causes significant VD, leading to chronic urinary retention, recurrent urinary tract infection (UTI), high detrusor voiding pressure, autonomic dysreflexia, vesicoureteral reflux, and possible renal damage [34]. Alpha-blockers have been used to decrease outlet resistance, but the results of urodynamic studies have not been convincing [35]. Clean intermittent catheterization (CIC) is an effective alternative for patients to empty their bladder, but some patients are not able to tolerate it well due to upper limb impairment or psychological unwillingness [36]. Surgical sphincterotomy is another drastic option for those who fail in the treatments mentioned above, however, many of such patients experience a worsened quality of life due to persistent incontinence and a high long-term failure rate [37]. BoNT-A is thought to be an alternative, as it can block the release of acetylcholine from presynaptic vesicles at the neuromuscular junction, which causes temporary, reversible chemo-denervation of the external EUS [38].

Dykstra et al. [5] first described both transperineal and transurethral injections of BoNT-A to the EUS in 1988 as a new therapeutic approach for 11 male patients with SCI and DSD. In this preliminary study, weekly injections using different dosages of BoNT-A effectively decreased the MUP and post-void residual (PVR) urine volume. Electromyography (EMG) further confirmed sphincter denervation in all patients. The authors then conducted a small sample, randomized, double-blind placebo-control trial in five SCI male patients with DSD to compare low dose BoNT-A with normal saline by weekly injections for three weeks. They concluded that the therapeutic effects were found only in the BoNT-A injection group [39].

Instead of a once-weekly injection, a once-monthly dose has also been confirmed to effectively improve sphincter function as well as to decrease PVR [40]. In addition, a single transurethral dose of BoNT-A was further evaluated by Petit et al. [41] in 17 male patients with SCI and DSD. Their results showed similar clinical improvements in approximately 70% of the cases with an average therapeutic effect of two to six months. Phelan et al. [42] first confirmed the effectiveness of sphincteric BoNT-A injections in both male and female patients with various etiologies of DSD, including SCI, TM, and MS. De Sèze et al. [43] carried out a randomized, double-blind control trial to compare the efficacy of and tolerability to BoNT-A with a lidocaine single transperineal injection in patients with DSD. Higher patient satisfaction scores and significant decreases in PVR, MUP, and EMG activity were found only in the BoNT-A group. Most of the patients tolerated the treatment well without major complications.

Recently, more data describing the clinical experiences related to sphincteric BoNT-A injections in patients with DSD have been reported. Both transperineal injections [5,40,43–47] and transurethral injections using cystoscopy [5,40–42,48–53] showed promising outcomes in terms of reducing sphincteric activity. Although transurethral injections have been reported to be more effective in terms of decreasing the MUP than the use of a transperineal route [40], no further trials have ever directly compared these two injection methods. Most of the recent publications on this topic involve the use of a sphincteric injection of 100 units of Botox in DSD patients since a more prolonged therapeutic effect was found, as compared to 50 units, in a previous randomized control trial [54].

Urodynamic parameters were commonly used as measurements of objective outcomes after sphincteric BoNT-A injections in patients with DSD. As expected, a significant reduction in EMG activity [5,39,43] and a decrease in MUP [5,40,41,43,44] during the voiding phase have been found. Improvements in PVR [5,40–43,49], detrusor contraction pressure [5,44,48,49], and maximal flow rate (Qmax) [42,48] were also reported as a result of decreased sphincteric resistance. However, unlike SCI patients, a randomized, double-blind, placebo-control trial in 86 patients with MS and DSD showed that a single injection of BoNT-A did not decrease the PVR [44]. The authors posited that the unchanged PVR could be attributed to the lower baseline detrusor contraction pressure. In addition to the outcome measurement, urodynamic parameters have also been used to predict therapeutic outcomes. Several pre-treatment urodynamic parameters, including higher baseline detrusor contraction pressure [41,53], lower baseline sphincteric tone [48,50,55], and a synergic bladder neck [53,55] have been confirmed as predictors of a favorable outcome.

Although objective urodynamic results have been improved after EUS BoNT-A injection, Kuo et al. [52] reported inconsistencies between urodynamic outcomes and patient satisfaction. Even though the PVR and detrusor contraction pressure were improved, patients were not satisfied with the outcomes mainly because of the increased incontinence grade [51]. Notably, for patients with SCI and DSD, a detrusor BoNT-A injection provided a much better quality of life than the case with an EUS injection [52] This result emphasized the importance of continence in a patient's quality of life. Other causes of patient dissatisfaction included persistent difficult urination [51], increases in urgency episodes [51], and the need for repeated injections [45]. For therapeutic outcomes, patient satisfaction was mainly due to improved voiding conditions and fewer autonomic dysreflexia (AD) episodes [52,53]. To summarize the subjective outcomes of sphincteric BoNT-A injections for patients with DSD, 61–88% experienced clinical improvement [5,40–42,48,51] for a therapeutic duration lasting two to six months [40–42,44], more than 80% could regain spontaneous voiding and successfully remove the indwelling catheter or stop CIC [42,48,49], and episodes of autonomic dysreflexia were reduced in more than 50% of the cases [5,43,50,51]. Table 1 summarizes the clinical studies on efficacy and adverse events related to sphincteric BoNT-A injections in the treatment of patients with DSD.

In spite of the benefits of sphincteric BoNT-A injections in patients with DSD based on the literature, the use of different injection protocols among various etiologies makes intergroup comparisons difficult. Further randomized control trials with large case numbers focusing on a single etiology of DSD are necessary to evaluate the therapeutic impacts on both objective and subjective parameters, quality of life, duration of effect, and long-term durability after repetitive injections.

Table 1. Summary of clinical studies using sphincteric botulinum toxin A (BoNT-A) injections for patients with detrusor sphincter dyssynergia (DSD).

Author (Year)	Sex (No.)	Cause of DSD (No.)	Injection Method and Dose	UDS Improvements	Clinical Improvements (Events/Total Cases)	Adverse Events (Events/Total Cases)	Effective Duration
Randomized control trials							
Dykstra and Sidi (1990) [39]	M (5)	SCI (5)	Transurethral low dose BoNT-A, weekly Transurethral N/S, weekly	PVR, MUP, EMG activity [a]	NA	Nil	NA
de Sèze et al. (2002) [43]	M (12) F (1)	SCI (9), MS (3), Congenital (1)	Transperineal 100U Botox Transperineal Lidocaine	PVR, MUP, EMG activity [a]	Higher satisfaction score in the Botox group Voiding function improved in the Botox group Less AD (3/4) in the Botox group	Nil	<3 months: 31% =3 months: 46% >3 months: 23%
Gallien et al. (2005) [44]	M (28) F (58)	MS (86)	Transperineal 100U Botox Transperineal N/S	MUP, Pdet, VV [a]	No between-group differences No improvement in IPSS and VAS	UTI (16/45) Incontinence (2/45) Fecal incontinence (1/45)	2 months
Kuo (2007) [54]	M or F (66)	DSD (6), Non-DSD (60)	Transurethral (M) or periurethral (F) 50U Botox Transurethral (M) or periurethral (F) 100U Botox	PVR, MUP, Pdet, QmaX	Excellent outcome (5/6) for DSD patients No differences between 50U and 100U	Nil	50U: 6.4 months 100U: 8.4 months
Nonrandomized control trial							
Kuo (2013) [52]	M or F (55)	SCI (47), MS (6), TM (2)	Transurethral (M) or periurethral (F) 100U Botox Intradetrusor 200U Botox	PVR, Pdet, Qmax [a]	Greater QoL improvement with detrusor injection than with sphincter injection	Incontinence is the major cause of dissatisfaction for sphincter injection	NA
Non-control open label trials							
Dykstra et al. (1988) [5]	M (11)	SCI (11)	Transperineal 20-80U BoNT-A, weekly Transurethral 80-240U BoNT-A, weekly	PVR, MUP, EMG activity	Less AD (5/7)	Nil	50 days
Schurch et al. (1996) [40]	M (24)	SCI (24)	Transperineal 250U Dysport, monthly Transurethral 100U Botox, monthly	PVR, MUP	Sphincter function improved (21/24)	Nil	3–9 months
Petit et al. (1998) [41]	M (17)	SCI (17)	Transurethral 150U Dysport	PVR, MUP, Pdet	Modality of voiding improved (10/17)	Urethral bleeding (1) Incontinence (5)	2–6 months
Phelan et al. (2001) [42]	M (8) F (13)	SCI (1), MS (9), TM (2), Non-DSD (9)	Transurethral 80-100U Botox	PVR, Qmax	Voiding pattern improved (14/21) Regain of spontaneous voiding (19/21)	Nil	3 months

Table 1. *Cont.*

Author (Year)	Sex (No.)	Cause of DSD (No.)	Injection Method and Dose	UDS Improvements	Clinical Improvements (Events/Total Cases)	Adverse Events (Events/Total Cases)	Effective Duration
Kuo (2003) [48]	M (48) F (55)	DSD (29), Non-DSD (74)	Transurethral (M) or periurethral (F) 100U Botox	Pdet, Qmax	Excellent outcome (8/29) Improved outcome (15/29)	NA [b]	2–6 months
Smith et al. (2005) [49]	M or F (68)	SCI (9), MS (32), Non-DSD (27)	Transurethral 80-200U Botox	PVR, Pdet, Capacity	Regain of spontaneous voiding (34/41)	Incontinence (3/68)	6 months
Liao and Kuo (2007) [55]	M (112) F (88)	DSD (48), Non-DSD (152)	Transurethral (M) or periurethral (F) 50-100U Botox	NA	Excellent outcome (19/48) Improved outcome (26/48)	Nil	NA
Kuo (2008) [51]	M (22) F (11)	SCI (26), MS (5), TM (2)	Transurethral (M) or periurethral (F) 100U Botox	PVR, Pdet, Qmax	Improved IIQ-7 and UDI-6 Voiding function improved (26/33) Less AD (3/6)	Incontinence (16/33) Increase urgency (5/33) De novo frequency (3/33)	Patients received repeat injection at 4–9 months
Chen et al. (2008) [50]	M (17) F (3)	SCI (20)	Transurethral 100U Botox	MUP, EMG activity	Vesico-ureteral reflux resolved (1/1) Less AD (4/4)	Mild hematuria (2/20)	NA
Tsai et al. (2009) [46]	M (18)	SCI (18)	Transperineal 100U Botox	PVR, MUP, Pdet	Less symptomatic UTI (11/13) Modality of voiding improved (17/18) Hydronephrosis resolved (7/9) Vesico-ureteral reflux resolved (1/1) Less AD (6/7)	Nil	3 months
Chen et al. (2010) [47]	M (18)	SCI (18)	Transperineal 100U Botox	PVR, MUP, EMG activity	Less AD (5/5)	Mild hematuria (1/20)	2–6 months
Huang et al. (2016) [53]	65	SCI (65)	Intradetrusor 200U and transurethral 100U Botox	MUP, Pdet, VV	Urgency incontinence improved (59/59) Incontinence resolved (25/59) Less symptomatic UTI (6/14) Less AD (11/18)	Nil	NA
Soler et al. (2016) [45]	M (72) F (27)	SCI (99)	Transperineal 100U Botox	PVR	Excellent outcome (48/99) Modality of voiding improved (25/99) Vesico-ureteral reflux resolved (6/11) Less AD (69/82)	Nil	6.5 months

AD = Autonomic dysreflexia; BoNT-A = Botulinum toxin A; DSD = Detrusor sphincter dyssynergia; EMG = Electromyogram; F = Female; IIQ-7 = Incontinence Impact Questionnaire–Short Form; IPSS = International prostate symptom score; M = Male; MS = Multiple sclerosis; MUP = Maximal urethral pressure; NA = data not accessible from the study; Nil = none; No. = Number; N/S = Normal saline; Pdet = Detrusor contraction pressure; PVR = Post-void residual urine volume; Qmax = Maximal flow rate; QoL = Quality of life index; SCI = Spinal cord injury; TM = Transverse myelitis; UDI-6 = Urogenital Distress Inventory–Short Form; UDS = Urodynamic study; UTI = Urinary tract infection; VAS = Visual analog scale; VV = Voided volume. Sphincteric injections used with preparation other than the typical BoNT-A commercial form, including Botox or Disport, were denoted as "BoNT-A". [a] UDS improvements were found in the urethral Botox group. [b] Individual results in specific disease groups were not available.

4. Urethral Sphincter BoNT-A Injections in Children with Dysfunctional Voiding

DV is characterized by an intermittent or fluctuating flow rate, owing to intermittent contractions of the periurethral striated muscles or pelvic floor muscles during voiding in neurologically normal patients [56]. In 1973, Hinman and Baumann first described the symptom complex including enuresis, daytime wetting, UTI, and upper tract dilatation in 14 boys without neurologic defects and suggested that the condition is a functional discoordination between detrusor contraction and external sphincter relaxation [57]. This syndrome was then described by other authors as Hinman syndrome, occult neuropathic bladder, non-neurogenic neurogenic bladder, learned voiding dysfunction, and dysfunctional voiding [58–60]. In children, the typical symptoms of DV include urinary incontinence, recurrent UTI, voiding difficulty, urinary retention, and hydronephrosis [61]. To establish the diagnosis, uroflowmetry with an EMG is required to confirm that a sudden change in flow rate in the form of a staccato or intermittent pattern is related to sphincter contraction. Also, a "spinning-top" urethra can also be seen in a video-urodynamic study (vUDS) or voiding cystourethrography, indicating discoordination of the EUS and detrusor contraction during voiding [56].

The conventional treatments for children with DV include non-pharmacological urotherapy [62,63] and alpha-blockers [64]. Since DV and DSD share similar pathophysiology in terms of abnormal sphincteric activity during voiding, applying BoNT-A to the EUS seems to be a reasonable therapeutic option. A sphincteric BoNT-A injection was first introduced as a novel treatment for children with DV by Steinhardt et al. [65], who successfully improved incontinence and recurrent UTI in a 7-year-old girl, and also demonstrated a marked improvement in the degree of urethral dilatation.

Several case series with small samples also discussed the therapeutic outcome of BoNT-A in children with DV who failed traditional urotherapy and medical management [66–70]. According to these data, 80–85% of patients showed improvement in daytime incontinence or enuresis [68,69], total dryness was found in 45–80% of patients after sphincteric BoNT-A injections [67–70], and approximately 45–75% of patients were free from recurrent UTI even without prophylaxis antibiotics [68–70]. A small case series reported by Mokhless et al. [66] revealed that nine children who were catheterized preoperatively experienced recovery of spontaneous voiding after sphincteric BoNT-A injections. In the case of urodynamic parameters, PVR improvement was found in most of the studies, and a flow pattern changed to bell-shaped curve was also reported [69,70]. Unlike the usual dose of 50 to 100 units of Botox in pediatric sphincter injections, Franco et al. [67] used a higher dose ranging from 200 to 300 units in 16 children with DV. They reported long-lasting improvements in PVR at six months, and the majority of their patients did not require repeated injections. The authors hypothesized that BoNT-A could block sensory feedback of overactive guarding reflex, making it possible to retrain these children to void appropriately. No acute complications, including nausea, dysphagia, respiratory distress, or paralysis, were found in any of these studies. Clinical studies of sphincteric BoNT-A injections for children with DV are summarized in Table 2.

Although the effects and safety of BoNT-A use in children with DV seem to be convincing, we should remember that all these study designs were nonrandomized, without controlled variables, and comprised small samples. Further better-designed trials with longer follow up are necessary to arrive at an accurate conclusion.

Table 2. Summary of clinical studies using sphincteric BoNT-A injections for children and adults with dysfunctional voiding (DV).

Author (Year)	Sex (No.)	Disease (No.)	Injection Method and Dose	UDS Improvements	Clinical Improvements (Events/Total Cases)	Adverse Events (Events/Total Cases)	Effective Duration
Studies regarding BoNT-A injection in children DV							
Mokhless et al. (2006) [66]	M (6) F (4)	DV (10)	Transurethral 50-100U Botox	PVR, Qmax, EMG activity	Regain of spontaneous voiding (9/9) Hydronephrosis resolved (2/4) Hydronephrosis downgraded (2/4) Vesico-ureteral reflux resolved (1/1)	Nil	6 months
Petronijevic et al. (2007) [70]	F (9)	DV (9)	Transperineal 500U Dysport	PVR, VV, voiding pattern	Improved voiding function (7/9) Incontinence resolved (4/5) Recurrent UTI resolved (6/8)	Nil	6 months
Franco et al. (2007) [67]	M or F (16)	DV (16)	Transurethral 200-300U Botox	PVR	Incontinence resolved (13/16) Recurrent epididymo-orchitis resolved (3/3)	Nil	>6 months
Vricella et al. (2014) [68]	M (8) F (4)	DV (12)	Transurethral (M) or periurethral (F) 100U Botox	PVR, Qmax	Voiding condition improved (8/12) Incontinence resolved (4/7), improved (2/7) Hydronephrosis resolved (1/2) Vesico-ureteral reflux resolved (1/3) Recurrent UTI resolved (4/7) Discontinued anticholinergics (6/6)	Nil	Repeat injection at 6–21 months
't Hoen et al. (2015) [69]	M (4) F (16)	DV (20)	Transurethral (M) or periurethral (F) 100U Botox	PVR, voiding pattern	Incontinence resolved (9/20), improved (7/20) Recurrent UTI resolved (5/11), improved (6/11)	Sudden increase of incontinence (9/20) Gluteus maximus muscle numbness (1/20)	Repeat injection after 13 months in average
Studies regarding BoNT-A injection in adult DV							
Kuo (2003) [48]	M (48) F (55)	DV (20) Non-DV (83)	Transurethral (M) or periurethral (F) 50-100U Botox	Pdet, Qmax	Excellent outcome (6/20) Improved outcome (14/20)	NA [a]	2–6 months
Liao and Kuo (2007) [55]	M (112) F (88)	DV (60) Non-DV (140)	Transurethral (M) or periurethral (F) 50-100U Botox	NA	Excellent outcome (37/60) Improved outcome (15/60)	Nil	NA
Kuo (2007) [b] [54]	M or F (66)	DV (21) Non-DV (45)	Transurethral (M) or periurethral (F) 50U Botox Transurethral (M) or periurethral (F) 100U Botox	NA	Excellent outcome (13/21) for DV patients Improved outcome (6/21) for DV patients No difference between 50U and 100U	Nil	50U: 6.4 months 100U: 8.4 months
Jiang et al. (2016) [b] [71]	M or F (62)	DV (38) Non-DV (24)	Transurethral (M) or periurethral (F) 100U Botox Transurethral (M) or periurethral (F) N/S	Pdet, Qmax, VV [c]	IPSS, QoL, and PPBC improved in both groups Success outcome (7/16) for Botox	De novo UUI (3/62) UTI (3/62) Micturition pain (2/62) Hematuria (2/62)	NA

BoNT-A = Botulinum toxin A; DV: dysfunctional voiding; EMG = Electromyogram; F = Female; IPSS = international prostate symptom score; M = Male; NA: data not accessible from the study; Nil = none; No. = Number; N/S = normal saline; Pdet = Detrusor contraction pressure; PPBC = Patient perception of bladder condition; PVR = Post-void residual urine volume; Qmax = Maximal flow rate; QoL = Quality of life index; UDS = Urodynamic study; UTI = Urinary tract infection; UUI = Urgency urinary incontinence; VV = Voided volume. [a] Individual results toward specific disease group were not assessable. [b] Both studies were designed as randomized control trials. [c] UDS improvements were found in the urethral Botox injection group for patients with DV.

5. Urethral Sphincter BoNT-A Injections in Adults with Dysfunctional Voiding

The precise prevalence of DV in the adult population is still unknown. In a urodynamic database review of 1015 adults who were evaluated for voiding symptoms, around 2% could be defined as having DV using strict vUDS criteria [60]. Adult DV may come from persistent disease since childhood or adult-onset symptoms due to non-neurological etiologies [72]. Although adults and children with DV share similar characteristics and are defined similarly [56,73], the clinical characteristics of these two groups are quite different. Unlike children, adult patients typically present with obstructive symptoms, followed by frequency, nocturia, and urgency. Recurrent UTI and urinary incontinence are less prominent in adults [60].

Data discussing the therapeutic effect of sphincteric BoNT-A injections in adults with DV are limited and are mostly provided by Kuo and his colleagues [48,55,71]. In a prospective nonrandomized study without controlled variables, the authors performed sphincteric injections using 50 to 100 units of Botox in 20 adults with DV and reported a subjectively excellent outcome in 30% of the patients, where the remaining 70% showed improvement [48]. Liao and Kuo also reported an overall success rate of 86.7% in adults with DV by sphincteric injections with 50 to 100 units of Botox in a five-year retrospective review. DU with low abdominal straining pressure, spastic EUS, and bladder neck obstruction were the most common causes of treatment failure [55].

A randomized, double-blind, placebo-controlled study was conducted in 31 adults with DV to compare the therapeutic effect of 100 units of Botox with normal saline [71]. Even though the detrusor voiding pressure and voided volume were significantly improved in the BoNT-A group, there were no significant between-group differences in the subjective success rate. The author hypothesized that the local injection itself might have some unknown therapeutic effects on the relaxation of the EUS [71]. This concept is similar to the dry needling effect on myofascial trigger point pain, which can relax the actin-myosin bonds and normalize muscle tone [74]. Additional well-designed studies to enroll more adult patients with DV are necessary to elucidate the therapeutic effect of sphincteric BoNT-A injections, normal saline injections, or even the dry needle effect. Clinical studies of sphincteric BoNT-A injections for adults with DV are summarized in Table 2.

6. Urethral Sphincter BoNT-A Injections in Patients with Fowler Syndrome

Fowler's syndrome (FS), a specific cause of unexplained urinary retention in young women, was first described by Fowler in 1986 [75]. The condition is characterized by EUS relaxation failure with unique components of complex repetitive discharges and decelerating bursts presented in concentric needle EMG [3]. The typical feature of FS in vUDS include a large bladder capacity, reduced bladder sensation in the storage phase, decreased or no detrusor contraction with a patent bladder neck, and narrowing in the midurethra with or without ballooning of the proximal urethra [76]. The decrease in sensation and motor function in the bladder were thought to be a result of abnormally strong urethra afferent activity, which inhibits the bladder afferent signals to reach the brain as a spinal 'pro-continence' mechanism [77]. These findings are different from the pattern of the typical pattern of high-pressure low-flow in DV also caused by involuntary EUS or pelvic floor muscle contraction during voiding [78]. Whether FS is a subgroup of DV or a totally different entity remains currently unanswered.

Few studies have evaluated the effect of BoNT-A on the management of FS [55,79,80]. The first study was performed by Fowler and colleagues in 1992, where six women with FS were enrolled [79]. Two hundred units of BoNT-A (Division of Biologics, Porton Down, Salisbury, UK) were given to one side of the EUS under EMG guiding via a hollow cannula electrode. No improvements in voiding function were noted in any of the patients. One patient even developed transient stress urinary incontinence. In 2007, Liao and Kuo also reported no restoration of efficient voiding in two patients suspected to have FS with high MUP lacking a typical abnormal needle EMG pattern after injections with 100 units of Botox in four to eight EUS sites [55]. However, decreases in MUP and abdominal voiding pressure by 20 to 25 cm H_2O after injections were noted by vUDS during follow up. In contrast to the poor outcome in the aforementioned studies, a 10-patient open-level pilot study in 2016 did find promising outcomes in the management of FS using BoNT-A [80]. The injections were done with 1 mL 2% lidocaine on either side of the external urethral meatus, followed by 100 units of Botox equally divided on either side of the EUS under EMG guidance. Four of five women with complete urine retention could void spontaneously four weeks after injections. Seven of the 10 women stopped CIC ten weeks after injections. Significant improvement in the Qmax, PVR, International Prostate Symptom Score (IPSS), and urethral pressure profile were also noted at ten weeks. No serious adverse effects were reported. Clinical studies on sphincteric BoNT-A efficacy and adverse FS events are summarized in Table 3.

Due to the rarity of the disease, the difficulties associated with arriving at a definitive diagnosis that needs special equipment, the techniques required for performance, and interpretation of concentric needle EMG, these studies were all limited to a small number of patients without adequate control groups. Further large cohort studies are needed to validate these outcomes. The contradictory findings might be the result of different BoNT-A injection techniques or the different etiology behind this disease. Compared to sacral neuromodulation, BoNT-A urethra injections might serve as a less invasive, low resource, safer alternative to other methods used to treat this disease.

Table 3. Summary of clinical studies using sphincteric BoNT-A injections for patients with Fowler's syndrome (FS) and poor relaxation of the external urethral sphincter (PRES).

Author (Year)	Sex (No.)	Disease (No.)	Injection Method and Dose	UDS Improvements	Clinical Improvements (Events/Total Cases)	Adverse Events (Events/Total Cases)	Effective Duration
Studies regarding BoNT-A injection in FS							
Fowler et al. (1992) [79]	F (6)	FS (6)	Transperineal 200U BoNT-A	NA	No women restored normal micturition reflex	SUI (1/6)	NA
Liao and Kuo (2007) [55]	M (112) F (88)	FS (2) [a] Non-FS (198)	Transperineal 100U Botox	MUP	No improvement in voiding efficiency	Nil	NA
Panicker et al. (2016) [80]	F (10)	FS (10)	Transperineal 1 mL 2% lidocaine followed by 100U Botox	PVR, Qmax, MUP	IPSS improvement (8/10) Stopped CIC (7/10)	Nil	12–14 weeks
Studies regarding BoNT-A injection in PRES							
Kuo (2003) [48]	M (48) F (55)	PRES (19) Non-PRES (84)	Transurethral (M) or periurethral (F) 100U Botox	PVR	Excellent outcome (8/19) Improved outcome (7/19)	NA [b]	2–6 months
Liao and Kuo (2007) [55]	M (112) F (88)	PRES (23) Non-PRES (177)	Transurethral (M) or periurethral (F) 100U Botox	NA	Excellent outcome (12/23) Improved outcome (10/23)	Nil	NA
Kuo (2007) [25]	M (22) F (5)	PRES (5) Non-PRES (22)	Transurethral (M) or periurethral (F) 50-100U Botox	PVR, Pdet, Qmax	Significant voiding and QoL improvement [b]	Nil	NA [b]
Lee et al. (2019) [81]	M or F (155)	PRES (17) Non-PRES (138)	Transurethral (M) or periurethral (F) 100U Botox	Voiding efficiency	Improved voiding efficiency and global response assessment (8/17)	NA [b]	NA

BoNT-A = Botulinum toxin A; CIC = Clean intermittent catheterization; F = Female; FS = Fowler's syndrome; IPSS = international prostate symptom score; M = Male; MUP = Maximal urethral pressure; NA = data not accessible from the study; Nil = none; No. = number; Pdet = Detrusor contraction pressure; PRES = Poor relaxation of the external urethral sphincter; PVR = Post-void residual urine volume; Qmax = Maximal flow rate; QoL = Quality of life index; SUI = Stress urinary incontinence; UDS = Urodynamic study. None of these studies were randomized or controlled. Sphincteric injections were given with preparation other than typical BoNT-A commercial form including Botox or Disport denoted as "BoNT-A". [a] The subjects enrolled were not typical FS patients. They had a very high baseline MUP but did not have typical patterns of FS presented in a concentric needle electromyographic study. [b] Data were analyzed using combined groups. Individual results for specific disease groups were not available.

7. Urethral Sphincter BoNT-A Injections in Patients with Poor Relaxation of The External Urethral Sphincter

PRES as a diagnosis was first described by Kuo in 2000 and was determined based on non-relaxed surface EMG activity combined with a narrow membranous urethra during the voiding phase in the vUDS [82]. It was believed to have a different pathophysiology beyond prostatic obstruction or bladder neck dysfunction in non-neurogenic male voiding dysfunction refractory to alpha-blocker or transurethral resection of prostate [83,84]. The concept was further applied to non-neurogenic females with the same EMG findings and narrowing of the distal urethra in vUDS [85]. The cause of PRES was posited to be multifactorial, including learned habituation, pelvic floor hypertonicity, increased bladder sensitivity, or occult neuropathy [86]. However, the exact etiology responsible for the poor relaxation of the EUS or pelvic floor remains to be elucidated [82].

The cardinal symptoms of PRES are hesitancy, small urine caliber, and terminal dribbling with an IPSS voiding-to-storage subscore ratio >1 [82,87]. PRES is characterized by relatively small but stable bladder [88] and low-pressure low-flow during voiding phase [89], which is different from the typical high-pressure low-flow presentation in DV or extremely large, compliant bladder in FS. The prevalence rates were 12–20% [87,89,90] and 17.6% [4] in male and female non-neurogenic VD refractory to medication patients, respectively. The incidence increased in young males [89] in patients with bladder pain syndrome [88] and in idiopathic DU patients [91]. Sphincteric BoNT-A injections might provide chemo-denervation of the EUS by inhibition of acetylcholine release in the neuromuscular junction to relieve the USD in PRES [23].

The improvement rate in clinical or urodynamic parameters after injection of 100 units of BoNT-A in patients with PRES was reported to be 79 to 96% [48,55]. However, with a stricter definition of excellent outcome, only 42% of such patients had restored spontaneous voiding or had a >25% improvement in urodynamic parameters [48]. Great patient satisfaction was also reported to be approximately 47–52% [81]. It was concluded that the major predictive factors for a successful outcome were opening of the bladder neck and a higher baseline Qmax, but not the type of USD [81]. An increased recovery rate of detrusor contractility was further reported in idiopathic DU combined with PRES [25]. This result supported the hypothesis suggesting that the low-pressure low-flow dysfunction presented in PRES might be the result of detrusor suppression induced by non-relaxed EUS activity. With the aid of EUS relaxation after BoNT-A injections, the suppressed detrusor function was resumed. Clinical studies on sphincteric BoNT-A efficacy and adverse events of PRES are summarized in Table 3. Notably, most of the therapeutic effects of EUS BoNT-A injections in PRES came from studies conducted by Kuo's research group. Further work from other clinical facilities and laboratories might lead to more prudent inferences.

8. Conclusions

In recent decades, BoNT-A has been used in the treatment of VD caused by various types of USD. It has been reported to be effective in the management of DSD, DV, PRES, and has shown promise in treating FS. However, patient satisfaction might not correlate well with objective improvement. BoNT-A injections may serve as a less invasive and safer option in treatment of USD refractory to conventional medications. The mechanism by which BoNT-A improves USD is thought to be a result of a decrease in urethral resistance via inhibition of acetylcholine released in the presynaptic neuron of the EUS, and through the recovery of detrusor muscle contractility via neuromodulation. Studies focused on BoNT-A injections at the EUS have often been limited to distinct etiologies of USD. Further well-designed clinical and basic studies are needed to confirm its effect.

Author Contributions: Conceptualization, H.-C.K.; Investigation, Y.-C.O., Y.-L.K., & K.-H.H.; Project administration, Y.-L.K., Y.-C.O., & K.-H.H.; Supervision, Y.-C.O. & Y.-L.K.; Visualization, Y.-L.K. & Y.-C.O.; Writing—original draft preparation, Y.-C.O. & Y.-L.K.; Writing—review and editing, Y.-L.K., Y.-C.O., & H.-C.K.

Acknowledgments: The work was greatly enhanced by the assistance of Yung-Ming Lin.

References

1. Dmochowski, R.R. Bladder outlet obstruction: Etiology and evaluation. *Rev. Urol.* **2005**, *7* (Suppl. S6), S3–S13. [PubMed]
2. Stoffel, J.T. Detrusor sphincter dyssynergia: A review of physiology, diagnosis, and treatment strategies. *Transl. Urol.* **2016**, *5*, 127–135. [CrossRef]
3. Fowler, C.J.; Christmas, T.J.; Chapple, C.R.; Parkhouse, H.F.; Kirby, R.S.; Jacobs, H.S. Abnormal electromyographic activity of the urethral sphincter, voiding dysfunction, and polycystic ovaries: A new syndrome? *Br. Med. J. (Clin. Res. Ed.)* **1988**, *297*, 1436–1438. [CrossRef] [PubMed]
4. Peng, C.H.; Chen, S.F.; Kuo, H.C. Videourodynamic analysis of the urethral sphincter overactivity and the poor relaxing pelvic floor muscles in women with voiding dysfunction. *Neurourol. Urodyn.* **2017**, *36*, 2169–2175. [CrossRef]
5. Dykstra, D.D.; Sidi, A.A.; Scott, A.B.; Pagel, J.M.; Goldish, G.D. Effects of botulinum A toxin on detrusor-sphincter dyssynergia in spinal cord injury patients. *J. Urol.* **1988**, *139*, 919–922. [CrossRef]
6. Leippold, T.; Reitz, A.; Schurch, B. Botulinum toxin as a new therapy option for voiding disorders: Current state of the art. *Eur. Urol.* **2003**, *44*, 165–174. [CrossRef]
7. Eldred-Evans, D.; Dasgupta, P. Use of botulinum toxin for voiding dysfunction. *Transl. Urol.* **2017**, *6*, 234–251. [CrossRef]
8. Kuo, H.C. Botulinun A toxin urethral sphincter injection for neurogenic or nonneurogenic voiding dysfunction. *Tzu Chi Med. J.* **2016**, *28*, 89–93. [CrossRef]
9. Seth, J.; Rintoul-Hoad, S.; Sahai, A. Urethral Sphincter Injection of Botulinum Toxin A: A Review of Its Application and Outcomes. *Low. Urin. Tract Symptoms* **2018**, *10*, 109–115. [CrossRef]
10. Kreyden, O.P. Botulinum toxin: From poison to pharmaceutical. The history of a poison that became useful to mankind. *Curr. Probl. Dermatol.* **2002**, *30*, 94–100.
11. Br, D. Structures of botulinum neurotoxin, its functional domains, and perspectives on the cristalline type a toxin. In *Therapy with Botulinum Toxin*; Jankovic, J.H.M., Ed.; Marcel Dekker Inc.: New York, NY, USA, 1994; pp. 3–13.
12. Schantz, E.J.E. Preparation and characterization of botulinum toxin type A for human treatment. In *Therapy with Botulinum Toxin*; Jankovic, J.H.M., Ed.; Marcel Dekker Inc.: New York, NY, USA, 1994; pp. 41–49.
13. Nigam, P.K.; Nigam, A. Botulinum toxin. *Indian J. Dermatol.* **2010**, *55*, 8–14. [CrossRef] [PubMed]
14. Aoki, K.R. Pharmacology and immunology of botulinum toxin serotypes. *J. Neurol.* **2001**, *248* (Suppl. S1), 3–10. [CrossRef] [PubMed]
15. Mangera, A.; Andersson, K.E.; Apostolidis, A.; Chapple, C.; Dasgupta, P.; Giannantoni, A.; Gravas, S.; Madersbacher, S. Contemporary management of lower urinary tract disease with botulinum toxin A: A systematic review of botox (onabotulinumtoxinA) and dysport (abobotulinumtoxinA). *Eur. Urol.* **2011**, *60*, 784–795. [CrossRef]
16. Grosse, J.; Kramer, G.; Stohrer, M. Success of repeat detrusor injections of botulinum a toxin in patients with severe neurogenic detrusor overactivity and incontinence. *Eur. Urol.* **2005**, *47*, 653–659. [CrossRef]
17. Maria, G.; Cadeddu, F.; Brisinda, D.; Brandara, F.; Brisinda, G. Management of bladder, prostatic and pelvic floor disorders with botulinum neurotoxin. *Curr. Med. Chem.* **2005**, *12*, 247–265. [CrossRef]
18. Wenzel, R.; Jones, D.; Borrego, J.A. Comparing two botulinum toxin type A formulations using manufacturers' product summaries. *J. Clin. Pharm. Ther.* **2007**, *32*, 387–402. [CrossRef]
19. Dong, M.; Yeh, F.; Tepp, W.H.; Dean, C.; Johnson, E.A.; Janz, R.; Chapman, E.R. SV2 is the protein receptor for botulinum neurotoxin A. *Science* **2006**, *312*, 592–596. [CrossRef]
20. Yoshimura, N. Bladder afferent pathway and spinal cord injury: Possible mechanisms inducing hyperreflexia of the urinary bladder. *Prog. Neurobiol.* **1999**, *57*, 583–606. [CrossRef]
21. Chapple, C.; Patel, A. Botulinum toxin–new mechanisms, new therapeutic directions? *Eur. Urol.* **2006**, *49*, 606–608. [CrossRef]
22. Moore, D.C.; Cohn, J.A.; Dmochowski, R.R. Use of Botulinum Toxin A in the Treatment of Lower Urinary Tract Disorders: A Review of the Literature. *Toxins* **2016**, *8*, 88. [CrossRef]

23. Jhang, J.F.; Kuo, H.C. Botulinum Toxin A and Lower Urinary Tract Dysfunction: Pathophysiology and Mechanisms of Action. *Toxins* **2016**, *8*, 120. [CrossRef] [PubMed]
24. Smith, C.P.; Franks, M.E.; McNeil, B.K.; Ghosh, R.; de Groat, W.C.; Chancellor, M.B.; Somogyi, G.T. Effect of botulinum toxin A on the autonomic nervous system of the rat lower urinary tract. *J. Urol.* **2003**, *169*, 1896–1900. [CrossRef] [PubMed]
25. Kuo, H.C. Recovery of detrusor function after urethral botulinum a toxin injection in patients with idiopathic low detrusor contractility and voiding dysfunction. *Urology* **2007**, *69*, 57–61. [CrossRef] [PubMed]
26. De Groat, W.C.; Fraser, M.O.; Yoshiyama, M.; Smerin, S.; Tai, C.; Chancellor, M.B.; Yoshimura, N.; Roppolo, J.R. Neural control of the urethra. *Scand. J. Urol. Nephrol. Suppl.* **2001**, *35*, 35–43.
27. Panicker, J.N.; Game, X.; Khan, S.; Kessler, T.M.; Gonzales, G.; Elneil, S.; Fowler, C.J. The possible role of opiates in women with chronic urinary retention: Observations from a prospective clinical study. *J. Urol.* **2012**, *188*, 480–484. [CrossRef] [PubMed]
28. Blaivas, J.G.; Sinha, H.P.; Zayed, A.A.; Labib, K.B. Detrusor-external sphincter dyssynergia. *J. Urol.* **1981**, *125*, 542–544. [CrossRef]
29. Blaivas, J.G. The neurophysiology of micturition: A clinical study of 550 patients. *J. Urol.* **1982**, *127*, 958–963. [CrossRef]
30. Weld, K.J.; Dmochowski, R.R. Association of level of injury and bladder behavior in patients with post-traumatic spinal cord injury. *Urology* **2000**, *55*, 490–494. [CrossRef]
31. Kalita, J.; Shah, S.; Kapoor, R.; Misra, U.K. Bladder dysfunction in acute transverse myelitis: Magnetic resonance imaging and neurophysiological and urodynamic correlations. *J. Neurol. Neurosurg. Psychiatry* **2002**, *73*, 154–159. [CrossRef]
32. Litwiller, S.E.; Frohman, E.M.; Zimmern, P.E. Multiple sclerosis and the urologist. *J. Urol.* **1999**, *161*, 743–757. [CrossRef]
33. De Seze, M.; Ruffion, A.; Denys, P.; Joseph, P.A.; Perrouin-Verbe, B. The neurogenic bladder in multiple sclerosis: Review of the literature and proposal of management guidelines. *Mult. Scler.* **2007**, *13*, 915–928. [CrossRef] [PubMed]
34. Gerridzen, R.G.; Thijssen, A.M.; Dehoux, E. Risk factors for upper tract deterioration in chronic spinal cord injury patients. *J. Urol.* **1992**, *147*, 416–418. [CrossRef]
35. Abrams, P.; Amarenco, G.; Bakke, A.; Buczynski, A.; Castro-Diaz, D.; Harrison, S.; Kramer, G.; Marsik, R.; Prajsner, A.; Stohrer, M.; et al. Tamsulosin: Efficacy and safety in patients with neurogenic lower urinary tract dysfunction due to suprasacral spinal cord injury. *J. Urol.* **2003**, *170*, 1242–1251. [CrossRef] [PubMed]
36. Dmochowski, R.R.; Ganabathi, K.; Leach, G.E. Non-operative management of the urinary tract in spinal cord injury. *Neurourol. Urodyn.* **1995**, *14*, 47–55. [CrossRef]
37. Yang, C.C.; Mayo, M.E. External urethral sphincterotomy: Long-term follow-up. *Neurourol. Urodyn.* **1995**, *14*, 25–31. [CrossRef]
38. Mahfouz, W.; Corcos, J. Management of detrusor external sphincter dyssynergia in neurogenic bladder. *Eur. J. Phys. Rehabil. Med.* **2011**, *47*, 639–650.
39. Dykstra, D.D.; Sidi, A.A. Treatment of detrusor-sphincter dyssynergia with botulinum a toxin: A double-blind study. *Arch. Phys. Med. Rehabil.* **1990**, *71*, 24–26.
40. Schurch, B.; Hauri, D.; Rodic, B.; Curt, A.; Meyer, M.; Rossier, A.B. Botulinum-A toxin as a treatment of detrusor-sphincter dyssynergia: A prospective study in 24 spinal cord injury patients. *J. Urol.* **1996**, *155*, 1023–1029. [CrossRef]
41. Petit, H.; Wiart, L.; Gaujard, E.; Le Breton, F.; Ferriere, J.M.; Lagueny, A.; Joseph, P.A.; Barat, M. Botulinum A toxin treatment for detrusor-sphincter dyssynergia in spinal cord disease. *Spinal Cord* **1998**, *36*, 91–94. [CrossRef]
42. Phelan, M.W.; Franks, M.; Somogyi, G.T.; Yokoyama, T.; Fraser, M.O.; Lavelle, J.P.; Yoshimura, N.; Chancellor, M.B. Botulinum toxin urethral sphincter injection to restore bladder emptying in men and women with voiding dysfunction. *J. Urol.* **2001**, *165*, 1107–1110. [CrossRef]
43. De Seze, M.; Petit, H.; Gallien, P.; de Seze, M.P.; Joseph, P.A.; Mazaux, J.M.; Barat, M. Botulinum a toxin and detrusor sphincter dyssynergia: A double-blind lidocaine-controlled study in 13 patients with spinal cord disease. *Eur. Urol.* **2002**, *42*, 56–62. [CrossRef]

44. Gallien, P.; Reymann, J.M.; Amarenco, G.; Nicolas, B.; de Seze, M.; Bellissant, E. Placebo controlled, randomised, double blind study of the effects of botulinum A toxin on detrusor sphincter dyssynergia in multiple sclerosis patients. *J. Neurol. Neurosurg. Psychiatry* **2005**, *76*, 1670–1676. [CrossRef] [PubMed]
45. Soler, J.M.; Previnaire, J.G.; Hadiji, N. Predictors of outcome for urethral injection of botulinum toxin to treat detrusor sphincter dyssynergia in men with spinal cord injury. *Spinal Cord* **2016**, *54*, 452–456. [CrossRef] [PubMed]
46. Tsai, S.J.; Ying, T.H.; Huang, Y.H.; Cheng, J.W.; Bih, L.I.; Lew, H.L. Transperineal injection of botulinum toxin A for treatment of detrusor sphincter dyssynergia: Localization with combined fluoroscopic and electromyographic guidance. *Arch. Phys. Med. Rehabil.* **2009**, *90*, 832–836. [CrossRef] [PubMed]
47. Chen, S.L.; Bih, L.I.; Chen, G.D.; Huang, Y.H.; You, Y.H.; Lew, H.L. Transrectal ultrasound-guided transperineal botulinum toxin a injection to the external urethral sphincter for treatment of detrusor external sphincter dyssynergia in patients with spinal cord injury. *Arch. Phys. Med. Rehabil.* **2010**, *91*, 340–344. [CrossRef] [PubMed]
48. Kuo, H.C. Botulinum A toxin urethral injection for the treatment of lower urinary tract dysfunction. *J. Urol.* **2003**, *170*, 1908–1912. [CrossRef]
49. Smith, C.P.; Nishiguchi, J.; O'Leary, M.; Yoshimura, N.; Chancellor, M.B. Single-institution experience in 110 patients with botulinum toxin A injection into bladder or urethra. *Urology* **2005**, *65*, 37–41. [CrossRef]
50. Chen, S.L.; Bih, L.I.; Huang, Y.H.; Tsai, S.J.; Lin, T.B.; Kao, Y.L. Effect of single botulinum toxin A injection to the external urethral sphincter for treating detrusor external sphincter dyssynergia in spinal cord injury. *J. Rehabil. Med.* **2008**, *40*, 744–748. [CrossRef]
51. Kuo, H.C. Satisfaction with urethral injection of botulinum toxin A for detrusor sphincter dyssynergia in patients with spinal cord lesion. *Neurourol. Urodyn.* **2008**, *27*, 793–796. [CrossRef]
52. Kuo, H.C. Therapeutic outcome and quality of life between urethral and detrusor botulinum toxin treatment for patients with spinal cord lesions and detrusor sphincter dyssynergia. *Int. J. Clin. Pract.* **2013**, *67*, 1044–1049. [CrossRef]
53. Huang, M.; Chen, H.; Jiang, C.; Xie, K.; Tang, P.; Ou, R.; Zeng, J.; Liu, Q.; Li, Q.; Huang, J.; et al. Effects of botulinum toxin A injections in spinal cord injury patients with detrusor overactivity and detrusor sphincter dyssynergia. *J. Rehabil. Med.* **2016**, *48*, 683–687. [CrossRef] [PubMed]
54. Kuo, H.-C. Comparison of the Therapeutic Effects of Urethral Injections of 50 and 100 Units of Botulinum A Toxin for Voiding Dysfunction. *Tzu Chi Med. J.* **2007**, *19*, 134–138. [CrossRef]
55. Liao, Y.M.; Kuo, H.C. Causes of failed urethral botulinum toxin a treatment for emptying failure. *Urology* **2007**, *70*, 763–766. [CrossRef]
56. Austin, P.F.; Bauer, S.B.; Bower, W.; Chase, J.; Franco, I.; Hoebeke, P.; Rittig, S.; Walle, J.V.; von Gontard, A.; Wright, A.; et al. The standardization of terminology of lower urinary tract function in children and adolescents: Update report from the standardization committee of the International Children's Continence Society. *Neurourol. Urodyn.* **2016**, *35*, 471–481. [CrossRef]
57. Hinman, F.; Baumann, F.W. Vesical and ureteral damage from voiding dysfunction in boys without neurologic or obstructive disease. *J. Urol.* **1973**, *109*, 727–732. [CrossRef]
58. Allen, T.D. The non-neurogenic neurogenic bladder. *J. Urol.* **1977**, *117*, 232–238. [CrossRef]
59. Hinman, F., Jr. Nonneurogenic neurogenic bladder (the Hinman syndrome)–15 years later. *J. Urol.* **1986**, *136*, 769–777. [CrossRef]
60. Groutz, A.; Blaivas, J.G.; Pies, C.; Sassone, A.M. Learned voiding dysfunction (non-neurogenic, neurogenic bladder) among adults. *Neurourol. Urodyn.* **2001**, *20*, 259–268. [CrossRef]
61. Sinha, S. Dysfunctional voiding: A review of the terminology, presentation, evaluation and management in children and adults. *Indian J. Urol. IJU J. Urol. Soc. India* **2011**, *27*, 437–447. [CrossRef]
62. Chase, J.; Austin, P.; Hoebeke, P.; McKenna, P. The management of dysfunctional voiding in children: A report from the Standardisation Committee of the International Children's Continence Society. *J. Urol.* **2010**, *183*, 1296–1302. [CrossRef]
63. Nelson, J.D.; Cooper, C.S.; Boyt, M.A.; Hawtrey, C.E.; Austin, J.C. Improved uroflow parameters and post-void residual following biofeedback therapy in pediatric patients with dysfunctional voiding does not correspond to outcome. *J. Urol.* **2004**, *172*, 1653–1656. [CrossRef] [PubMed]
64. Austin, P.F.; Homsy, Y.L.; Masel, J.L.; Cain, M.P.; Casale, A.J.; Rink, R.C. alpha-Adrenergic blockade in children with neuropathic and nonneuropathic voiding dysfunction. *J. Urol.* **1999**, *162*, 1064–1067. [CrossRef]

65. Steinhardt, G.F.; Naseer, S.; Cruz, O.A. Botulinum toxin: Novel treatment for dramatic urethral dilatation associated with dysfunctional voiding. *J. Urol.* **1997**, *158*, 190–191. [CrossRef] [PubMed]
66. Mokhless, I.; Gaafar, S.; Fouda, K.; Shafik, M.; Assem, A. Botulinum A toxin urethral sphincter injection in children with nonneurogenic neurogenic bladder. *J. Urol.* **2006**, *176*, 1767–1770. [CrossRef]
67. Franco, I.; Landau-Dyer, L.; Isom-Batz, G.; Collett, T.; Reda, E.F. The use of botulinum toxin A injection for the management of external sphincter dyssynergia in neurologically normal children. *J. Urol.* **2007**, *178*, 1775–1779. [CrossRef]
68. Vricella, G.J.; Campigotto, M.; Coplen, D.E.; Traxel, E.J.; Austin, P.F. Long-term efficacy and durability of botulinum-A toxin for refractory dysfunctional voiding in children. *J. Urol.* **2014**, *191*, 1586–1591. [CrossRef]
69. 't Hoen, L.A.; van den Hoek, J.; Wolffenbuttel, K.P.; van der Toorn, F.; Scheepe, J.R. Breaking the vicious circle: Onabotulinum toxin A in children with therapy-refractory dysfunctional voiding. *J. Pediatric Urol.* **2015**, *11*, 119. [CrossRef]
70. Petronijevic, V.; Lazovic, M.; Vlajkovic, M.; Slavkovic, A.; Golubovic, E.; Miljkovic, P. Botulinum toxin type A in combination with standard urotherapy for children with dysfunctional voiding. *J. Urol.* **2007**, *178*, 2599–2602. [CrossRef]
71. Jiang, Y.H.; Wang, C.C.; Kuo, H.C. OnabotulinumtoxinA Urethral Sphincter Injection as Treatment for Non-neurogenic Voiding Dysfunction—A Randomized, Double-Blind, Placebo-Controlled Study. *Sci. Rep.* **2016**, *6*, 38905. [CrossRef]
72. Morin, F.; Akhavizadegan, H.; Kavanagh, A.; Moore, K. Dysfunctional voiding: Challenges of disease transition from childhood to adulthood. *Can. Urol. Assoc. J.* **2018**, *12*, S42–S47. [CrossRef]
73. D'Ancona, C.; Haylen, B.; Oelke, M.; Abranches-Monteiro, L.; Arnold, E.; Goldman, H.; Hamid, R.; Homma, Y.; Marcelissen, T.; Rademakers, K.; et al. The International Continence Society (ICS) report on the terminology for adult male lower urinary tract and pelvic floor symptoms and dysfunction. *Neurourol. Urodyn.* **2019**, *38*, 433–477. [CrossRef]
74. Unverzagt, C.; Berglund, K.; Thomas, J.J. Dry needling for myofascial trigger point pain: A clinical commentary. *Int. J. Sports Phys.* **2015**, *10*, 402–418.
75. Fowler, C.J.; Kirby, R.S. Electromyography of urethral sphincter in women with urinary retention. *Lancet (Lond. Engl.)* **1986**, *1*, 1455–1457. [CrossRef]
76. DasGupta, R.; Fowler, C.J. Urodynamic study of women in urinary retention treated with sacral neuromodulation. *J. Urol.* **2004**, *171*, 1161–1164. [CrossRef]
77. Osman, N.I.; Chapple, C.R. Fowler's syndrome—A cause of unexplained urinary retention in young women? *Nat. Rev. Urol.* **2014**, *11*, 87–98. [CrossRef]
78. Haylen, B.T.; de Ridder, D.; Freeman, R.M.; Swift, S.E.; Berghmans, B.; Lee, J.; Monga, A.; Petri, E.; Rizk, D.E.; Sand, P.K.; et al. An International Urogynecological Association (IUGA)/International Continence Society (ICS) joint report on the terminology for female pelvic floor dysfunction. *Neurourol. Urodyn.* **2010**, *29*, 4–20. [CrossRef]
79. Fowler, C.J.; Betts, C.D.; Christmas, T.J.; Swash, M.; Fowler, C.G. Botulinum toxin in the treatment of chronic urinary retention in women. *Br. J. Urol.* **1992**, *70*, 387–389. [CrossRef]
80. Panicker, J.N.; Seth, J.H.; Khan, S.; Gonzales, G.; Haslam, C.; Kessler, T.M.; Fowler, C.J. Open-label study evaluating outpatient urethral sphincter injections of onabotulinumtoxinA to treat women with urinary retention due to a primary disorder of sphincter relaxation (Fowler's syndrome). *BJU Int.* **2016**, *117*, 809–813. [CrossRef]
81. Lee, Y.K.; Kuo, H.C. Therapeutic Effects of Botulinum Toxin A, via Urethral Sphincter Injection on Voiding Dysfunction Due to Different Bladder and Urethral Sphincter Dysfunctions. *Toxins* **2019**, *11*, 487. [CrossRef]
82. Kuo, H.C. Pathophysiology of lower urinary tract symptoms in aged men without bladder outlet obstruction. *Urol. Int.* **2000**, *64*, 86–92. [CrossRef]
83. Ke, Q.S.; Jiang, Y.H.; Kuo, H.C. Role of Bladder Neck and Urethral Sphincter Dysfunction in Men with Persistent Bothersome Lower Urinary Tract Symptoms after alpha-1 Blocker Treatment. *Low. Urin. Tract Symptoms* **2015**, *7*, 143–148. [CrossRef]
84. Kuo, H.C. Analysis of the pathophysiology of lower urinary tract symptoms in patients after prostatectomy. *Urol. Int.* **2002**, *68*, 99–104. [CrossRef] [PubMed]
85. Hsiao, S.M.; Lin, H.H.; Kuo, H.C. Videourodynamic Studies of Women with Voiding Dysfunction. *Sci. Rep.* **2017**, *7*, 6845. [CrossRef] [PubMed]

86. Shao, I.H.; Kuo, H.C. Role of poor urethral sphincter relaxation in men with voiding dysfunction refractory to alpha-blocker therapy: Clinical characteristics and predictive factors. *Low. Urin. Tract Symptoms* **2019**, *11*, 8–13. [CrossRef] [PubMed]
87. Liao, C.H.; Chung, S.D.; Kuo, H.C. Diagnostic value of International Prostate Symptom Score voiding-to-storage subscore ratio in male lower urinary tract symptoms. *Int. J. Clin. Pract.* **2011**, *65*, 552–558. [CrossRef]
88. Kuo, Y.C.; Kuo, H.C. Videourodynamic characteristics of interstitial cystitis/bladder pain syndrome-The role of bladder outlet dysfunction in the pathophysiology. *Neurourol. Urodyn.* **2018**, *37*, 1971–1977. [CrossRef]
89. Kuo, H.C. Videourodynamic analysis of pathophysiology of men with both storage and voiding lower urinary tract symptoms. *Urology* **2007**, *70*, 272–276. [CrossRef]
90. Jiang, Y.H.; Liao, C.H.; Kuo, H.C. Role of Bladder Dysfunction in Men with Lower Urinary Tract Symptoms Refractory to Alpha-blocker Therapy: A Video-urodynamic Analysis. *Low. Urin. Tract Symptoms* **2018**, *10*, 32–37. [CrossRef]
91. Jiang, Y.H.; Kuo, H.C. Video-urodynamic characteristics of non-neurogenic, idiopathic underactive bladder in men—A comparison of men with normal tracing and bladder outlet obstruction. *PLoS ONE* **2017**, *12*, e0174593. [CrossRef]

12

Promise and the Pharmacological Mechanism of Botulinum Toxin A in Chronic Prostatitis Syndrome

Chien-Hsu Chen [1], Pradeep Tyagi [2] and Yao-Chi Chuang [1,*]

1 Department of Urology 1, Kaohsiung Chang Gung Memorial Hospital, Chang Gung University College of Medicine, Kaohsiung 83301, Taiwan; kenkochen@yahoo.com.tw
2 Department of Urology, University of Pittsburgh School of Medicine2, Pittsburgh, PA 15213, USA; tyagpradeep@gmail.com
* Correspondence: chuang82@ms26.hinet.net

Abstract: Chronic prostatitis/chronic pelvic pain syndrome (CP/CPPS) has a negative impact on the quality of life, and its etiology still remains unknown. Although many treatment protocols have been evaluated in CP/CPPS, the outcomes have usually been disappointing. Botulinum neurotoxin A (BoNT-A), produced from *Clostridium botulinum*, has been widely used to lower urinary tract dysfunctions such as detrusor sphincter dyssynergia, refractory overactive bladder, interstitial cystitis/bladder pain syndromes, benign prostatic hyperplasia, and CP/CPPS in urology. Here, we review the published evidence from animal models to clinical studies for inferring the mechanism of action underlying the therapeutic efficacy of BoNT in CP/CPPS. Animal studies demonstrated that BoNT-A, a potent inhibitor of neuroexocytosis, impacts the release of sensory neurotransmitters and inflammatory mediators. This pharmacological action of BoNT-A showed promise of relieving the pain of CP/CPPS in placebo-controlled and open-label BoNT-A and has the potential to serve as an adjunct treatment for achieving better treatment outcomes in CP/CPPS patients.

Keywords: botulinum toxin; chronic prostatitis

Key Contribution: This article reviewed basic research and the clinical results of botulinum toxin A in patients with CP/CPPS and suggested the potential to improve the therapeutic outcome.

---

1. Introduction

Chronic prostatitis describes a constellation of complaints such as pain in the perineum, genitalia, pelvis, or lower abdomen, ejaculation pain, or irritative/voiding urinary symptoms [1,2]. In 1995, National Institutes of Health (NIH) developed a consensus on the general definition and classification of prostatitis, chronic prostatitis/chronic pelvic pain syndrome (CP/CPPS) as the "presence of genitourinary pain in the absence of uropathogenic bacteria as detected by standard microbiologic methodology" [3]. This disease has negatively affected the quality of life in 5–10% of the adult males of North America; however, the etiology is still largely unknown [4,5].

2. Current Understanding of CP/CPPS Pathophysiology

Considering that CP/CPPS symptoms are not localized to a singular organ, there is mounting evidence to support that symptoms emanate from the interplay between multiple organ systems. Several possible mechanisms are postulated to cause referred pain of CP/CPPS, prominent among them is neurogenic inflammation that describes activation of prostate afferent nerves by prostate inflammation [6]. The constellation of CP/CPPS symptoms necessitates multimodal treatment approaches including α-blockers, antimuscarinics, anti-inflammatory agents, or muscle relaxants [7]. However, the failure of most approaches to effectively treat patients with chronic prostatitis is a source of great frustration. Thus, it is necessary to develop new therapy for patients with refractory CP/CPPS. The clinicians should not only pay attention to urological complaints but also evaluate if the co-existence of nonurological symptoms in the anorectal area, genital region or beyond these areas. Previous studies demonstrated the possible association between chronic pelvic pain and other chronic pain conditions such as irritable bowel syndrome. There are three proposed explanations for these conditions, including physiological dysfunction, victimization, and psychological distress [8,9]. Examining these factors perhaps can clarify the relationship between these comorbidities.

3. Botulinum Neurotoxin (BoNT)

BoNT is a potent toxin isolated from *Clostridium botulinum*, which can cleave SNAP-25 and block the release of some neurotransmitters (e.g., acetylcholine) from pre-junctional nerves at the neuromuscular junction. This toxin has been widely used to treat muscle dysfunction, such as strabismus [10]. In urology, more and more studies have focused on the application of BoNTs in detrusor sphincter dyssynergia (DSD) [11,12], overactive bladder (OAB) [13,14], interstitial cystitis/bladder pain syndromes [15,16], benign prostatic hyperplasia (BPH) [17–20], and CP/CPPS [14,16,21] over the past decade. Growing evidence suggests that inhibition of exocytotic machinery by BoNT-A could modulate sensory processing, inflammation and glandular function [22–26]. To date, BoNT-A have been listed as a third-line treatment for refractory OAB [27] and fourth-line for interstitial cystitis/bladder pain syndromes [28] in the American Urology Association (AUA) guidelines. However, the application of BoNT-A for patients with prostate disorders is still under off-label use. In this article, we reviewed published literature documenting mechanisms of action, basic research and the clinical use of botulinum toxin in CP/CPPS from Pubmed and used botulinum toxin, chronic prostatitis, and chronic pelvic pain as search terms. In addition to published studies, we also gathered some abstracts presented at international meetings.

4. Mechanisms of Botulinum Neurotoxins (BoNTs)

BoNT is produced by *Clostridium botulinum*, a Gram-positive anaerobic bacterium. BoNT includes seven kinds of antigenically distinct neurotoxins (A~G) [29,30]. Among them, BoNT-A is the most commonly used serotype in clinics with the most durable effect [13].

BoNT-A is synthesized as an inactive form of 1285 amino acids and becomes activated when it is cleaved into a light chain (50-kDa) and a heavy chain (100-kDa). Unique binding of BoNT to nerve terminals occurs due to their ability to interact with two independent receptors of the presynaptic membrane: a polysialoganglioside (PSG) and a glycosylated luminal domain of a synaptic vesicle protein that mediates BoNT internalization [30]. The mechanism of denervation by BoNT is divided into five steps: (1) binding to nerve terminals, (2) internalization within an endocytic compartment, (3) low pH-driven translocation of the L chain across the vesicle membrane, (4) release of the L chain in the cytosol by reduction of the interchain disulfide bond, and (5) cleavage of SNAREs for ensuing the blockade of neurotransmitter release and consequent neuroparalysis [29–31].

5. The Rationale for BoNT-A Application in Chronic Prostatitis

BoNT-A causes muscle relaxation by blocking the release of acetylcholine.

BoNT-A has been well known to have paralyzing effects via the blockage of acetylcholine release at the presynaptic cholinergic neuromuscular junction. The inhibitory effects of BoNT-A on both somatic and autonomic nerves have been used to treat a variety of conditions associated with muscularhypercontractility. Intramuscular injection of BoNT-A could lead to temporary chemodenervation and muscle relaxation in both striated and smooth muscles [29,30]. In 1988, Dykstra et al. first treated 11 patients with DSD due to spinal cord injury (SCI) by using urethral sphincter injection of BoNT-A [11]. In a prospective study using 100 U of BoNT-A injection into the urethral sphincter to treat patients with spinal cord lesions and DSD, decreased voiding detrusor pressure and increased maximum flow rate were observed [12]; 60.6% of patients felt satisfied with the outcomes but post-injection urinary incontinence was another concern.

Huang et al. conducted a prospective multicentre trial with a total of 59 SCI patients having both detrusor overactivity (DO) and DSD. All the patients simultaneously received intravesical (200 U) and urethral sphincter (100 U) injections of BoNT-A [32]. This trial demonstrated significant reductions in maximum detrusor pressure, urinary incontinence episode, and improvement in voiding volume after treatment. All patients could achieve complete dryness at the follow-up point of 2 weeks. In view of the effect of BoNT-A on smooth muscle relaxation, the therapeutic response in DO has been widely studied. In 2000, Schurch et al. first reported the injection of BoNT-A (200 to 300 U) into detrusor muscle to treat patients with neurogenic DO [33]. At the 6-week follow up, 17 of 19 (89%) patients achieved complete continence. Significantly increased maximum bladder capacity and decreased maximum detrusor voiding pressure were observed after injection. To date, intravesical BoNT-A injection has become the preferred option for refractory OAB and neurogenic DO.

In addition to the role in blocking motor neurons, BoNT-A also has effects on the modulation of sensory nerves and inflammation as evinced by animal studies (Figure 1). A large body of evidence now supports that BoNT-A achieves analgesic effect by hindering the release of mediators responsible for painful sensation, including nerve growth factor (NGF), substance P, calcitonin gene-related peptide (CGRP), glutamate, as well as adenosine triphosphate (ATP) involved in afferent neurotransmission [22,23]. Therefore, it is postulated that BoNT-A may relieve the pain associated with chronic prostatitis by inhibiting the abnormal nociceptive neurotransmission conveyed by prostatic afferent nerves. Sensory dysfunction may be one of the postulated causes driving the symptoms of chronic prostatitis [6].

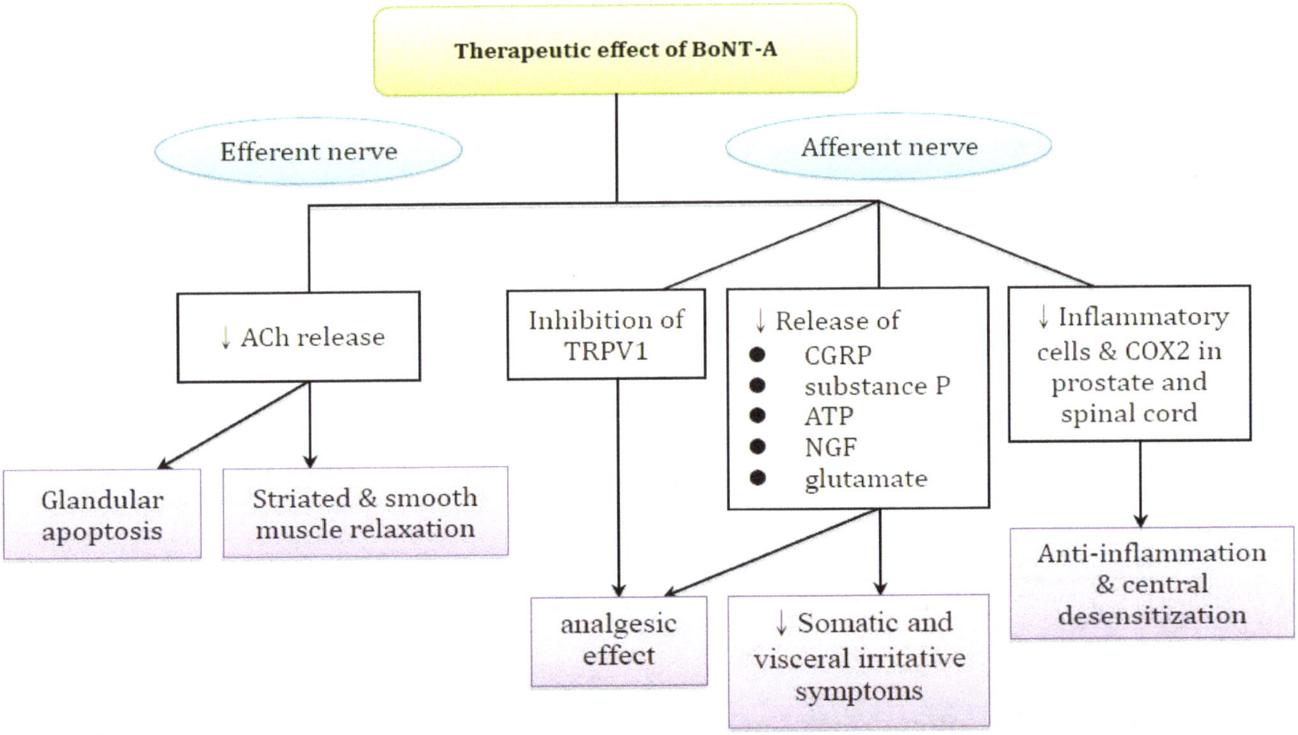

Figure 1. Conceivable mechanisms of BoNT-A in the treatment of CP/CPPS.

Transient Receptor Potential Vanilloid 1 (TRPV1), a non-selective cation channel, is expressed in some primary afferent neurons [34], especially in small and medium diameters (e.g., C-fibers) that are responsible for neurogenic pain and inflammation development [35]. In humans, TRPV1 activation might result in a burning pain sensation in the lower urinary tract [36]. Dinis et al. have demonstrated that abundant TRPV1 innervation are located on the prostatic urethral mucosa, verumontanum, and ejaculatory ducts [37]. Using rats in an adjuvant-arthritis pain model, Fan et al. reported that BoNT-A exerts its antinociceptive effect by reducing TRPV1 protein expression via the inhibition of plasma membrane trafficking [38]. Taken together, BoNT-A might play an important role in inhibiting TRPV1 expression in human prostate, which provides an alternative therapeutic strategy for CP/CPPS.

Regarding the anti-inflammatory effect, Chuang et al. reported that BoNT-A significantly decreased painful behavior, inflammatory cell accumulation, and cyclooxygenase (COX)-2 expression in the prostate and L6 spinal cord in dose-dependent fashion in a rat model of capsaicin-induced prostatitis [24,25]. This finding demonstrates the potential of BoNT-A in the treatment of prostate inflammation.

6. Clinical Studies in BoNT-A for CP/CPPS Treatment

Table 1 summarized the clinical studies of BoNT-A intraprostatic injection for chronic prostatitis. Maria el al. first reported the transperineal injection of 30 U BoNT-A into prostatic apex to treat the voiding problem in patients with chronic prostatitis in 1998 [39]. In their series, three of four patients obtained improvement in voiding without urinary incontinence with a mean follow-up duration of 12 months.

Table 1. Clinical studies of BoNT-A intraprostatic injection for chronic prostatitis.

	Maria et al. [39]	Park et al. [40]	Gottsch el al. [41]	Falahatkar et al. [42]	Abdel-Meguid et al. [43]	El-Enen et al. [44]
No. pts	4	84	29	60	43	63
Study design	prospective	prospective	randomized placebo-controlled	prospective, randomized, double-blind	Prospective two-group controlled	uncontrolled random-ised
Duration of followup (mo)	12	—	1	6	12	12
Patient criteria	spastic external urethral sphincter with poor respond to α-blocker for more than 4 months	CPPS, category IIIB	CPPS	NIH-CPSI scores ≥10 and pain subscores ≥8, refractory to 4–6 weeks' medical therapy	refractory CP/CPPS	CP/CPPS, aged <50years, symptom duration of >2 years
BONT dose (U)	30 U	transrectal (40 U) or transperineal (200 U)	100U	prostate volumes <30 mL (100 U), 30–60 mL (200 U)	200U	100U
Injection route	transperineal	transrectal (78), transperineal (6)	transperineal	transurethral	transurethral	transurethral (28), transrectal (35)
Needle gauge	26	—	—	23	—	22
Outcomes	decrease in times of urinary flow and maximum urinary flow	NIH-CPSI improvement: transrectal (59%) and transperineal (50%). Durations of effectiveness: 6 to 18 months	Global Response Assessment (GRA): 30% response rate at 1-month; Only CPSI pain subscore reached significant improvement compared with controls	NIH-CPSI pain subdomain and the VAS scores decreased by 79.9% and 82.1% at 6-month follow-up, respectively	≥ 6 points reductions of total score of NIH-CPSI were 72.1% and 37.2% at 3 and 12 mo, respectively	good response in small prostate, short symptom duration, or transrectal route

CP/CPPS, Chronic prostatitis/chronic pelvic pain syndrome; NIH-CPSI, National Institutes of Health Chronic Prostatitis Symptom Index; AUA-SS, American Urological Association-symptom score; VAS, visual analogue scale; QoL, quality of life; "—" indicates "not available"

Park et al. reported intraprostatic BoNT-A injection in 84 patients with CPPS using transrectal (40 U, $n = 78$) or transperineal (200 U, $n = 6$) route [40]. Symptom improvement was found in 59% of patients with transrectal injection and in 50% with transperineal route. By the National Institutes of Health Chronic Prostatitis Symptom Index (NIH-CPSI) questionnaire, the most significant improvement was in the pain domain, followed by ejaculation-related pain. The therapeutic effect was sustained for 6~18 months. The NIH-CPSI is a 13-item questionnaire developed to assess symptoms and quality of life (QoL) in men with CP/CPPS. This questionnaire includes three domains evaluating pain, urinary complaints, and QoL.

Gottsch el al. conducted a randomized placebo-controlled study to evaluate the effect of BoNT-A (100 U) injection into perineal body and bulbospongiosus muscle for CPPS treatment [41]. One month after treatment, the response rate assessed by Global Response Assessment (GRA) was significantly better in the BoNT-A group than the placebo group (30% vs. 13%, $p = 0.0002$). Although the NIH-CPSI pain subdomain was also significantly improved in the BoNT-A group, the total NIH-CPSI score did not improve.

In a prospective, randomized, double-blind, placebo-controlled trial on transurethral intraprostatic injection of BoNT-A (100 U) for men with chronic prostatitis, Falahatkar et al. demonstrated that BoNT-A treatment group significantly improved the NIH-CPSI total and subscale scores, the American Urological Association-symptom score (AUA-SS), visual analogue scale (VAS), quality of life, and frequencies of diurnal and nocturnal urinations when compared to baseline. The most noticeable improvement was the NIH-CPSI pain subdomain and the VAS scores, which decreased by 79.9% and 82.1% at 6-month follow-up, respectively [42].

Recently, another prospective controlled study using transurethral intraprostatic injection of BoNT-A (200 U) in 43 patients also showed encouraging response rates for refractory nonbacterial CP/CPPS [43]. However, the therapeutic effect gradually declined at 9–12 months.

As for the optimal injection route into the prostate, including transurethral, transperineal, and transrectal approaches, there is no definite suggestion so far. El-Enen et al. compared the transurethral route with transrectal intraprostatic BoNT-A injection for refractory CP/CPPS [44]. More significant improvement was observed in the transrectal group during the follow-up points. Their data also showed better results for BoNT-A injection in men with small prostates. Controversially, the aforementioned study showed that activation of TRPV1 might be one of the possible etiologies in CP/CPPS [36]. TRPV1-immunoreactive nerve fibers are distributed throughout the prostatic urethra mucosa, verumontanum, ejaculatory duct, and periurethral prostatic acini [37]. It is plausible that instead of transrectal injection, transurethral BoNT-A injection may be able to target TRPV1-immunoreactive nerve fibers as not only TRPV1-immunoreactive nerve fibers but other nerve fibers distributed in the transitional and peripheral zones may affect the efficacy of different injection routes. In addition, the drug extravasation out of the target site after injection is also an interesting issue to be discussed [45]. Further randomized and large-scale comparative studies are needed to evaluate the efficacy of different injection routes. The potential injection sites of BoNT-A for CP/CPPS treatment are shown in Figure 2.

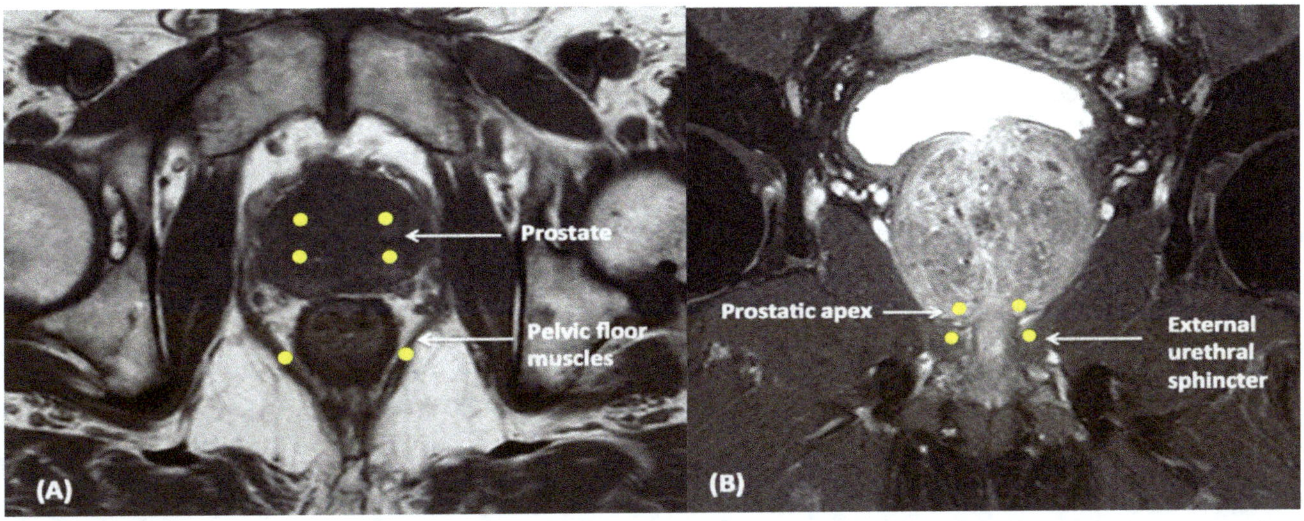

Figure 2. The potential injection sites of BoNT-A for CP/CPPS treatment: intraprostatic, prostatic apex, external urethral sphincter, and pelvic floor muscles. (**A**) MRI, axial view (**B**) MRI, coronal view.

BoNT-A injection targeting at prostate and surrounding tissue is a safe procedure when administered by an experienced injector. Side effects are always transient, like local pain, hematuria, and urinary tract infection, and in the majority of cases they are mild and tolerable [17,19,20].

7. Potential Impact of BoNT-A Injection on: The UPOINT Phenotype System

Clinically, it is challenging to achieve satisfactory outcomes for CP/CPPS treatment. In most cases, monotherapy has failed to successfully treat CP/CPPS, largely because of the heterogeneous nature due to multiple factors involved in the pathogenesis of CP/CPPS, such as pelvic floor muscle dysfunction, chemical irritants, as well as neurological and immunological factors. With these unsatisfactory treatment responses, combination therapies and individual consideration provide another way to improve the efficacy of treating patients with CP/CPPS. In 2009, Shoskes et al. developed the UPOINT system to classify patients with CP/CPPS to help clinicians understand the etiology and more importantly, to guide the treatment [46]. The UPOINT phenotype system includes six domains to evaluate and manage CP/CPPS: **U**rinary symptoms, **P**sychosocial dysfunction, **O**rgan-specific findings, **I**nfection, **N**eurologic/systemic complaints, and **T**enderness. Each domain has been related to specific mechanisms and treatments [7]. Patients with "urinary" complaints (storage, voiding symptoms or much post-void residual urine) can be treated with α-blocker, diet modification, and/or antimuscarinics. Intraprostatic BoNT-A can also relieve urinary symptoms [17,19,20]. "Psychosocial" patients with depression or catastrophizing evidence can be managed with counseling, cognitive behavioral therapy, antidepressants, or stress reduction. In the "organ-specific" group presenting with tenderness on prostate, increased leukocytes in prostatic fluid, blood in semen, or prostatic calcifications, some anti-inflammatory agents such as quercetin can be considered. BoNT-A has been shown to have effects on the inhibition of COX-2 expression in a preclinical prostatitis models [24,25], from which beneficial effects might reduce prostate inflammation in human CP/CPPS. Patients with "infection" (exclusion of NIH category I or II prostatitis) can be treated with antibiotics. "Neurologic/systemic" patients usually present with pain beyond abdomen and pelvis or other complaints, such as irritable bowel syndrome, fibromyalgia or chronic fatigue syndrome. In these kinds of patients, neuroleptic medications can be used to relieve symptoms. In the domain of "tenderness", trigger points may be noted in the abdomen or pelvic floor, and treatments may include muscle relaxants use, pelvic floor physical therapy (PFPT), low-intensity shock wave, or PFPT in combination with adjuvant trigger point injection [47,48]. BoNT-A injection targeting at the pelvic muscle or trigger point might ameliorate the symptom of tenderness. Using the UPOINT system in classifying patients with CP/CPPS can facilitate hypothesis testing for possible etiologies and treatment. Shoskes et al. found that the number of positive domains was associated with severity and duration of complaints [46]. Their group also conducted a prospective study using UPOINT approach in treating 100 patients with CPPS. Eighty-four percent of patients had at least a 6-point improvement in NIH-CPSI at a median follow-up of 50 weeks [49]. Similarly, another prospective study of 140 Chinese men with CP/CPPS based on the UPOINT approach also showed a 75% response rate with a follow-up of 6 months [50]. Taken together, increasing evidence has shown that the UPOINT phenotype system is feasible and effective to clinical physicians in treating CP/CPPS. The BoNT-A prostate and pelvic muscle injection might have direct or indirect effects on the domains of **U**rinary symptoms, **P**sychosocial dysfunction, **O**rgan-specific findings, **N**eurologic/systemic complaints, and **T**enderness.

8. Conclusions

From basic research, it is reasonable to treat CP/CPPS with intraprostatic BoNT-A injection, based on its effects on sensory neurotransmitters and inflammation. Clinical studies have shown that results of BoNT-A treatment for CP/CPPS are promising. The most prominent improvement was on the pain subdomain of NIH-CPSI. However, the evidence is still limited and the application of BoNT-A for CP/CPPS is off-label use. Further larger randomized and placebo-controlled studies with longer follow-up periods are necessary to draw a solid conclusion.

Author Contributions: C.-H.C. and Y.-C.C. conceived and designed the ideas and article structure; C.-H.C. analyzed the data; C.-H.C. wrote the paper. Y.-C.C. and P.T. revised the paper.

References

1. Magistro, G.; Wagenlehner, F.M.; Grabe, M.; Weidner, W.; Stief, C.G.; Nickel, J.C. Contemporary management of chronic prostatitis/chronic pelvic pain syndrome. *Eur. Urol.* **2016**, *69*, 286–297. [CrossRef] [PubMed]
2. Polackwich, A.S.; Shoskes, D.A. Chronic prostatitis/chronic pelvic pain syndrome: A review of evaluation and therapy. *Prostate Cancer Prostatic Dis.* **2016**, *19*, 132–138. [CrossRef] [PubMed]
3. Krieger, J.N.; Nyberg, L.; Nickel, J.C. NIH consensus definition and classification of prostatitis. *JAMA* **1999**, *282*, 236–237. [CrossRef] [PubMed]
4. Nickel, J.C.; Downey, J.; Hunter, D.; Clark, J. Prevalence of pros-tatitis-like symptoms in a population-based study employing the National Institute of Health chronic pros- tatitis symptom index. *J. Urol.* **2001**, *165*, 842–845. [CrossRef]
5. Schaeffer, A. Etiology and management of chronic pelvic pain syndrome in men. *Urology* **2004**, *63*, 75–84. [CrossRef] [PubMed]
6. Pontari, M.A.; Ruggieri, M.R. Mechanism in prostatitis/chronic pelvic pain syndrome. *J. Urol.* **2004**, *172*, 839–845. [CrossRef]
7. DeWitt-Foy, M.E.; Nickel, J.C.; Shoskes, D.A. Management of Chronic Prostatitis/Chronic Pelvic Pain Syndrome. *Eur. Urol. Focus.* **2019**, *5*, 2–4. [CrossRef]
8. Rodríguez, M.Á.B.; Afari, N.; Buchwald, D.S.; National Institute of Diabetes and Digestive and Kidney Diseases Working Group on Urological Chronic Pelvic Pain. Evidence for overlap between urological and nonurological unexplained clinical conditions. *J. Urol.* **2009**, *182*, 2123–2131.
9. Rodríguez, M.Á.B.; Afari, N.; Buchwald, D.S.; National Institute of Diabetes and Digestive and Kidney Diseases Working Group on Urological Chronic Pelvic Pain. Evidence for overlap between urological and nonurological unexplained clinical conditions. *J. Urol.* **2013**, *189*, S66–S74.
10. Scott, A.B. Botulinum toxin injection of eye muscles to correct strabismus. *Trans. Am. Ophthalmol. Soc.* **1981**, *79*, 734–770.
11. Dykstra, D.D.; Sidi, A.A.; Scott, A.B.; Pagel, J.M.; Goldish, G.D. Effects of botulinum A toxin on detrusor-sphincter dyssynergia in spinal cord injury patients. *J. Urol.* **1988**, *139*, 919–922. [CrossRef]
12. Kuo, H.C. Satisfaction with urethral injection of botulinum toxin A for detrusor sphincter dyssynergia in patients with spinal cord lesion. *Neurourol. Urodyn.* **2008**, *27*, 793–796. [CrossRef] [PubMed]
13. Chuang, Y.C.; Kuo, H.C.; Chancellor, M.B. Botulinum toxin for the lower urinary tract. *BJU Int.* **2010**, *105*, 1046–1058. [CrossRef] [PubMed]
14. Jhang, J.F.; Kuo, H.C. Novel Applications of OnabotulinumtoxinA in Lower Urinary Tract Dysfunction. *Toxins* **2018**, *10*, 260. [CrossRef] [PubMed]
15. Jabbari, B. Pelvic and Urogenital Pain. In *Botulinum Toxin Treatment of Pain Disorders*; Springer: New York, NY, USA, 2015; pp. 123–136.
16. Jhang, J.F.; Kuo, H.C. Novel Treatment of Chronic Bladder Pain Syndrome and Other Pelvic Pain Disorders by OnabotulinumtoxinA Injection. *Toxins* **2015**, *7*, 2232–2250. [CrossRef] [PubMed]
17. Chuang, Y.C.; Chancellor, M.B. The application of botulinum toxin in the prostate. *J. Urol.* **2006**, *176*, 2375–2382. [CrossRef] [PubMed]
18. Thomas, C.A.; Guercini, F.; Chuang, Y.C.; Chancellor, M.B. Botulinum-A toxin: An exciting new treatment option for prostatic disease. *Int. J. Clin. Pract.* **2006**, *60*, 33–37. [CrossRef] [PubMed]
19. de Kort, L.M.; Kok., E.T.; Jonges, T.N.; Rosier, P.F.; Bosch, J.L. Urodynamic effects of transrectal intraprostatic Ona botulinum toxin A injections for symptomatic benign prostatic hyperplasia. *Urology* **2012**, *80*, 889–893. [CrossRef]
20. Hsu, Y.C.; Wang, H.J.; Chuang, Y.C. Intraprostatic Botulinum Neurotoxin Type A Injection for Benign Prostatic Hyperplasia-A Spotlight in Reality. *Toxins* **2016**, *8*, 126. [CrossRef]
21. Zhang, Y.; Smith, C.P. Botulinum toxin to treat pelvic pain. *Toxicon* **2018**, *147*, 129–133. [CrossRef]

22. Chuang, Y.C.; Yoshimura, N.; Huang, C.C.; Chiang, P.H.; Chancellor, M.B. Intravesical botulinum toxin a administration produces analgesia against acetic acid induced bladder pain responses in rats. *J. Urol.* **2004**, *172*, 1529–1532. [CrossRef] [PubMed]
23. Aoki, K.R. Review of a proposed mechanism for the antinociceptive action of botulinum toxin type A. *Neurotoxicology* **2005**, *26*, 785–793. [CrossRef] [PubMed]
24. Chuang, Y.C.; Yoshimura, N.; Huang, C.C.; Chiang, P.H.; Wu, M.; Chancellor, M.B. Intraprostatic capsaicin injection as a novel model for non-bacteria prostatitis. *Eur. Urol.* **2007**, *51*, 1119–1127. [CrossRef] [PubMed]
25. Chuang, Y.C.; Yoshimura, N.; Huang, C.C.; Chiang, P.H.; Wu, M.; Chancellor, M.B. Intraprostatic botulinum toxin A injection inhibits Cyclooxygenase-2 expression and suppresses prostatic pain on capsaicin induced prostatitis model in rat. *J. Urol.* **2008**, *180*, 742–748. [CrossRef] [PubMed]
26. Chuang, Y.C.; Huang, C.C.; Kang, H.Y.; Chiang, P.H.; Demiguel, F.; Yoshimura, N.; Chancellor, M.B. Novel action of botulinum toxin on the stromal and epithelial components of the prostate gland. *J. Urol.* **2006**, *175*, 1158–1163. [CrossRef]
27. Gormley, E.A.; Lightner, D.J.; Faraday, M.; Vasavada, S.P.; American Urological Association; Society of Urodynamics, Female Pelvic Medicine. Diagnosis and treatment of overactive bladder (non-neurogenic) in adults: AUA/SUFU guideline amendment. *J. Urol.* **2015**, *193*, 1572–1580. [CrossRef] [PubMed]
28. Hanno, P.M.; Erickson, D.; Moldwin, R.; Faraday, M.M.; American Urological Association. Diagnosis and treatment of interstitial cystitis/bladder pain syndrome: AUA guideline amendment. *J. Urol.* **2015**, *193*, 1545–1553. [CrossRef]
29. Rummel, A. The long journey of botulinum neurotoxins into the synapse. *Toxicon* **2015**, *107*, 9–24. [CrossRef] [PubMed]
30. Pirazzini, M.; Rossetto, O.; Eleopra, R.; Montecucco, C. Botulinum Neurotoxins: Biology, Pharmacology, and Toxicology. *Pharmacol. Rev.* **2017**, *69*, 200–235. [CrossRef]
31. Dolly, J.O.; O'Connell, M.A. Neurotherapeutics to inhibit exocytosis from sensory neurons for the control of chronic pain. *Curr. Opin. Pharmacol.* **2012**, *12*, 100–108. [CrossRef]
32. Huang, M.; Chen, H.; Jiang, C.; Xie, K.; Tang, P.; Ou, R.; Zeng, J.; Liu, Q.; Li, Q.; Huang, J.; et al. Effects of botulinum toxin A injections in spinal cord injury patients with detrusor overactivity and detrusor sphincter dyssynergia. *J. Rehabil. Med.* **2016**, *48*, 683–687. [CrossRef] [PubMed]
33. Schurch, B.; Stöhrer, M.; Kramer, G.; Schmid, D.M.; Gaul, G.; Hauri, D. Botulinum-A toxin for treating detrusor hyperreflexia in spinal cord injured patients: A new alternative to anticholinergic drugs? Preliminary results. *J. Urol.* **2000**, *164*, 692–697. [CrossRef]
34. Caterina, M.J.; Schumacher, M.A.; Tominaga, M.; Rosen, T.A.; Levine, J.D.; Julius, D. The capsaicin receptor: A heat-activated ion channel in the pain pathway. *Nature* **1997**, *389*, 816–824. [CrossRef] [PubMed]
35. Richardson, J.D.; Vasko, M.R. Cellular mechanisms of neurogenic inflammation. *J. Pharmacol. Exp. Ther.* **2002**, *302*, 839–901. [CrossRef] [PubMed]
36. Cruz, F.; Guimaraes, M.; Silva, C.; Rio, M.E.; Coimbra, A.; Reis, M. Desensitization of bladder sensory fibers by intravesical capsaicin has long lasting clinical and urodynamic effects in patients with hyperactive or hypersensitive bladder dysfunction. *J. Urol.* **1997**, *157*, 585–589. [CrossRef]
37. Dinis, P.; Charrua, A.; Avelino, A.; Nagy, I.; Quintas, J.; Ribau, U.; Cruz, F. The distribution of sensory fibers immunoreactive for the TRPV1 (capsaicin) receptor in the human prostate. *Eur. Urol.* **2005**, *48*, 162–167. [CrossRef]
38. Fan, C.; Chu, X.; Wang, L.; Shi, H.; Li, T. Botulinum toxin type A reduces TRPV1 expression in the dorsal root ganglion in rats with adjuvant-arthritis pain. *Toxicon* **2017**, *133*, 116–122. [CrossRef]
39. Maria, G.; Destito, A.; Lacquaniti, S.; Bentivoglio, A.R.; Brisinda, G.; Albanese, A. Relief by botulinum toxin of voiding dysfunction due to prostatitis. *Lancet.* **1998**, *352*, 625. [CrossRef]
40. Park, D.S.; Shin, S.M. Intraprostatic injection of botulinum toxin for men with chronic pelvic pain syndrome. *Eur. Urol. Suppl.* **2006**, *5*, 249. [CrossRef]
41. Gottsch, H.P.; Yang, C.C.; Berger, R.E. A pilot study of botulinum toxin A for male chronic pelvic pain syndrome. *Scand. J. Urol. Nephrol.* **2011**, *45*, 72–76. [CrossRef]
42. Falahatkar, S.; Shahab, E.; Gholamjani Moghaddam, K.; Kazemnezhad, E. Transurethral intraprostatic injection of botulinum neurotoxin type A for the treatment of chronic prostatitis/chronic pelvic pain syndrome: Results of a prospective pilot double-blind and randomized placebo-controlled study. *BJU Int.* **2015**, *116*, 641–649. [CrossRef] [PubMed]

43. Abdel-Meguid, T.A.; Mosli, H.A.; Farsi, H.; Alsayyad, A.; Tayib, A.; Sait, M.; Abdelsalam, A. Treatment of refractory category III nonbacterial chronic prostatitis/chronic pelvic pain syndrome with intraprostatic injection of onabotulinumtoxinA: A prospective controlled study. *Can. J. Urol.* **2018**, *25*, 9273–9280. [PubMed]
44. El-Enen, M.A.; Abou-Farha, M.; El-Abd, A.; El-Tatawy, H.; Tawfik, A.; El-Abd, S.; Rashed, M.; El-Sharaby, M. Intraprostatic injection of botulinum toxin-A in patients with refractory chronic pelvic pain syndrome: The transurethral vs. transrectal approach. *Arab J. Urol.* **2015**, *13*, 94–99. [CrossRef] [PubMed]
45. Mehnert, U.; Boy, S.; Schmid, M. A morphological evaluation of botulinum neurotoxin A injections into the detrusor muscle using magnetic resonance imaging. *World J. Urol.* **2009**, *27*, 397–403. [CrossRef] [PubMed]
46. Shoskes, D.A.; Nickel, J.C.; Dolinga, R.; Prots, D. Clinical phenotyping of patients with chronic prostatitis/chronic pelvic pain syndrome and correlation with symptoms severity. *Urology* **2009**, *73*, 538–542. [CrossRef]
47. Guu, S.J.; Geng, J.H.; Chao, I.T.; Lin, H.T.; Lee, Y.C.; Juan, Y.S.; Liu, C.C.; Wang, C.J.; Tsai, C.C. Efficacy of low-intensity extracorporeal shock wave therapy on men with chronic pelvic pain syndrome refractory to 3-As therapy. *Am. J. Men's Health* **2018**, *12*, 441–452. [CrossRef] [PubMed]
48. Tadros, N.N.; Shah, A.B.; Shoskes, D.A. Utility of trigger point injection as an adjunct to physical therapy in men with chronic prostatitis/chronic pelvic pain syndrome. *Transl. Androl. Urol.* **2017**, *6*, 534–537. [CrossRef] [PubMed]
49. Shoskes, D.A.; Nickel, J.C.; Kattan, M.W. Phenotypically directed multi-modal therapy for chronic prostatitis/chronic pelvic pain syndrome: A prospective study using UPOINT. *Urology* **2010**, *75*, 1249–1253. [CrossRef] [PubMed]
50. Guan, X.; Zhao, C.; Ou, Z.Y.; Wang, L.; Zeng, F.; Qi, L.; Tang, Z.Y.; Dun, J.G.; Liu, L.F. Use of the UPOINT phenotype system in treating Chinese patients with chronic prostatitis/chronic pelvic pain syndrome: A prospective study. *Asian J. Androl.* **2015**, *17*, 120–123. [PubMed]

13

Can Botulinum Toxin A Play a Role in Treatment of Chronic Pelvic Pain Syndrome in Female Patients?—Clinical and Animal Evidence

Chin-Li Chen and En Meng *

Division of Urology, Department of Surgery, Tri-Service General Hospital, National Defense Medical Center, 325, Section 2, Cheng-Gung Road, Taipei 114, Taiwan; j0921713355@gmail.com

* Correspondence: en.meng@gmail.com

Abstract: Chronic pelvic pain (CPP) is defined as chronic pain and inflammation in the pelvic organs for more than six months. There are wide ranges of clinical presentations, including pelvic pain, painful intercourse, irritable bowel syndrome, and pain during urinating. Chronic pelvic pain syndrome (CPPS) is a subdivision of CPP, and the pain syndrome may be focused within a single organ or more than one pelvic organ. As there is uncertain pathogenesis, no standard treatment is currently available for CPPS. Botulinum toxin A (BoNT-A) is a potent neurotoxin that blocks acetylcholine release to paralyze muscles. Intravesical BoNT-A injection can reduce bladder pain in patients with interstitial cystitis/bladder pain syndrome. BoNT-A injected into the pelvic floor muscles of women has also been reported to improve chronic pain syndrome. Due to the reversible effect of BoNT-A, repeated injection appears to be necessary and effective in reducing symptoms. Adverse effects of BoNT-A may worsen the preexisting conditions, including constipation, stress urinary incontinence, and fecal incontinence. This review summarizes the evidence of BoNT-A treatment for CPPS in animal studies and clinical studies regarding the therapeutic effects of BoNT-A for CPPS in female patients.

Keywords: botulinum toxin A; chronic pelvic pain syndrome; pelvic pain

Key Contribution: We have reviewed the current basic and clinical evidence of BoNT-A injections for treating CPPS in female patients. This treatment is safe and effective and should be considered as a standard treatment for female CPPS.

---

1. Introduction

Chronic pelvic pain (CPP) is chronic or persistent pain perceived in pelvic structures for more than six months with continuous or recurrent pelvic pain as well as with symptoms suggestive of the lower urinary tract, sexual, bowel, pelvic floor or gynecological dysfunction in men and women [1]. CPP may be divided into situations with well-defined classical pathology (such as infection or cancer) and those without confirmed etiology [1]. According to this classification, the former is considered to be "specific disease-associated pelvic pain," and the latter is described as "chronic pelvic pain syndrome" (CPPS) [1]. The incidence rate of CPP in women is around 6% to 27% worldwide [2]. CPP in women is reported to affect 18–50-year-old women, mostly [3].

CPPS is a subdivision of CPP and the pain syndrome may be focused within a single organ or more than one pelvic organ, including bladder, urethra, vagina, rectum, anus and whole pelvic musculatures [1]. When the pain is localized to a single organ, some specialists use an end organ term such as Bladder Pain Syndrome (BPS), and use "syndrome" to indicate pain localized in more than one organ site [1]. However, some specialists sub-divide pelvic pain through psychological and functional symptoms rather than anatomy [1].

CPPS of women can exhibit different symptoms, including dyspareunia, dysmenorrhea, dyschezia, and non-menstrual pelvic pain. It may also cause lower urinary tract symptoms, such as frequency, urgency, difficulty urinating, and pain with urination. The most important evaluations for diagnosis of CPPS are medical history and physical examinations. [4]. Vaginal examination is critical to diagnose pelvic floor spasm due to the easily palpable taut muscles. Electromyography, perineometry, vaginal manometry, and digital assessment of pelvic floor muscle (PFM) are also conducted for diagnosis [5]. There are limited laboratory testing and imaging for diagnosis, and it should be considered to be evaluated by laparoscopic or urologic evaluation according to the clinical findings [4].

There is no single definitive etiology or standard management for CPPS. It is supposed that CPPS results from a combination of risk factors, such as neurological, mechanical, and biochemical factors. More than one-half of CPP patients live with interstitial cystitis/painful bladder syndrome (IC/BPS), endometriosis, irritable bowel syndrome, or pelvic adhesions [6,7]. Spasticity of the PFMs, which leads to an increase in muscle tone, has been proposed to play one of the important pathogenic factors of CPPS [8]. PFMs spasm may result from a primary event on the pelvic floor musculatures or secondary to other diseases related to psychological or pathological disorders. It is another significant problem that may decrease quality of life and increase health care costs.

The European Association of Urology (EAU) proposed comprehensive guidelines about the diagnosis and management of CPPS [1]. Management for CPPS remains limited, and the treatment points are usually symptom relief [9]. Secondary disease processes associated with CPPS in women should receive targeted treatment first. The etiologies of CPPS involve multiple mechanisms, so treatments for CPPS need a holistic approach including behavioral, physical, psychological, and sexual components. Modalities of treatments for CPP involve behavioral interventions, physical therapy, medications, surgical interventions, and alternative therapies [4]. The EAU guidelines suggest simple analgesics, such as nonsteroidal anti-inflammatory drugs, to be the first-line therapy of general management. Opioids and neuropathic analgesics, such as tricyclic antidepressants, anticonvulsants, and gabapentin, should be used as further medications if simple analgesics fail. If medications fail to provide symptom relief, nonpharmacologic managements, such as nerve blocks, suprapubic transcutaneous electrical nerve stimulation, sacral neuromodulation, and injection with Botulinum toxin A (BoNT-A) should be considered to help treat CPPS.

Botulinum neurotoxin (BoNT) comprises seven different serotypes (A to G) and more than 40 subtypes [10]. These serotypes have a similar mechanism to inhibit the release of acetylcholine (ACh), but they have different potency of actions. Among different subtypes of BoNT-A, A1 is the only isoform for the therapeutic purpose because of the high potency and long duration of paralysis [11]. The only subtypes of BoNT for clinical purposes are A1 and B1 [12]. However, the paralytic effect of BoNT-B is not as efficient as the function of BoNT-A according to the results of Sloop et al. [13]. The most studied BoNT for clinical treatment is BoNT-A.

BoNT-A injection can reduce spasms and pressure in the PFMs of women with CPPS [14]. Many women with CPPS reported diminution of pelvic pain symptoms after BoNT-A injection. Reduction in pelvic pain can improve quality of life, social activity, working performance, sexual relationships, urinating pain, and mood situations [15]. BoNT-A injected into the pelvic floor musculature of women with CPPS has been reported to improve chronic pelvic pain symptoms and spasms of PFMs [14]. The organ specificity of pelvic pain syndrome in CPPS includes urology, gynecology, gastroenterology, neurology, sexology, and the pelvic floor [1]. This review will focus on the BoNT-A treatment in female CPPS, especially in PFMs pain, IC/BPS, and sexual pain syndrome.

2. Mechanisms of BoNT-A for Treating CPPS

Bacterium *Clostridium botulinum* was first isolated in 1895. BoNT-A was first purified from bacterium *Clostridium botulinum* in 1928 and its off-label use started in the 70s [16].

There are three major mechanisms of BoNT-A that function on the muscles, neural system, and inflammation to relieve pain symptoms [17]. BoNT-A plays an important function in the reduction of pain symptoms. It is believed that spasms and tenderness of the PFMs are highly associated with CPPS in women [18,19]. BoNT-A injection has been used to paralyze muscles, and its effect is localized, partial, and reversible. After injecting to the PFMs, BoNT-A can reduce the hypertonic pressure and improve pelvic muscle spasms.

BoNT-A is a selective neurotoxin that acts on neuromusculatures. After binding to terminal receptors on the motor neuron, it can inhibit the release of ACh to cause muscle paralysis. BoNT-A inhibits ACh vesicles releasing to the synaptic cleft by cleaving particular proteins, such as SNAP-25 or VAMP, which are essential for binding with ACh vesicles at the presynaptic membrane. Due to the effect of BoNT-A, there is no release of ACh in the synaptic cleft, and it can paralyze the innervated muscles subsequently [20]. This mechanism has been used to relieve the storage of lower urinary tract symptoms of IC/BPS such as frequency and urgency.

Animal studies reported that BoNT-A could inhibit the delivery of several neurotransmitters, such as calcitonin gene-related peptide (CGRP), glutamate, adenosine triphosphate (ATP), and substance P [21–25].

BoNT-A may block these neurotransmitters from releasing muscular nociceptors, and reduce the symptom of muscle pain in patients with CPPS [26]. BoNT-A could also inhibit the contraction of muscles via alpha and gamma motor neurons and block spasms of pelvic floor musculature, which results in relieving the pelvic pain caused by muscle spasms [26]. Current literature has shown that the use of BoNT-A can reduce the hypertonicity of PFMs to improve pain scores from CPPS patients.

In addition, BoNT-A has the analgesic effect of relieving pain symptoms. From the animal and human studies, increased expression of cell membranes receptors, such as the TRPV1 and P2 × 3, in the nociceptors may up-regulate the symptoms of neuralgia [27,28]. BoNT-A has been reported to reduce the expression of TRPV1 in rats with neuropathic pain [29].

After the injection of BoNT-A, paralysis of muscle occurs after 2–5 days [5]. The functional effects can typically last from three to six months [14]. The clinical efficacy of BoNT-A injection for CPPS in women was durable to 24 weeks [30]. This long-term but reversible effect has made BoNT-A an important therapy for a wide variety of neuromuscular diseases.

After formation of antibodies against BoNT-A, the duration of the BoNT-A effect and the therapeutic extent of the maximal treatment effect are usually reduced after a few BoNT-A applications (partial therapy failure) before complete therapy failure occurs [5].

3. Clinical Evidence of BoNT-A for Pelvic Floor Muscle Pain in CPPS Women

BoNT-A was first used for therapeutic purposes in the 1960s when Dr. Alan B. Scott, an ophthalmologist, injected BoNT-A into extraocular muscles of rhesus monkies to treat strabismus. His results were successfully replicated in humans [31]. BoNT-A has been widely studied in several therapeutic applications and different diseases. However, previous studies and clinical trials have not confirmed the effect of BoNT-A for relieving myofascial pain in the neck, shoulders, or trunk [17,32].

Although BoNT-A has been widely used for muscular disorders, its role in treating CPPS has yet to be established. Present literature suggests that injecting BoNT-A into the PFMs may improve symptoms in women with CPPS. Joo et al. reported a 50% success rate of BoNT-A injection in anismus for a long-term period [33]. Brin and Vapnek first reported the injection of BoNT-A to treat vaginismus in 1997 [34].

A systematic review including five studies supports that BoNT-A treatment was beneficial for relieving spasms of PFMs due to CPPS [17,35]. BoNT-A administration could relieve symptoms of dyspareunia, dysmenorrhea, non-menstrual pain and dyschezia. After BoNT-A treatment, it also improved the quality of life and sexual activity. The improvement may because of BoNT-A injection causing localized, partial denervation of the PFMs resulting in muscle weakness and reduction of pressure.

CPP can occur at several muscles in the pelvic region such as pubococcygeus, ischiococcygeus, iliococcygeus, piriformis, transverse perinei muscles, and obturator internus. Preliminary studies have reported that BoNT-A injection could be able to decrease levator ani muscle spasms in women with CPP [14,36,37]. Halder et al. reported 200 U of BoNT-A injections into the trigger points of the perineum in 50 women with CPP [38]. The outcomes showed a significant decrease in pelvic pain scores (3.7 ± 4.0 vs. 6.4±1.8, $p = 0.005$), and fewer trigger points (44% vs. 100%, $p < 0.001$). There was an improvement (20.7%) in patients with the previous placement of incontinence sling versus no improvement (0%) in pain ($p = 0.003$).

The major factor of pelvic pain in women with a spasm of PFMs appears to be ischemia due to vessel compression of the muscles, which leads to the release of bradykinin and sensitization or excitation of nociceptors [5]. BoNT-A injection can improve symptoms of CPP by the antispasticity effect on a spasm of PFMs rather than the result of the antinociceptive activity [17]. Injected BoNT-A into PFMs in women with CPP has been reported to improve the overall quality of life significantly, specifically to improve dyspareunia and female sexual function [30].

Because of the reversible effect and natural metabolism by the body, treatment with repeated BoNT-A injection for CPPS is frequently required. A low dosage of BoNT-A was injected in other muscle groups of the body at three-month intervals, as it was unlikely to produce significant side effects [14].

Injection of 300 U of BoNT-A into PFMs may be safe, especially administered to the regions of hyper-spastic muscles [30]. However, the timing for repeat injection, the optimal dilution, and injected dosage are still challenging to maximize the therapeutic effects of BoNT-A in CPPS of women. It is unclear how significantly the pain will be relieved after BoNT-A injection. The outcome of BoNT-A in relieving CPPS needs more large prospective, randomized, controlled studies.

Table 1 lists important clinical studies of BoNT-A injection for relieving pain symptoms of PFMs.

Table 1. Study of BoNT-A for pelvic floor muscle pain in CPPS women.

Study	Javis [14]	Adelowo [36]	Nesbitt-Hawes [37]	Halder [38]	Morrissey [30]
Numbers	12	29	37 (single injection: 26; multiple injection: 11)	50	21
Age	31.1 (18–55)	55 (38–62)	Single injection: 30 Multiple injection: 31 (21–52 years)	44.5	35.1 (22–50)
Study Model	Prospective cohort study	Retrospective cohort study	Prospective cohort study	Retrospective case series	Prospective pilot open-label study
Follow-Up	12 weeks	Visit 1: <6 weeks post-injection Visit 2: ≥6 weeks post injection	26 weeks	6 weeks (2–192 weeks)	6 months
Criteria	Objective hypertonicity of PFM and 2-year history of CPP at least	Refractory myofascial pelvic pain	Objective overactivity of PFM and a two-year history of pelvic pain	CPP, trigger points of pelvic floor on examinations, and failure (with subsequent discontinuation) of one treatment modality at least including outpatient physical treatment and/or oral analgesics	CPP and HTPFD who have failed conventional therapy
Dose of BoNT-A	40 U	100–300 U	100 U	–	Up to 300 U
Injection Sites	Bilateral puborectalis and pubococcygeus muscles	PFMs (coccygeus, iliococcygeus, pubococcygeus, puborectalis, obturator, and pyriformis muscles)	Puborectalis and pubococcygeous muscles	Multiple areas of the perineum	Spastic PFM trigger points and deeper PFMs (pubococcygeus, iliococcygeus, coccygeus, and obturator internus muscles)
Outcomes	• Median VAS scores presented improvements on dyspareunia (80 vs. 28, p = 0.01) and dysmenorrhea (67 vs. 28, p = 0.03). • PFMs manometry showed a 37% reduction in resting pressure at week 4 and a 25% reduction maintained at week 12 (p < 0.0001). • It showed significant improvements of sexual activity scores, with a reduction in discomfort (4.8 vs. 2.2, p = 0.02) and improvement in habit (0.2 vs. 1.9, p = 0.03).	• 79.3% improvement in pain. • 51.7% female patients elected to have a second BoNT-A injection. • The median time of the first injection to the second injection was 4.0 months (3.0–7.0 months).	• 26 (70%) women had one injection of BoNT-A and 11 (30%) had 2 or more injections. • The median number of repeat injections was 3. • The second injection was performed at the earliest at 26 weeks after the first, with subsequent injections having a median time to re-injection of 33.4 weeks (range 9.4–122.7 weeks). Single and repeated injections both significantly reduced dyspareunia by VAS scores (54 to 30, and 51 to 23, p = 0.001), non-menstrual pelvic pain VAS (37 to 25, p = 0.04), as well as vaginal pressures (40 vs. 34 cm H_2O (p = 0.02).	• Posttreatment, patients had lower average pelvic pain scores (6.4 to 3.7, p = 0.005), and fewer trigger pints (44% vs. 100%, p < 0.001)	• 61.9% improvement on GRA at 4 weeks. • 80.9% improvement on GRA at 8, 12, and 24 weeks. • Dyspareunia VAS significantly improved at weeks 12 (5.6, p = 0.011) and 24 (5.4, p = 0.004). • Sexual dysfunction as measured by the FSDS significantly improved at 8 weeks (27.6, p = 0.005), 12 weeks (27.9, p = 0.006), and 24 weeks (22.6, p < 0.001) compared with baseline (34.5). • Vaginal manometry demonstrated a significant decrease in resting pressures and in maximum contraction pressures at all follow-up visits (p < 0.05).

CPP: chronic pelvic pain. PFM: pelvic floor muscle. HTPFD: high-tone pelvic floor dysfunction GRA: global response assessment. FSDS: Female Sexual Distress Scale.

4. Clinical Application of BoNT-A in IC/BPS Women

The etiology and pathophysiology of IC/BPS are still unclear. There are many treatments for relieving IC/BPS including analgesic medicine, changing habits of lifestyle, pentosan polysulfate sodium, cystoscopy with hydrodistention, or instillation of dimethyl sulfoxide in the bladder.

Smith et al. first reported that submucosal BoNT-A injection into 20 to 30 sites of the trigone and bladder floor for a total of 100 to 200 U would result in a 69% improvement of IC/BPS patients, including daytime frequency episodes, nocturia, pain, and bladder capacity [39]. In 2009, Kuo et al. reported a prospective, randomized, and controlled study including 67 patients with IC/BPS who failed conventional treatments, comparing intravesical BoNT-A injection in 100 U or 200 U plus hydrodistention with hydrodistention alone. The IC/BPS symptom score significantly improved in all three groups. However, it only showed a significant reduction of pain visual analogue scale (VAS), an increase of functional bladder capacity (FBC) and cystometric bladder capacity in the BoNT-A group [40].

In 2016, a multicenter, randomized, double-blind, placebo-controlled trial compared hydrodistention plus 100 U of BoNT-A injections at 20 sites with injections of normal saline at 20 sites in 60 patients with refractory IC/BPS. A significantly greater reduction of bladder pain symptoms and increased bladder capacity under cystoscopy were observed in the group with BoNT-A injection, with 63% of overall success rates versus 15% in the normal saline group [41].

Compared to single intravesical BoNT-A injection for IC/BPS patients, there were long-term therapeutic effects in repeated injections, such as pain relief, improved bladder capacity, and better success rates for a long-term period. Kuo et al. reported a repeated intravesical injection of 100 U of BoNT-A every six months for up to four times or until symptoms improved in 81 patients with refractory IC/BPS. It showed significant improvement in pain relief, FBC, and daytime frequency after repeated therapy with different BoNT-A injections. Compared to one single injection, it also reported significantly better success rates for four repeated injections ($p = 0.0242$) and three repeated injections ($p = 0.050$) [42]. In a recent prospective study, 104 patients received an intravesical injection of 100 U of BoNT-A and cystoscopic hydrodistention for refractory IC/BPS. Repeated BoNT-A injections were done every six months for two years. The study showed that 56.7% of patients received four injections of BoNT-A and 34% of patients received another fifth injection because of progressive IC symptoms. It showed a better success rate in those patients who completed repeated BoNT-A injections and significant improvements of O'Leary-Sant IC symptom and problem indexes (ICSI, ICPI, OSS), painful VAS, FBC, frequency, and global response assessment (GRA) during 79 months of follow-up [43].

Liu et al. reported the levels of nerve growth factor (NGF) in the bladder tissue were significantly increased in 19 patients with IC/BPS compared with 12 healthy patients. After injections with 100 U or 200 U of BoNT-A followed by cystoscopic hydrodistention two weeks later, they showed a decrease of the NGF mRNA levels and no significant difference compared with the healthy controls [44]. Intravesical BoNT-A injections could improve chronic bladder inflammation, decrease apoptosis, and decrease the level of bladder vascular endothelial growth factor in patients with IC/BPS [45 46].

The injection sites and the numbers of injections are controversial. It has been reported to inject BoNT-A into the trigone and the posterior bladder wall simultaneously, only the trigone, and sites excluding out the trigone. Pinto et al. reported injecting 100 U of BoNT-A into ten trigonal sites compared to saline injections for refractory IC/BPS patients. They showed significant improvements in bladder pain and quality of life [47]. Jiang et al. injected 100 U of BoNT-A into 20 bladder body sites or 10 trigonal sites in 39 IC/BPS patients. After eight weeks from baseline, they showed no significant difference in changes in urinary frequency, voided volume, post-void residual volume, and bladder capacity. No significant difference in decreasing VAS, symptom improvement, and dysuria were also noted [48].

Kuo et al. investigated the therapeutic predictors, such as ICSI, ICPI, FBC, frequency, and first desire to void for successful treatment of BoNT-A injection in the bladder for refractory IC/BPS patients. Successful treatment was defined as GRA ≥ 2 at six months. The success rate was 45.54% at six months. Multivariate logistic regression showed the only therapeutic predictor for successful management was the baseline ICSI. Patients with an ICSI ≥ 12 may indicate a poorer therapeutic outcome of BoNT-A injections [49]. For refractory IC/BPS, the effectiveness and success of BoNT-A injections has been shown.

To summarize, BoNT-A injection has been widely studied for IC/BPS patients and it has become a promising treatment for refractory IC/BPS patients with the combination with hydrodistention (Table 2), although repeated injection may be needed for long-term therapeutic effects.

Table 2. Study of BoNT-A for IC/BPS women.

Reference	Study Design	Diagnosis	Numbers	Age	Follow-Up	BoNT-A Dose	Assessment	Outcomes
Kuo HC [41]	Multicenter, randomized, double-blind, placebo-controlled trial	IC/BPS refractory to conventional treatment	60 (52 women, 8 men)	50.8	8 weeks	100U (cystoscopic hydrodistention plus intravesical injections of 100 U BoNT-A)	Pain VAS, 3-day voiding diary, ICSI, ICPI, VUDS GRA	• Δ pain VAS of BoNT-A group vs. control group: −2.6 vs. −0.9 ($p = 0.021$). • 8 weeks after BoNT-A injection, ICSI, ICPI, OSS, GRA, and FBC all showed significant improvement in both groups. • At 3 months, GRA in BoNT-A group vs. saline group: 62% vs. 15% ($p = 0.028$).
Kuo HC [42]	Prospective interventional study	IC/BPS refractory to conventional treatment	81 (71 women, 10 men)	Women: 48; Men 48.2	24 months	100 U (injected into bladder walls at posterior and lateral sites) followed by cystoscopic hydrondistention and repeated injections every 6 months up to 4 times	Pain VAS, 3-day voiding diary, ICSI, ICPI, VUDS, GRA	• It showed significant improvement in ICSI, ICPI, VAS, FBC, and daytime frequency after repeated treatment of BoNT-A with different injections. • It showed better success rates in patients with 3 ($p = 0.050$) and 4 ($p = 0.0242$) repeated injections of BoNT-A, compared to those with a single injection. • Dysuria after each injection: 30%. • UTI after each injection: 4.9–19%.
Lee CL [43]	Prospective study	Refractory IC/BPS	104 (88 women, 16 men)	Women: 48.5; Men: 46.6	79 months	100 U (delivered at 20 suburothelial locations at posterior and lateral bladder walls) followed by cystoscopic hydrodistention and repeated injections every 6 months up to 4 times or until symptoms resolved	Pain VAS, 3-day voiding diary, ICSI, ICPI, VUDS, GRA	• At 6 months after one single injection, improvement of symptoms include overall OSS (23.7 ± 6.1 vs. 16.6 ± 8.9), pain VAS (5.2 ± 2.4 vs. 3.5 ± 2.5), FBC (129.1 ± 75.0 vs. 177.7 ± 85.0), daytime frequency episodes (15.3 ± 7.7 vs. 11.3 ± 6.3), and all of the p value <0.0001. • Improvement of GRA (1.31 ± 0.97, $p < 0.0001$). • After fourth injection of BoNT-A, OSS (24.6 ± 6.1 vs. 15.2 ± 8.9), VAS (5.4 ± 2.2 vs. 2.9 ± 2.3), FBC (133.5 ± 74.0 vs. 226.9 ± 108.8), and daytime frequency (15.2 ± 7.1 vs. 10.3 ± 5.3) all showed improvement with p value < 0.0001. • After each injection of BoNT-A, the most frequently reported symptom is dysuria (32.7% to 41.7%). • After each injection of BoNT-A, 5.9% to 13.9% of patients. occurred urinary tract infection.
Liu HT [44]	Prospective study	Refractory IC	19 (14 women, 5 men)	Women: 37; Men: 41	3 months	100 U (14 patients) or 200 U (5 patients) followed by cystoscopic hydrodistension 2 weeks later	Pain VAS, 3-day voiding diary, VUDS	• The FBC of the overall patients increased by 1.4 times the baseline value. • After BoNT-A treatment, the pain VAS score decreased from 5.16 ± 2.09 to 2.53 ± 1.43 ($p < 0.0001$), and the daily frequency episodes decreased from 12.6 ± 4.3 to 8.8 ± 2.5 ($p = 0.001$). • NGF mRNA levels at baseline: IC patients vs. control=0.65 ± 0.33 vs. 0.42 ± 0.25, p = 0.046). • At 2 weeks after BoNT-A injections, the levels of NGF mRNA had decreased to 0.47 ± 0.23 ($p = 0.002$). • The overall success rate: 74%.

Table 2. *Cont.*

Reference	Study Design	Diagnosis	Numbers	Age	Follow-Up	BoNT-A Dose	Assessment	Outcomes
Shie JH [45]	Prospective study	IC/BPS and glomerulations after cystoscopic hydrodistention	23 women (11 received three repeated injections every 6 months)	46.6	18 months	100 U (40 suburothelial injections at the lateral and posterior bladder walls) followed by cystoscopic hydrodistention	Pain VAS, 3-day voiding diary, OSS, UDS, GRA	• After single BoNT-A treatment, it showed improvements in clinical symptoms, pain VAS, and daytime frequency. • After single injection of BoNT-A, tryptase decreased significantly. • 11 patients who received three repeated injections of BoNT-A showed significantly lower pain VAS (mean: 5.8 vs. 3.03, $p = 0$), glomerulation degree (mean: 1.8 vs. 1.2, $p = 0.026$) and GRA (mean: 0.3 vs. 1.2, $p = 0$). • SNAP-25 decreased after repeated injections with BoNT-A.
Peng CH [46]	Prospective study	Refractory IC/BPS	21 (20 women, 1 man)	44.8	24 weeks	100 U (20 suburothelial injection at posterior and lateral bladder walls) with cystoscopic hydrodistention and repeated every 6 months for 4 times	Pain VAS, 3-day voiding diary, OSS, UDS, GRA	• After BoNT-A treatment, it showed significantly decreased in OSS (15.1 ± 8.65 vs. 21.1 ± 7.92, $p = 0.009$) and VAS (3.0 ± 2.92 vs. 5.14 ± 2.46, $p = 0.003$). • Decreased VEGF level: after BoNT-A treatment vs. baseline = 0.83 ± 0.28 vs. 1.0; $p = 0.016$. • After BoNT-A treatment, apoptotic cell count decreased from 1.76 ± 1.69 to 0.86 ± 1.00 ($p = 0.026$) and mast cell activity decreased from 5.82 ± 4.97 to 1.81 ± 2.29 ($p = 0.009$).
Pinto RA [47]	Single center, randomized, double-blind, placebo controlled, phase 2 study	IC/BPS	19 women	45.8	12 weeks	100U (10 trigonal sites)	Pain VAS, 3-day voiding diary, OSS, QoL score	• At week 12 BoNT-A treatment, it showed significantly reduced pain compared with saline (−3.8 ± 2.5 vs. −1.6 ± 2.1, $p < 0.05$). • The mean change in OSS from baseline to week 12: BoNT-A group vs. saline group = −9 ± 4.7 vs. −7.1 ± 4.6, $p < 0.05$). • Reductions in voiding frequency were observed at BoNT-A group.
Jiang YH [48]	Single center, randomized, double-blind study	Refractory IC/BPS for at least 6 months	39 women (bladder body, n = 20; trigone, n = 19)	53.9 (bladder body group), 55.1 (trigone group)	12 weeks	100U (comparative group: 20 bladder body sites at the posterior and lateral walls; treatment group: 10 trigonal sites) followed by cystoscopic hydrodistention	Pain VAS, 3-day voiding diary, OSS, VUDS, GRA	• After BoNT-A injections, thirteen (65.0%) patients in bladder body group and 10 (52.6%) patients in trigone group had improvement of VAS more than 2 points ($p = 0.43$). • After BoNT-A treatment, nine (45%) patients in bladder body group and 10 (52.6%) patients in trigone group had GRA ≥ 2 ($p = 0.63$) and dysuria ($p = 0.52$).
Kuo YC [49]	Prospective study	Refractory IC/BPS	101 (88 women, 13 men)	48.45 (Women: 48.81; Men: 46.0)	6 months	100U (20 suburothelial injection at posterior and lateral walls) immediately followed by cystoscopic hydrodistention	Pain VAS, 3-day voiding diary, OSS, ICSI, ICPI, VUDS, GRA	• Significant improvements observed in OSS, ICSI, ICPI, pain VAS, FBC, daytime frequency, nocturia, GRA at 3 months after BoNT injections, and these improvements could exist at 6 months. • Overall successful rate at 6 months: 45.54% (women: 46.59%; men: 38.46%). • Baseline ICSI score was the only significant predictor for a therapeutic outcome (cutoff value of ICSI to predict treatment failure: ICSI ≥ 12).

GRA: global response assessment. VAS: visual analog scale. OSS: O'Leary-Sant symptom score. ICSI: O'Leary-Sant symptom indexes. ICPI: O'Leary-Sant problem indexes. UDS: Urodynamic study. VUDS: videourodynamic study. FBC: functional bladder capacity. NGF: nerve growth factor. SNAP-25: 25-kD synaptosomal-associated protein. VEGF: vascular endothelial growth factor. QoL: quality of life.

5. Animal Evidence of BoNT-A for IC/BPS

Although there is currently no definite animal model for CPPS, several chemical-induced cystitis animal models have been used to investigate the pathophysiology and develop a new treatment strategy for this disease. Lucioni et al. explored the effect of BoNT-A on the sensory neurotransmitters in chronic and acute injury models of the rat bladder by intraperitoneal injection of cyclophosphamide (CYP) and incubation of the bladder preparation with hydrochloric acid (HCl). The study found that a greater release of neuropeptides substance P (SP) and CGRP caused by acute injury with HCl and suggested that there is a potential therapeutic effect of BoNT-A in the treatment of neurogenic inflammation of the bladder [50].

Cayan et al. used 41 female Sprague-Dawley rats with intravesical instillation of HCl monthly to induce chemical cystitis and maintain chronic inflammation. These rats injected with 2-3 units of BoNT-A into the bladder detrusor and saline as the control group. Urodynamic studies showed that BoNT-A treatments increase the maximum bladder capacity and bladder compliance compared to the control group at the beginning and end of the study. The histological examinations reported similar counts of mast cells and leukocyte infiltration in these two groups. In this animal model of chemical cystitis, injected BoNT-A into the bladder detrusor led to improvements in vesical function which may be an alternative, minimally invasive treatment compared to other surgical modalities for a chronic inflammatory condition to improve deteriorated bladder function [51].

Smith et al. demonstrated intraperitoneally injected 150 mg/kg CYP to induce chronic cystitis in female Sprague-Dawley rats. It showed an increase of voiding frequency and hyperactivity of bladder. Treatment with CYP or BoNT-A did not affect the release of ATP in resting urothelium. Injection of CYP led to hypoosmotic stimulation and an increase of ATP release in chronic cystitis. After BoNT-A treatment, hypoosmotic shock-induced ATP decreased significantly. Cystometry revealed that CYP injection increased non-voiding bladder contraction. BoNT-A instillation markedly reduced non-voiding contraction frequency that was induced by CYP injection. However, neither CYP nor BoNT-A nor a combination of CYP + BoNT-A had any effect on the contraction frequency of bladder voiding. Furthermore, intravesical instillation of BoNT-A did not affect the release of ATP from the serosal side, implying that its effects were confined to the urothelial side of the bladder preparation [52].

Vemulakonda et al. studied the inhibitory function of BoNT-A on afferent pathways of chronic inflammation in the bladder. Among four groups of female Sprague-Dawley rats, namely group 1: saline-treated, group 2: BoNT-A treated, group 3: CYP treated, group 4: BoNT-A and CYP treated, all animals received intravesical protamine sulfate (1%), followed by intravesical BoNT-A or saline, and subsequently CYP or saline-injected intraperitoneally. Compared to saline controls, the study showed an increase of L6 and S1 c-fos immunoreactive cells after CYP treatment. BoNT-A/CYP treated group presented with a significant decrease of L6 and S1 c-fos immunoreactive cells compared with the CYP group. There was no significant difference in presentation between these two groups of saline and BoNT-A alone. Cystometrogram revealed that the increase of the non-voiding intercontractile interval in the BoNT-A/CYP group was more than 10-fold in CYP group. Conclusively, in a CYP animal model of chronic bladder inflammation, intravesical BoNT-A significantly inhibits the afferent neural response without impairing efferent bladder function [53]. Table 3 concludes the animal studies of applying BoNT-A for IC/BPS treatment.

Table 3. Study of BoNT-A treatment for IC/BPS in the animal.

Reference	Animal Numbers	Models	Dose of BoNT-A	Outcomes
Lucioni [50]	18 male Sprague-Dawley rats (300–350 g)	Intraperitoneal injection with CYP or saline for 10-day	Harvested bladders were incubated in 10 U BoNT-A for 1 h	• Neuropeptides SP in saline group vs. CYP group: 1060 vs. 605 pg/g ($p < 0.005$) • SP in CYP group: before BTX vs. after BTX: 1060 vs. 709 pg/g ($p < 0.05$)
Smith [52]	21 female Sprague–Dawley rats (200–250 g)	Intravesical instillation and intraperitoneal injection into four groups (n = 5–6 per group): (1) Control (intravesical saline/intraperitoneal saline) (2) BoNT-A (intravesical BoNT-A/intraperitoneal saline) (3) CYP (intravesical saline/intraperitoneal CYP) (4) CYP + BoNT-A (intravesical BoNT-A/intraperitoneal CYP)	Bladder was instilled with 1 mL of 20 U BoNT-A for 30 min	• BoNT-A instillation markedly reduced bladder hyperactivity induced by CYP by reducing non-voiding contraction frequency by 91%.
Cayan [51]	41 female Sprague-Dawley rats (200–300 g)	Intravesical instillation of HCl (0.2 mL of 0.4 N HCl) induced chemical cystitis	2–3 U (0.2–0.3 mL) BoNT-A was injected into the detrusor at the 3, 6, 9 and 12 o'clock positions (10–12 sites)	• Increases in the maximum bladder capacity and compliance were significantly higher in the BoNT-A group compared to the control group ($p = 0.000$ and $p = 0.025$).
Vemulakonda [53]	24 female Sprague-Dawley rats (200–250 g)	Intravesical instillation and intraperitoneal injection into four groups: (1) Saline (intravesical saline/intraperitoneal saline) (2) BoNT-A (intravesical BoNT-A/intraperitoneal saline) (3) CYP (intravesical saline/intraperitoneal CYP) (4) CYP/BoNT-A (intravesical BoNT-A/intraperitoneal CYP)	Bladder was instilled with 20 U BoNT-A for 30 min	• After CYP treated, expression of c-fos increased significantly in L6 and S1 (78% and 107%) compared to saline control ($p < 0.001$). • Compared to the CYP group, it showed a significant decrease of c-fos expression in L6 and S1 (50% and 52%) in the BoNT-A/CYP group ($p < 0.001$). • Compared to CYP group, the increase of nonvoiding intercontractile interval was more than 10-fold in BoNT-A/CYP group ($p < 0.01$).

Cystitis of rats was induced by chronic CYP model that reported by Vizzard [54]. Intraperitoneal injection with CYP (150 mg/kg) was administered every third day to a total of three doses to achieve chronic inflammation. CYP: cyclophosphamide. HCl: hydrochloric acid. SP: substance P.

6. Clinical Use of BoNT-A for Sexual Pain Syndrome

Women with sexual pain disorders experience genital pain during sexual intercourse occurring at the periods including before, in the process, or after the sexual activity that involves the clitoris, vulva, vagina, and/or perineum, thus causing difficulty in sexual intercourse and personal distress. Dyspareunia is painful sexual intercourse, in which pain can occur over the external genitalia, inside the vagina or deeper pelvis due to numerous medical, physical, social, or psychological causes. Generally, the prevalence of dyspareunia was reported to affect between 8%–21.1% of women [55]. More sexual pain disorders were reported in female patients with CPP than women without CPP [1]. Morrissey et al. reported a prospective pilot open-label study of 21 women with CPP and refractory high-tone pelvic floor dysfunction (HTPFD) under needle electromyography (EMG) guidance with BoNT-A injections [30]. They prepared 300 U of BoNT-A with nonpreserved saline in a 10-mL syringe and attached it to a 12.5 cm disposable monopolar EMG needle electrode. BoNT-A was injected into the spastic PFM trigger point (30 U), other deeper PFMs including pubococcygeus, iliococcygeus, and coccygeus (30 U each as needed), and obturator internus muscles (up to 60 U into each side). Of these 21 female patients, 66.7% had vulvodynia. After treatment, the dyspareunia VAS score showed significant improvement at weeks 12 (5.6, $p = 0.011$) and 24 (5.4, $p = 0.004$) than baseline (7.8). The Female Sexual Distress Scale (FSDS) showed significant improvement of sexual function at 8 weeks (27.6, $p = 0.005$), 12 weeks (27.9, $p = 0.006$), and 24 weeks (22.6, $p < 0.001$) compared with baseline

(34.5). Resting pressures and maximum contraction pressures of the vagina as measured by vaginal manometry significantly decreased during all follow-up examinations ($p < 0.05$).

Vulvodynia is characterized as genital pain without clear etiology that may have resulted from sexual intercourse and causes sexual pain disorder. In the general population, the estimated prevalence of vulvodynia ranges from 10% to 28% in reproductive-aged women [56]. Aberrant increase in the number of nociceptors, which causes peripheral hypersensitivity, leads to intraepithelial neural hyperplasia and strong pain in the vestibule, which may be the cause of vulvodynia [12]. Approximately 7–8% of women have experienced vulvodynia by age 40 that limited sexual intercourse [57]. BoNT-A can inhibit the release of ACh from sympathetic neurons and parasympathetic neurons to relieve vulvodynia and improve dyspareunia. A retrospective study recruited seven women aged 28–61 years with intractable genital pain that was refractory to conventional treatment [58]. Twenty units of BoNT-A was injected into the pain sites including the vestibule, levator ani muscle and the perineal body. If the symptoms had not subsided totally, 40 U of BoNT-A was injected repeatedly every two weeks. After BoNT-A injections, pain decreased or disappeared in all patients. The mean VAS score decreased to 1.4 from 8.3 before the treatment, with no recurrence. The study showed improvement of sexual life without significant pain or discomfort during or after sexual activity.

Hedebo et al. used BoNT-A to treat vulvodynia refractory to conventional treatment for at least six months [59]. The cohort consisted of 79 women and each received 100 U of BoNT-A injections. The results showed significant improvements in dyspareunia (7.82 to 5.82, $p < 0.01$), Negative Interference in Quality of Life (NIQL) (7.88 to 6.19, $p < 0.01$) and the cotton swab test (6.81 to 5.50, $p < 0.01$).

High doses of BoNT-A injection seem to have effectiveness in the treatment of vulvodynia related to sexual pain syndrome. A randomized, double-blind, three-arm, placebo-controlled study from June 2008 to September 2014 included 32 women aged 23–35 years with provoked vestibulodynia [60]. They subcutaneously injected BoNT-A 50 U (arm A), 100 U (arm B) or saline (arm C) into the dorsal vulvar vestibulum and evaluated pain scores after three months. They injected 100 U of BoNT-A for persistently symptomatic women. At the 6-month visit, symptomatic patients received a second injection of BoNT-A 100 U in arm C. The results showed no significant differences in pain between these three groups after three months from the initial injection. However, significant improvements were observed among all three arms using the von Frey filaments test. Exploratory analyses reported that repeat injections with 100 U of BoNT-A over six months had a significant reduction of pain including VAS and von Frey filaments. Fifty-eight percent of patients assessable after repeat BoNT-A injections with 100 U had symptom-free or ≥ 2 points improvement of VAS score.

In 2016 Pelletier et al. evaluated in a prospective cohort study the long-term effectiveness of BoNT-A injection for more than two years in 19 women with provoked vestibulodynia [61]. Fifty units of BoNT-A were diluted in 1.0 mL saline solution followed by injection into bilateral bulbospongiosus muscles for a total dose of 100 U. After 24 months, 37% of participants had no pain. After treatment, they showed significant improvements in the VAS, Dermatology Life Quality Index (DLQI) and Female Sexual Function Index (FSFI) scores at 24 months compared to baseline ($p < 0.0001$). Eighteen women (95%) were able to have sexual intercourse after 24 months.

BoNT-A was successfully used in sexual pain syndrome and appeared to have long-term beneficial effects for sexual activity (Table 4). It is important to continue further research for investigating the novel treatments in the sexual pain syndrome of women.

Table 4. Studies of BoNT-A injection for sexual pain syndrome in women.

Paper	Study Model	Patients	Treatment	Injection Sites	Result Measures	Duration	Outcomes
Yoon [58]	Retrospective study	7	Dilution: 20 U of BoNT-A diluted in isotonic saline. Dose: 20 to 40 U of BoNT-A	Vestibule, levator ani muscle, perineal body	VAS	4–24 months	• After BoNT-A injections, it showed disappear of pain in all patients. • Two patients needed only one injection; the other five patients received a 2nd injections • VAS score improved from 8.3 to 1.4, with no recurrence. • Improvement of sexual activity without significant discomfort during or after sexual intercourse.
Hebedo [59]	Prospective study	79	Dilution: 100 U of BoNT-A diluted into 1 mL isotonic saline. Dose: 100 U of BoNT-A	Bilaterally (50 units each site) and levator ani pars pubo rectalis	NRS NIQL Cotton swab test Active vita sexualis	6 months	• Dyspareunia: 7.81 to 5.82 ($p < 0.01$) • NIQL: 7.88 to 6.19 ($p < 0.01$) • Cotton swab test: 6.81 to 5.50 ($p < 0.01$) • Active Vitae Sexualis: no significances ($p = 0.25$)
Pelletier [61]	Prospective study	19	Dilution: 50 U of BoNT-A diluted into 1 mL saline. Dose: 100 U of BoNT-A	Bilateral bulbospongiosus muscles	VAS FSFI DLQI	24 months	• Cured: 37% • Mean VAS: 8.69 to 3.07 ($p < 0.0001$) • Mean DLQI: 19.2 to 9.05 ($p = 0.0005$) • Mean FSFI: 6.01 to 22.68 ($p < 0.0001$) • Able to have sexual intercourse: 95%
Diomande [60]	Randomized, double-blind, placebo-controlled study	32	• Dilution: 50 U (arm A) or 100 U (arm B) of BoNT-A diluted in 1 mL saline. • Dose: • Baseline: Arm A: 50 U Arm B: 100 U Arm C: saline • 3 month-visit: Arm A & B & C: 100 U (for symptomatic patients) • 6 month-visit: Arm A & B: - Arm C: 100 U (for symptomatic patients)	Subcutaneous layers of the dorsal vestibulum (each side 0.5 mL)	Cotton swab-provoked VASVon Frey filamentsMarinoff dyspareunia scale	6–9 months	• Improvement of cotton swab provoked VAS score: no significant difference between 3 groups and intragroup at 3 months. • Improvement of von Frey filaments: significantly reduced pain level in all treatment groups including placebo arm after 3 months. • It showed significant improvements of Marinoff dyspareunia scale between baseline and 3 months in arm A. • Success rate (≥ 2 VAS point improvement): 58%

NRS: Numerical rating scale. NIQL: Negative interference in quality of life. FSFI: Female Sexual Function Index. DLQI: Dermatology Life Quality Index.

7. Adverse Events of BoNT-A on CPPS

The common adverse events of BoNT-A injection into the bladder for IC/BPS are slow urinary flow rate, decreased detrusor pressure, and dysuria [39,62,63].

The most common adverse event of BoNT-A injection into PFMs for CPPS is dysuria. Increasing flatus has also been reported after BoNT-A injection into bilateral puborectalis and pubococcygeus muscles in women with chronic pelvic floor muscle spasms [14].

Adelowo et al. reported several adverse events, including retention of urine, fecal incontinence, constipation, and rectal pain after BoNT-A injection into PFMs (including coccygeus, iliococcygeus, pubococcygeus, puborectalis, obturator, and pyriformis muscles), which would be resolved spontaneously [36]. This might be because the injection sites were close to the sphincters of the urethra and anus.

Since the urethral sphincter and anal sphincter are adjacent to PFMs, BoNT-A injected into PFMs may result in disruption of urethral and/or anal sphincter mechanisms [30]. The adverse effects after BoNT-A injections reported progression of the following preexisting conditions: constipation (28.6%), stress urinary incontinence (4.8%), fecal incontinence (4.8%), and new-onset stress urinary incontinence (4.8%) [30]. Under electromyography (EMG) guidance, a needle provides more precise delivery of BoNT-A to highly spastic trigger points of the PFMs and helps with the avoidance of neighboring sphincter muscles [30].

Dressler et al. reported atrophy of target muscles after repeated injections of BoNT-A into a hyperactive muscle [64]. However, more serious side effects on systemic organs, such as respiratory failure, heart failure, weakness of muscles, or fatigue have not been reported [17].

Although most of the adverse events resulting from BoNT-A treatment are usually self-repairing, it should be clearly explained to the patient before BoNT-A injection. It is important to discuss with the patient the possibility of mild, transient, and reversible adverse effects on musculatures before BoNT-A injection.

There is still no guidelines about single injections or repeat injections, frequencies of repeat injections, an acceptable interval during repeat injections, injected sites and numbers, and maximum dosage of BoNT-A.

8. Conclusions

It is challenging to treat female CPPS patients because of the uncertainty of this disorder. There is currently no definite animal model for CPPS, although the chemical-induced cystitis rat model has been used to investigate the treatment strategy for this disease. Combination management, including physical therapy, biofeedback, behavioral modifications, and medicines may improve CPPS in women. Current literature suggests BoNT-A injection provides promising results in relieving symptoms of pelvic floor pain and muscle spasms in female patients. Intravesical injection of BoNT-A plus hydrodistension also helps to improve symptoms in refractory IC/BPS patients. BoNT-A injection appeared to have long-term beneficial effects for sexual activity in patients with sexual pain syndrome. It is safe for BoNT-A injection with limited adverse effects. However, more double-blind, randomized, eontrolled clinical studies and well-designed animal studies are needed to support the beneficial fficacy of BoNT-A injection in female patients with CPPS.

Author Contributions: C.-L.C. and E.M. wrote the paper; E.M. supervised and revised the paper. All authors have read and agreed to the published version of the manuscript.

References

1. Engeler, D.; Baranowski, A.P.; Berghmans, B.; Borovicka, J.; Cottrell, A.M.; Elneil, P.S.; Hughes, J.; Messelink, E.; de C Williams, A.C. EAU guidelines on chronic pelvic pain. 2019. Available online: https://uroweb.org/guideline/chronic-pelvic-pain/ (accessed on 1 December 2019).
2. Ahangari, A. Prevalence of chronic pelvic pain among women: an updated review. *Pain Physician* **2014**, *17*, E141–E147. [PubMed]
3. Mathias, S.D.; Kuppermann, M.; Liberman, R.F.; Lipschutz, R.C.; Steege, J.F. Chronic pelvic pain: prevalence, health-Related quality of life, and economic correlates. *Obstet. Gynecol.* **1996**, *87*, 321–327. [CrossRef]
4. Speer, L.M.; Mushkbar, S.; Erbele, T. Chronic Pelvic Pain in Women. *Am. Fam. Physician* **2016**, *93*, 380–387.
5. Purwar, B.; Khullar, V. Use of botulinum toxin for chronic pelvic pain. *Women's Health (Lond. Engl.)* **2016**, *12*, 293–296. [CrossRef] [PubMed]
6. Williams, R.E.; Hartmann, K.E.; Sandler, R.S.; Miller, W.C.; Steege, J.F. Prevalence and characteristics of irritable bowel syndrome among women with chronic pelvic pain. *Obstet. Gynecol.* **2004**, *104*, 452–458. [CrossRef] [PubMed]
7. Haggerty, C.L.; Peipert, J.F.; Weitzen, S.; Hendrix, S.L.; Holley, R.L.; Nelson, D.B.; Randall, H.; Soper, D.E.; Wiesenfeld, H.C.; Ness, R.B. Predictors of chronic pelvic pain in an urban population of women with symptoms and signs of pelvic inflammatory disease. *Sex. Transm. Dis.* **2005**, *32*, 293–299. [CrossRef]
8. Latthe, P.; Mignini, L.; Gray, R.; Hills, R.; Khan, K. Factors predisposing women to chronic pelvic pain: Systematic review. *BMJ (Clin. Res. ed.)* **2006**, *332*, 749–755. [CrossRef]
9. Cheong, Y.C.; Smotra, G.; Williams, A.C. Non-Surgical interventions for the management of chronic pelvic pain. *Cochrane Database Syst. Rev.* **2014**. [CrossRef]
10. Peck, M.W.; Smith, T.J.; Anniballi, F.; Austin, J.W.; Bano, L.; Bradshaw, M.; Cuervo, P.; Cheng, L.W.; Derman, Y.; Dorner, B.G.; et al. Historical Perspectives and Guidelines for Botulinum Neurotoxin Subtype Nomenclature. *Toxins* **2017**, *9*, 38. [CrossRef]
11. Moritz, M.S.; Tepp, W.H.; Bradshaw, M.; Johnson, E.A.; Pellett, S. Isolation and Characterization of the Novel Botulinum Neurotoxin A Subtype 6. *mSphere* **2018**, *3*. [CrossRef]
12. Moga, M.A.; Dimienescu, O.G.; Balan, A.; Scarneciu, I.; Barabas, B.; Ples, L. Therapeutic Approaches of Botulinum Toxin in Gynecology. *Toxins* **2018**, *10*, 169. [CrossRef] [PubMed]
13. Sloop, R.R.; Cole, B.A.; Escutin, R.O. Human response to botulinum toxin injection: type B compared with type A. *Neurology* **1997**, *49*, 189–194. [CrossRef] [PubMed]
14. Jarvis, S.K.; Abbott, J.A.; Lenart, M.B.; Steensma, A.; Vancaillie, T.G. Pilot study of botulinum toxin type A in the treatment of chronic pelvic pain associated with spasm of the levator ani muscles. *Aust. N. Z. J. Obstet. Gynaecol.* **2004**, *44*, 46–50. [CrossRef] [PubMed]
15. Stones, R.W.; Selfe, S.A.; Fransman, S.; Horn, S.A. Psychosocial and economic impact of chronic pelvic pain. *Best Pract. Res. Clin. Obstet. Gynaecol.* **2000**, *14*, 415–431. [CrossRef]
16. Erbguth, F.J. Historical notes on botulism, Clostridium botulinum, botulinum toxin, and the idea of the therapeutic use of the toxin. *Mov. Disord. Off. J. Mov. Disord. Soc.* **2004**, *19* (Suppl. 8), S2–S6. [CrossRef]
17. Jhang, J.F.; Kuo, H.C. Novel Treatment of Chronic Bladder Pain Syndrome and Other Pelvic Pain Disorders by OnabotulinumtoxinA Injection. *Toxins* **2015**, *7*, 2232–2250. [CrossRef]
18. Montenegro, M.L.; Mateus-Vasconcelos, E.C.; Rosa e Silva, J.C.; Nogueira, A.A.; Dos Reis, F.J.; Poli Neto, O.B. Importance of pelvic muscle tenderness evaluation in women with chronic pelvic pain. *Pain Med. (Malden, Mass.)* **2010**, *11*, 224–228. [CrossRef]
19. Tu, F.F.; As-Sanie, S.; Steege, J.F. Prevalence of pelvic musculoskeletal disorders in a female chronic pelvic pain clinic. *J. Reprod. Med.* **2006**, *51*, 185–189.
20. Mense, S. Neurobiological basis for the use of botulinum toxin in pain therapy. *J. Neurol.* **2004**, *251* (Suppl. 1), I1–I7. [CrossRef]
21. Kaya, S.; Hermans, L.; Willems, T.; Roussel, N.; Meeus, M. Central sensitization in urogynecological chronic pelvic pain: a systematic literature review. *Pain Physician* **2013**, *16*, 291–308.
22. Aoki, K.R. Evidence for antinociceptive activity of botulinum toxin type A in pain management. *Headache* **2003**, *43* (Suppl. 1), S9–S15. [CrossRef]

23. Foran, P.G.; Mohammed, N.; Lisk, G.O.; Nagwaney, S.; Lawrence, G.W.; Johnson, E.; Smith, L.; Aoki, K.R.; Dolly, J.O. Evaluation of the therapeutic usefulness of botulinum neurotoxin B, C1, E, and F compared with the long lasting type A. Basis for distinct durations of inhibition of exocytosis in central neurons. *J. Biol. Chem.* **2003**, *278*, 1363–1371. [CrossRef] [PubMed]
24. Durham, P.L.; Cady, R.; Cady, R. Regulation of calcitonin gene-Related peptide secretion from trigeminal nerve cells by botulinum toxin type A: implications for migraine therapy. *Headache* **2004**, *44*, 35–42. [CrossRef] [PubMed]
25. Khera, M.; Somogyi, G.T.; Kiss, S.; Boone, T.B.; Smith, C.P. Botulinum toxin A inhibits ATP release from bladder urothelium after chronic spinal cord injury. *Neurochem. Int.* **2004**, *45*, 987–993. [CrossRef] [PubMed]
26. Arezzo, J.C. Possible mechanisms for the effects of botulinum toxin on pain. *Clin. J. Pain* **2002**, *18*, S125–S132. [CrossRef] [PubMed]
27. Liu, B.L.; Yang, F.; Zhan, H.L.; Feng, Z.Y.; Zhang, Z.G.; Li, W.B.; Zhou, X.F. Increased severity of inflammation correlates with elevated expression of TRPV1 nerve fibers and nerve growth factor on interstitial cystitis/bladder pain syndrome. *Urol. Int.* **2014**, *92*, 202–208. [CrossRef] [PubMed]
28. Tempest, H.V.; Dixon, A.K.; Turner, W.H.; Elneil, S.; Sellers, L.A.; Ferguson, D.R. P2X and P2X receptor expression in human bladder urothelium and changes in interstitial cystitis. *BJU Int.* **2004**, *93*, 1344–1348. [CrossRef]
29. Xiao, L.; Cheng, J.; Dai, J.; Zhang, D. Botulinum toxin decreases hyperalgesia and inhibits P2 × 3 receptor over-Expression in sensory neurons induced by ventral root transection in rats. *Pain Med. (Malden, Mass.)* **2011**, *12*, 1385–1394. [CrossRef]
30. Morrissey, D.; El-Khawand, D.; Ginzburg, N.; Wehbe, S.; O'Hare, P., 3rd; Whitmore, K. Botulinum Toxin A Injections Into Pelvic Floor Muscles Under Electromyographic Guidance for Women With Refractory High-Tone Pelvic Floor Dysfunction: A 6-Month Prospective Pilot Study. *Female Pelvic Med. Reconstr. Surg.* **2015**, *21*, 277–282. [CrossRef]
31. Scott, A.B.; Rosenbaum, A.; Collins, C.C. Pharmacologic weakening of extraocular muscles. *Investig. Ophthalmol.* **1973**, *12*, 924–927.
32. Ho, K.Y.; Tan, K.H. Botulinum toxin A for myofascial trigger point injection: A qualitative systematic review. *Eur. J. Pain (Lond. Engl.)* **2007**, *11*, 519–527. [CrossRef] [PubMed]
33. Joo, J.S.; Agachan, F.; Wolff, B.; Nogueras, J.J.; Wexner, S.D. Initial North American experience with botulinum toxin type A for treatment of anismus. *Dis. Colon Rectum* **1996**, *39*, 1107–1111. [CrossRef] [PubMed]
34. Brin, M.F.; Vapnek, J.M. Treatment of vaginismus with botulinum toxin injections. *Lancet (Lond. Engl.)* **1997**, *349*, 252–253. [CrossRef]
35. Bhide, A.A.; Puccini, F.; Khullar, V.; Elneil, S.; Digesu, G.A. Botulinum neurotoxin type A injection of the pelvic floor muscle in pain due to spasticity: A review of the current literature. *Int. Urogynecol. J.* **2013**, *24*, 1429–1434. [CrossRef]
36. Adelowo, A.; Hacker, M.R.; Shapiro, A.; Modest, A.M.; Elkadry, E. Botulinum toxin type A (BOTOX) for refractory myofascial pelvic pain. *Female Pelvic Med. Reconstr. Surg.* **2013**, *19*, 288–292. [CrossRef]
37. Nesbitt-Hawes, E.M.; Won, H.; Jarvis, S.K.; Lyons, S.D.; Vancaillie, T.G.; Abbott, J.A. Improvement in pelvic pain with botulinum toxin type A-Single vs. repeat injections. *Toxicon Off. J. Int. Soc. Toxinol.* **2013**, *63*, 83–87. [CrossRef]
38. Halder, G.E.; Scott, L.; Wyman, A.; Mora, N.; Miladinovic, B.; Bassaly, R.; Hoyte, L. Botox combined with myofascial release physical therapy as a treatment for myofascial pelvic pain. *Investig. Clin. Urol.* **2017**, *58*, 134–139. [CrossRef]
39. Smith, C.P.; Radziszewski, P.; Borkowski, A.; Somogyi, G.T.; Boone, T.B.; Chancellor, M.B. Botulinum toxin a has antinociceptive effects in treating interstitial cystitis. *Urology* **2004**, *64*, 871–875. [CrossRef]
40. Kuo, H.C.; Chancellor, M.B. Comparison of intravesical botulinum toxin type A injections plus hydrodistention with hydrodistention alone for the treatment of refractory interstitial cystitis/painful bladder syndrome. *BJU Int.* **2009**, *104*, 657–661. [CrossRef]
41. Kuo, H.C.; Jiang, Y.H.; Tsai, Y.C.; Kuo, Y.C. Intravesical botulinum toxin-A injections reduce bladder pain of interstitial cystitis/bladder pain syndrome refractory to conventional treatment-A prospective, multicenter, randomized, double-blind, placebo-controlled clinical trial. *Neurourol. Urodyn.* **2016**, *35*, 609–614. [CrossRef]
42. Kuo, H.C. Repeated onabotulinumtoxin-A injections provide better results than single injection in treatment of painful bladder syndrome. *Pain Physician* **2013**, *16*, E15–E23. [PubMed]

43. Lee, C.L.; Kuo, H.C. Long-Term Efficacy and Safety of Repeated Intravescial OnabotulinumtoxinA Injections Plus Hydrodistention in the Treatment of Interstitial Cystitis/Bladder Pain Syndrome. *Toxins* **2015**, *7*, 4283–4293. [CrossRef] [PubMed]
44. Liu, H.T.; Kuo, H.C. Intravesical botulinum toxin A injections plus hydrodistension can reduce nerve growth factor production and control bladder pain in interstitial cystitis. *Urology* **2007**, *70*, 463–468. [CrossRef] [PubMed]
45. Shie, J.H.; Liu, H.T.; Wang, Y.S.; Kuo, H.C. Immunohistochemical evidence suggests repeated intravesical application of botulinum toxin A injections may improve treatment efficacy of interstitial cystitis/bladder pain syndrome. *BJU Int.* **2013**, *111*, 638–646. [CrossRef]
46. Peng, C.H.; Jhang, J.F.; Shie, J.H.; Kuo, H.C. Down regulation of vascular endothelial growth factor is associated with decreased inflammation after intravesical OnabotulinumtoxinA injections combined with hydrodistention for patients with interstitial cystitis-Clinical results and immunohistochemistry analysis. *Urology* **2013**, *82*, e1451–e1456. [CrossRef]
47. Pinto, R.A.; Costa, D.; Morgado, A.; Pereira, P.; Charrua, A.; Silva, J.; Cruz, F. Intratrigonal OnabotulinumtoxinA Improves Bladder Symptoms and Quality of Life in Patients with Bladder Pain Syndrome/Interstitial Cystitis: A Pilot, Single Center, Randomized, Double-Blind, Placebo Controlled Trial. *J. Urol.* **2018**, *199*, 998–1003. [CrossRef]
48. Jiang, Y.H.; Jhang, J.F.; Lee, C.L.; Kuo, H.C. Comparative study of efficacy and safety between bladder body and trigonal intravesical onabotulinumtoxina injection in the treatment of interstitial cystitis refractory to conventional treatment-A prospective, randomized, clinical trial. *Neurourol. Urodyn.* **2018**, *37*, 1467–1473. [CrossRef]
49. Kuo, Y.C.; Kuo, H.C. O'Leary-Sant Symptom Index Predicts the Treatment Outcome for OnabotulinumtoxinA Injections for Refractory Interstitial Cystitis/Bladder Pain Syndrome. *Toxins* **2015**, *7*, 2860–2871. [CrossRef]
50. Lucioni, A.; Bales, G.T.; Lotan, T.L.; McGehee, D.S.; Cook, S.P.; Rapp, D.E. Botulinum toxin type A inhibits sensory neuropeptide release in rat bladder models of acute injury and chronic inflammation. *BJU Int.* **2008**, *101*, 366–370. [CrossRef]
51. Cayan, S.; Coskun, B.; Bozlu, M.; Acar, D.; Akbay, E.; Ulusoy, E. Botulinum toxin type A may improve bladder function in a rat chemical cystitis model. *Urol. Res.* **2003**, *30*, 399–404. [CrossRef]
52. Smith, C.P.; Vemulakonda, V.M.; Kiss, S.; Boone, T.B.; Somogyi, G.T. Enhanced ATP release from rat bladder urothelium during chronic bladder inflammation: effect of botulinum toxin A. *Neurochem. Int.* **2005**, *47*, 291–297. [CrossRef] [PubMed]
53. Vemulakonda, V.M.; Somogyi, G.T.; Kiss, S.; Salas, N.A.; Boone, T.B.; Smith, C.P. Inhibitory effect of intravesically applied botulinum toxin A in chronic bladder inflammation. *J. Urol.* **2005**, *173*, 621–624. [CrossRef] [PubMed]
54. Vizzard, M.A. Alterations in neuropeptide expression in lumbosacral bladder pathways following chronic cystitis. *J. Chem. Neuroanat.* **2001**, *21*, 125–138. [CrossRef]
55. Latthe, P.; Latthe, M.; Say, L.; Gulmezoglu, M.; Khan, K.S. WHO systematic review of prevalence of chronic pelvic pain: a neglected reproductive health morbidity. *BMC Public Health* **2006**, *6*, 177. [CrossRef]
56. Sorensen, J.; Bautista, K.E.; Lamvu, G.; Feranec, J. Evaluation and Treatment of Female Sexual Pain: A Clinical Review. *Cureus* **2018**, *10*, e2379. [CrossRef]
57. Harlow, B.L.; Kunitz, C.G.; Nguyen, R.H.; Rydell, S.A.; Turner, R.M.; MacLehose, R.F. Prevalence of symptoms consistent with a diagnosis of vulvodynia: population-Based estimates from 2 geographic regions. *Am. J. Obstet. Gynecol.* **2014**, *210*, 40.e41–e48. [CrossRef]
58. Yoon, H.; Chung, W.S.; Shim, B.S. Botulinum toxin A for the management of vulvodynia. *Int. J. Impot. Res.* **2007**, *19*, 84–87. [CrossRef]
59. Hedebo Hansen, T.; Guldberg, R.; Meinert, M. Botulinum toxin-Treatment of localized provoked vulvodynia refractory to conventional treatment. *Eur. J. Obstet. Gynecol. Reprod. Biol.* **2019**, *234*, 6–9. [CrossRef]
60. Diomande, I.; Gabriel, N.; Kashiwagi, M.; Ghisu, G.P.; Welter, J.; Fink, D.; Fehr, M.K.; Betschart, C. Subcutaneous botulinum toxin type A injections for provoked vestibulodynia: A randomized placebo-Controlled trial and exploratory subanalysis. *Arch Gynecol. Obstet.* **2019**, *299*, 993–1000. [CrossRef]
61. Pelletier, F.; Girardin, M.; Humbert, P.; Puyraveau, M.; Aubin, F.; Parratte, B. Long-Term assessment of effectiveness and quality of life of OnabotulinumtoxinA injections in provoked vestibulodynia. *J. Eur. Acad. Dermatol. Venereol. JEADV* **2016**, *30*, 106–111. [CrossRef]

62. Chung, S.D.; Kuo, Y.C.; Kuo, H.C. Intravesical onabotulinumtoxinA injections for refractory painful bladder syndrome. *Pain Physician* **2012**, *15*, 197–202. [PubMed]
63. Giannantoni, A.; Porena, M.; Costantini, E.; Zucchi, A.; Mearini, L.; Mearini, E. Botulinum A toxin intravesical injection in patients with painful bladder syndrome: 1-Year followup. *J. Urol.* **2008**, *179*, 1031–1034. [CrossRef] [PubMed]
64. Dressler, D.; Adib Saberi, F. Botulinum toxin: Mechanisms of action. *Eur. Neurol.* **2005**, *53*, 3–9. [CrossRef] [PubMed]

14

Predictive Factors for a Satisfactory Treatment Outcome with Intravesical Botulinum Toxin A Injection in Patients with Interstitial Cystitis/Bladder Pain Syndrome

Hsiu-Jen Wang [1], Wan-Ru Yu [2], Hueih-Ling Ong [3] and Hann-Chorng Kuo [1,*]

1 Department of Urology, Hualien Tzu Chi Hospital, Buddhist Tzu Chi Medical Foundation and Tzu Chi University, Hualien 970, Taiwan
2 Department of Nursing, Hualien Tzu Chi Hospital, Buddhist Tzu Chi Medical Foundation and Tzu Chi University, Hualien 970, Taiwan
3 Department of Urology, Dalin Tzu Chi Hospital, Buddhist Tzu Chi Medical Foundation, Chiayi 622, Taiwan
* Correspondence: hck@tzuchi.com.tw

Abstract: A botulinum toxin A (BoNT-A) intravesical injection can improve the symptoms of interstitial cystitis/bladder pain syndrome (IC/BPS). Patients with IC/BPS have different clinical characteristics, urodynamic features, and cystoscopic findings. This study assessed the treatment outcomes of a BoNT-A intravesical injection and aimed to identify the predictive factors of a satisfactory outcome. This retrospective study included IC/BPS patients treated with 100 U BoNT-A. The treatment outcomes were assessed by global response assessment (GRA) at 6 months. We classified patients according to different clinical, urodynamic, and cystoscopic characteristics and evaluated the treatment outcomes and predictive factors. A total of 238 patients were included. Among these patients, 113 (47.5%) had a satisfactory outcome (GRA $\geq$ 2) and 125 (52.5%) had an unsatisfactory outcome. Improvements in the IC symptom score, IC problem score, O'Leary–Sant symptom score, and visual analog scale score for pain were significantly greater in patients with a satisfactory outcome than in patients with an unsatisfactory outcome (all $p = 0.000$). The IC disease duration and maximal bladder capacity (MBC) were significantly different between patients with and without a satisfactory outcome. Multivariate analysis revealed that only the MBC was a predictor for a satisfactory outcome. Patients with a MBC of ≥760 mL and glomerulations of 0/1 (58.7%) or glomerulations of 2/3 (75.0%) frequently had a satisfactory outcome. We found that BoNT-A intravesical injection can effectively improve symptoms among patients with IC/BPS, with a remarkable reduction in bladder pain. A MBC of ≥760 mL is a predictive factor for a satisfactory treatment outcome.

Keywords: bladder pain; botulinum toxin A; predictor; maximal bladder capacity; hydrodistention

Key Contribution: Single intravesical botulinum toxin A (BoNT-A) injection improved symptoms in 47.5% of IC/BPS patients. A maximal bladder capacity of ≥760 mL during cystoscopic hydrodistention predicts a satisfactory outcome, regardless of the glomerulation grade.

---

1. Introduction

Interstitial cystitis/bladder pain syndrome (IC/BPS) is a clinical symptom syndrome characterized by frequency, urgency, and nocturia, with or without bladder pain [1]. Although this mysterious disease has been documented for over 100 years, the underlying pathophysiology is still not well elucidated. IC/BPS is usually classified as ulcer type (with Hunner's lesion) or non-ulcer type (with glomerulations after cystoscopic hydrodistention) [1,2]. Among all symptoms, pelvic pain has been considered as the primary symptom of IC/BPS [3]. However, a previous study found that some patients presenting with similar indicative symptoms did not show remarkable glomerulations, and a hypersensitive bladder was considered [4].

Chronic inflammation of the bladder has been accepted as the fundamental cause of IC/BPS [5]; however, the reasons for inflammation are unclear. This unsolved bladder inflammation results in denudation of the urothelium, abnormal expression of tight junction proteins, deficiency of barrier proteins, altered differentiation of urothelial cells, and increased permeability of the bladder urothelium [6–11]. A previous study demonstrated that intravesical botulinum toxin A (BoNT-A) can reduce bladder pain in IC/BPS patients [12]. Additionally, repeated BoNT-A intravesical injections have been shown to increase functional bladder capacity and reduce bladder pain in responders [13]. In IC/BPS patients, BoNT-A treatment could gradually reduce bladder inflammation and improve urothelial repair, leading to symptomatic relief [14].

Clinically, not all IC/BPS patients have the same bladder characteristics and histological findings. Some IC/BPS patients have comorbid systemic diseases and mental illnesses [14,15]. Functional somatic syndrome has been found to be closely associated with IC/BPS [16]. IC/BPS might involve heterogeneous subgroups of patients who present with different clinical, urodynamic, and cystoscopic characteristics [17].

Although BoNT-A intravesical injection is listed as the third-line therapeutic option for IC/BPS, the treatment effect has not been well demonstrated in real-world practice, and the predictors for a satisfactory outcome have not been clarified. A previous study on BoNT-A injection for IC/BPS revealed excellent symptom improvement in approximately 60% of patients [18]. However, the long-term treatment efficacy of BoNT-A injections with regard to IC/BPS has not been established [19], and repeat intravesical BoNT-A injections are necessary to achieve a better long-term outcome [20]. The treatment efficacy of BoNT-A injections might differ depending on the IC/BPS phenotype.

The present study aimed to assess the treatment outcomes of an intravesical BoNT-A injection and identify the predictive factors for a satisfactory treatment outcome in patients with IC/BPS.

2. Results

A total of 238 patients (38 male and 200 female patients) were included in this study. The mean patient age at the diagnosis of IC/BPS was 40.2 ± 13.5 years, and the mean duration of their treatment course for IC/BPS was 15.1 ± 9.5 years. According to the definition of treatment outcome, a satisfactory outcome (global response assessment (GRA) ≥ 2) was noted in 113 (47.5%) patients and an unsatisfactory outcome (GRA ≤ 1) was noted in 125 (52.5%) patients. In the beginning, we used receiver operation characteristics to analyze the cut-off value for a satisfactory treatment outcome. According to the treatment outcome, the result revealed that a maximal bladder capacity (MBC) of ≥760 mL had the greatest area under the curve (AUC = 0.547). Patients with a satisfactory outcome had a significantly greater MBC than those with an unsatisfactory outcome (684.5 ± 197.5 mL vs. 619.1 ± 192.3 mL, $p = 0.010$). The clinical characteristics, urodynamic findings, and cystoscopic findings of the satisfactory and unsatisfactory groups are listed in Table 1. The IC/BPS duration was significantly shorter and the rate of MBC ≥ 760 mL was significantly higher in the satisfactory group than in the unsatisfactory group ($p = 0.017$ and $p = 0.002$, respectively). The other variables showed no significant differences between the groups. Therefore, we further classified the patients into five subgroups according to the glomerulation grade (0/1, 2/3, and Hunner's lesion) and MBC (≥760 mL or <760 mL) during cystoscopic hydrodistention. Patients with glomerulation grade 2/3 and MBC ≥ 760 mL had a satisfactory rate of 75%, and those with glomerulation grade 0/1 and MBC ≥ 760 mL had a satisfactory rate of 58.7%, the satisfactory rates of the other subgroups were approximately 40% ($p = 0.024$) (Table 2). Multivariate analysis revealed that a MBC ≥ 760 mL ($p = 0.000$) and the IC/BPS phenotype ($p = 0.012$) were predictive factors for a satisfactory outcome.

Table 1. Characteristics of the study patients according to the treatment outcome.

Characteristics	Item	Unsatisfactory Outcome GRA ≤ 1 (n = 125)	Satisfactory Outcome GRA ≥ 2 (n = 113)	Univariate *p*-Value	Multivariate *p*-Value
Sex (male:female)		18:107	20:93	0.488	
Age at IC symptom (years)		39.8 ± 13.6	42.7 ± 13.7	0.127	
IC duration (years)		16.6 ± 10.7	13.5 ± 8.64	0.017	
Comorbidity	≥2	64 (52.0%)	59 (48.0%)	0.532	
	≤1	61 (55.7%)	54 (44.3%)		
Bladder pain	Yes	86 (56.2%)	67 (43.8%)	0.126	
	no	39 (45.9%)	46 (54.1%)		
Increased bladder sensation	Yes	107 (52.2%)	98 (47.8%)	0.802	0.292
	No	18 (50.5%)	15 (45.5%)		
Detrusor overactivity	Yes	16 (53.3%)	14 (46.7%)	0.924	0.904
	No	109 (52.4%)	99 (47.6%)		
Bladder neck dysfunction	Yes	4 (40.4%)	6 (60.0%)	0.524	0.732
	No	121 (53.1%)	107 (46.9%)		
Dysfunctional voiding	Yes	9 (52.9%)	8 (47.1%)	0.971	0.619
	No	116 (52.5%)	105 (47.5%)		
Poor PFM relaxation	Yes	62 (56.9%)	47 (43.1%)	0.216	0.206
	No	63 (48.8%)	66 (51.2%)		
Intrinsic sphincter deficiency	Yes	4 (66.7%)	2 (33.3%)	0.686	0.087
	No	121 (52.2%)	111 (47.8%)		
Maximal bladder capacity (mL)	Mean	619.1 ± 192.3	684.5 ± 197.5	0.010	
	≥760	24 (36.4%)	42 (63.6%)	0.002	0.000
	<760	101 (58.7%)	71 (41.3%)		
Glomerulation	0/1	47 (51.1%)	45 (48.9%)	0.940	0.537
	2/3	71 (53.4%)	62 (46.6%)		
	ulcer	7 (53.8%)	6 (46.2%)		
IC phenotype		125 (52.5%)	113 (47.5%)	0.024	0.012

GRA, global response assessment; IC, interstitial cystitis; PFM, pelvic floor muscle.

Table 2. Cystoscopic phenotype distribution according to the treatment outcome.

Phenotype	Unsatisfactory Outcome GRA ≤ 1	Satisfactory Outcome GRA ≥ 2	Total
Glomerulation 0/1, MBC ≥ 760 mL	19 (41.3%)	27 (58.7%)	46 (19.3%)
Glomerulation 0/1, MBC < 760 mL	28 (60.9%)	18 (39.1%)	46 (19.3%)
Glomerulation 2/3, MBC ≥ 760 mL	5 (25.0%)	15 (75.0%)	20 (8.4%)
Glomerulation 2/3, MBC < 760 mL	66 (58.4%)	47 (41.6%)	113 (47.5%)
With Hunner's lesion	7 (53.8%)	6 (46.2%)	13 (5.5%)
Total	125 (52.5%)	113 (47.5%)	238 (100%)

GRA, global response assessment; MBC, maximal bladder capacity.

The changes in clinical symptoms and the urodynamic parameters after BoNT-A injections are shown in Table 3. Both the satisfactory and unsatisfactory groups showed improvements in the interstitial cystitis symptom index (ICSI), interstitial cystitis problem index (ICPI), O'Leary–Sant symptom score (OSS), and visual analog scale (VAS) score after BoNT-A treatment. However, the improvements in symptomatic variables were significantly greater in the satisfactory group than those in the unsatisfactory group. The urodynamic parameters revealed that both the satisfactory and unsatisfactory groups had an increase in the bladder capacity of first sensation of bladder filling (FSF) and post-void residual (PVR) volume, while the voided volume did not change; however, a significant change in the detrusor pressure after a BoNT-A intravesical injection was noted only in the patients with a satisfactory outcome.

Table 3. Changes in symptom scores and urodynamic parameters from baseline to 6 months after intravesical Botox injection according to the treatment outcome.

Urodynamic Parameters	Time Point	Unsatisfactory Outcome GRA ≤ 1 (n = 125)	Satisfactory Outcome GRA ≥ 2 (n = 113)	Total (n = 238)
ICSI	BL	12.2 ± 3.70	12.6 ± 3.77	
	FU	9.41 ± 4.71 *	4.97 ± 3.88 *#	
ICPI	BL	11.5 ± 3.07	12.0 ± 3.39	
	FU	9.45 ± 4.41 *	4.59 ± 4.23 *#	
OSS	BL	23.7 ± 6.39	24.6 ± 6.64	
	FU	18.9 ± 8.56 *	9.56 ± 7.77 *#	
VAS score	BL	4.48 ± 32.42	5.19 ± 2.77	
	FU	3.87 ± 3.38	2.15 ± 2.74 *#	
First sensation (mL)	BL	112 ± 50.5	117 ± 51.9	115 ± 51.2
	FU	126 ± 67.9 *	130 ± 58.2 *	128 ± 63.2 *
Full sensation (mL)	BL	177 ± 74.2	184 ± 73.3	180 ± 7.7
	FU	190 ± 91.1	205 ± 90.0	197 ± 90.6 *
Urge sensation (mL)	BL	216 ± 86.6	229 ± 90.1	222 ± 88.4
	FU	222 ± 110	238 ± 110	230 ± 110
Detrusor pressure (cmH_2O)	BL	20.4 ± 12.7	21.9 ± 14.9	21.1 ± 13.
	FU	21.4 ± 25.7	18.2 ± 14.4 *	819.9 ± 20.9
Maximum flow rate (mL/s)	BL	12.0 ± 6.51	12.5 ± 4.94	12.3 ± 5.79
	FU	10.5 ± 5.97	12.4 ± 6.30	11.4 ± 6.19
Voided volume (mL)	BL	232 ± 113	268 ± 130	249 ± 123
	FU	227 ± 139	253 ± 131	240 ± 135
Post-void residual volume (mL)	BL	39.4 ± 71.3	26.9 ± 53.4	33.2 ± 63.3
	FU	70.4 ± 106 *	48.0 ± 82.1 *	59.3 ± 95.2 *
Cystometric bladder capacity (mL)	BL	273 ± 109	297 ± 126	285 ± 11
	FU	290 ± 147	304 ± 126	8297 ± 137
Bladder compliance (mL/cmH_2O)	BL	63.4 ± 67.0	60.0 ± 61.	61.7 ± 64.4
	FU	62.7 ± 60.0	879.7 ± 88.5	71.1 ± 75.7

* $p < 0.05$ in variables between baseline and follow-up within group; # $p < 0.05$ in the change of variables from baseline to follow-up between group. GRA, global response assessment; ICSI, interstitial cystitis symptom index; ICPI, interstitial cystitis problem index; OSS, O'Leary–Sant symptom score; VAS, visual analog scale; BL, baseline; FU, follow-up.

Adverse events were hematuria after injection in 12 (5%) patients, urinary tract infection in 18 (7.6%), and mild dysuria in 24 (10.1%). No urinary retention was reported in any of the patients treated.

3. Discussion

The results of this study demonstrated that an intravesical BoNT-A injection greatly improved symptoms in 47.5% of IC/BPS patients with a long disease duration and refractory to medical treatment. Patients with an unsatisfactory outcome also showed symptomatic improvement, but the urodynamic parameters did not change after treatment. A MBC ≥ 760 mL during cystoscopic hydrodistention predicts a satisfactory outcome, regardless of the glomerulation grade.

A BoNT-A intravesical injection for the treatment of IC/BPS has been attempted for the last 15 years. An intravesical BoNT-A (100–200 U) injection into the detrusor plus hydrodistention has been shown to be effective for alleviating bladder pain and decreasing frequency nocturia in IC/BPS patients [21]. Additionally, a previous randomized, double-blind clinical trial demonstrated that BoNT-A (100 U) is effective and safe for the treatment of IC/BPS [18]. The bladder pain reduction and bladder capacity improvement were significantly greater in the patients receiving BoNT-A treatment than in the placebo group [18]. In this study, we only found that a single BoNT-A injection increased the FSF, but not the voided volume. A BoNT-A injection in IC/BPS bladders has been found to inhibit noxious neurotransmitter releases, including calcitonin gene-related peptide, glutamate, adenosine triphosphate, and substance P from neurons [22]. Therefore, the therapeutic effect of BoNT-A on sensory afferents could reduce the sensory urgency and increase FSF. With solid evidence, an intravesical BoNT-A injection has been listed as a fourth-line therapeutic option in the clinical guidelines for IC/BPS in the American Urological Association [23].

The clinical presentations of IC/PBS are frequency and urgency with or without bladder and lower abdominal pain, glomerulations developed after cystoscopic hydrodistention, and denudation of the bladder urothelium [5]. As the actual pathophysiology of IC/BPS has not been well elucidated, there could be different underlying pathologies in IC/BPS bladders, resulting in heterogeneous clinical phenotypes. Among the different clinical characteristics of IC/BPS, Hunner's lesion, bladder pain symptoms, glomerulation grade, and MBC after cystoscopic hydrodistention might imply different pathophysiologies in the diseased bladder. A bladder with a Hunner's lesion usually has chronic inflammation at the lesion, and it causes severe pain when the bladder is distended. High expressions of T-cell and B-cell makers in the submucosa and high urinary immunoglobulin levels have been noted in Hunner's lesion [24]. Urothelial dysfunction due to abnormal urothelial cell differentiation, loss of E-cadherin and zonula occluden-1 expression, and deficient differentiation makers are remarkable in IC/BPS bladders [24]. High acute and chronic bladder inflammation, high lymphocyte infiltration, but not mast cell activation, limit the bladder capacity during cystoscopic hydrodistention and cause a low anesthetic bladder capacity [25]. High sensory afferent nerve activity causes an increase in bladder pain and a small functional capacity in daily life [26].

The previous classification usually divided IC/BPS into Hunner's lesion and non-ulcer IC/BPS. This classification was based on histopathologic findings, distinct clinical characteristics, and underlying pathophysiology [27]. Recent Asian IC guidelines added the hypersensitive bladder subtype to define a subgroup of patients with IC clinical symptoms but no glomerulation [4]. In real-world practice, we noted that the glomerulation grade and MBC might have different combinations during cystoscopic hydrodistention. In this study, a MBC $\geq$ 760 mL was found to have a significantly better treatment outcome after the intravesical BoNT-A injection. The glomerulation grade does not have a predictive value for the BoNT-A treatment outcome. If glomerulation and MBC are combined for IC/BPS, a satisfactory treatment outcome is still mainly based on a MBC $\geq$ 760 mL, suggesting that a larger MBC indicates a better response to a BoNT-A injection.

BoNT-A has been demonstrated to have anti-inflammatory effects on the chronic cystitis rat model and to reduce the expression of nerve growth factors in IC/BPS bladders, with satisfactory pain relief [28,29]. In addition, a BoNT-A injection relaxes the smooth muscles and increases functional bladder capacity through the inhibition of acetylcholine release. After a BoNT-A injection, both motor and sensory nerves are affected and patients experience symptomatic relief [18]. The results of this study demonstrate that patients with a satisfactory outcome showed a great decrease in detrusor pressure after the BoNT-A intravesical injection, suggesting a strong response of the detrusor muscle to the BoNT-A injection in patients with a satisfactory outcome. Although the PVR volume increased significantly after the BoNT-A injection in both patients with a satisfactory outcome and those with an unsatisfactory outcome, there was no significant difference between group. The increased PVR was not clinically significant, because only 10.1% of patients complained of dysuria after the BoNT-A injection. Moreover, no patient reported acute urinary retention after the BoNT-A injection, indicating that BoNT-A is a safe and effective treatment for IC/BPS refractory to lifestyle modification and medical treatment. Although the satisfactory rate is not high after one single BoNT-A injection, our previous study showed that repeated BoNT-A injections could improve the satisfactory rate [20].

4. Conclusions

The present study showed that a BoNT-A injection is effective for pain relief and symptom improvement among IC/BPS patients. The improvement in bladder pain is remarkable in patients with a satisfactory treatment outcome. A MBC $\geq$ 760 mL is a predictive factor for a satisfactory treatment outcome, whereas glomerulation grade and urodynamic parameters do not have predictive value for the IC/BPS treatment outcome.

5. Materials and Methods

This retrospective study included IC/BPS patients who had been treated for the first time with 100 U of BoNT-A (BOTOX, Allergan, Irvine, CA, USA) in 10 mL saline injected at 20 sites. All patients had been diagnosed to have IC/BPS based on the characteristic IC symptoms and cystoscopic findings of glomerulations, petechiae, or mucosal fissures on hydrodistention under anesthesia [30]. Among the IC/BPS patients, at least two treatment modalities had been tried, including lifestyle modification, cystoscopic hydrodistention, intravesical hyaluronic acid instillation, or painkiller medication, but the IC symptoms were persistent or had relapsed.

All patients received a thorough investigation at enrollment and were not included if they failed to meet the inclusion criteria of the National Institute of Diabetes and Digestive and Kidney Diseases (NIDDK) [31]. The treatment outcomes were assessed by the global response assessment (GRA) at 6 months after an intravesical BoNT-A injection. In addition, the IC symptoms were assessed by the O'Leary–Sant symptom score (OSS), including the IC symptom index (ICSI) and IC problem index (ICPI) [32]. The bladder pain was also reported by a self-assessed 10-point visual analog scale (VAS).

This study had been approved by the Research Ethics Committee of Hualien Tzu Chi Hospital, Buddhist Tzu Chi Medical Foundation (IRB 105-25-B, date of approval: 2 June 2018). The written informed consent was waived due to the nature of retrospective analysis.

A videourodynamic study (VUDS) was performed before the BoNT-A injection, using standard procedures. The VUDS involved the infusion of normal saline at a rate of 20 mL/min. All descriptions and terminologies used in this study were according to the recommendations of the International Continence Society [33]. The reported urodynamic parameters included: FSF, urge sensation, cystometric bladder capacity, pressure, maximum flow rate (Qmax) and detrusor pressure at Qmax during voiding, and post-void residual (PVR) volume. According to the characteristic VUDS findings, the urodynamic diagnosis was recorded as increased bladder sensation, detrusor overactivity, dysfunctional voiding, poor pelvic floor muscle relaxation, or intrinsic sphincter deficiency [34]. The potassium chloride (KCl) test (infusion of 0.4 M KCl in normal saline) was performed after evacuation of the PVR urine. The KCl test was considered positive if there was bladder pain or a severe urge to void during the KCl infusion [35]. The VUDS was performed at baseline to confirm the diagnosis of IC/BPS and search for other bladder conditions mimicking IC/BPS. A repeat VUDS was performed at 6 months after the first BoNT-A injection to evaluate the bladder condition after treatment and as a guide for the selection of the next step treatment.

The injected BoNT-A solution constituted a vial of onabotulinumtoxinA (100 U) diluted with 10 mL of normal saline. Each 1.0 mL solution contained 10 U of BoNT-A in saline. A total of 20 injections were performed with this BoNT-A solution, resulting in 5 U of BoNT-A in each injection site. The injection technique was reported in our previous article [18]. In brief, the BoNT-A solution was injected in four rows (each row with 5 injection sites) from the interureteric ridge to the bladder dome to cover the lateral and posterior wall, at a bladder capacity of 100 mL. The trigone was spared, because glomerulations are usually not involved in this region. After the BoNT-A injections, cystoscopic hydrodistention was routinely performed by a slow infusion of normal saline to an 80 cm H_2O intravesical pressure for 15 min. The maximal bladder capacity (MBC) at the end of the infusion and the degree of glomerulations developed after bladder drainage were also recorded [18]. The glomerulation grade was classified as 0, 1, 2, and 3 based on the appearance of glomerulations at none, less than half, more than half, and more than half of the bladder wall and severe waterfall bleeding, respectively. Patients were classified as ulcer type IC/BPS if a Hunner's lesion was present with and without glomerulations [4]. After BoNT-A treatment, patients were indwelled with a 14-Fr Foley catheter overnight and discharged the next day. An antibiotic (cephalexin 500 mg every 6 h) was routinely prescribed for seven days and patients visited the outpatient clinic at 2, 4, and 8 weeks after treatment, followed by monthly visits in the outpatient clinic for outcome assessment. The primary end-point was 6 months after the BoNT-A injection.

We classified patients into five subgroups according to different clinical, urodynamic, and cystoscopic characteristics (MBC and glomerulations) and evaluated the treatment outcome (GRA ≥ 2 or GRA ≤ 1), symptom change (with and without bladder pain), urodynamic findings, and comorbidity coexistence. Predictive factors for a satisfactory outcome were also assessed.

The continuous variables reported in this study are expressed as means ± standard deviations (SDs). The Wilcoxon rank-sum test was used for statistical comparisons of continuous variables between groups, and the Wilcoxon sign-rank test was used to evaluate the difference of the variables between baseline and post-treatment. All statistical assessments were performed by two-sided analysis, and significant differences were considered at a p-value < 0.05. SPSS version 15.0 statistical software (SPSS Inc., Chicago, IL, USA) was used in all statistical analyses.

Author Contributions: Conceptualization, H.-C.K.; methodology, H.-J.W., W.-R.Y. and H.-L.O.; formal analysis, H.-L.O., H.-J.W. and W.-R.Y.; writing manuscript-draft, H.-J.W. and W.-R.Y.; writing—review and editing, H.-C.K.; supervision, H.-C.K.

References

1. Bouchelouche, K.; Nordling, J. Recent developments in the management of interstitial cystitis. *Curr. Opin. Urol.* **2003**, *13*, 309–313. [CrossRef] [PubMed]
2. Hanno, P.M.; Sant, G.R. Clinical highlights of the National Institute of Diabetes and Digestive and Kidney Diseases/Interstitial Cystitis Association scientific conference on interstitial cystitis. *Urology* **2001**, *57*, 2–6. [CrossRef]
3. Hanno, P.M.; Burks, D.A.; Clemens, J.Q.; Dmochowski, R.R.; Erickson, D.; Fitzgerald, M.P.; Forrest, J.B.; Gordon, B.; Gray, M.; Mayer, R.D.; et al. AUA guideline for the diagnosis and treatment of interstitial cystitis/bladder pain syndrome. *J. Urol.* **2011**, *185*, 2162–2170. [CrossRef] [PubMed]
4. Homma, Y.; Ueda, T.; Tomoe, H.; Lin, A.T.; Kuo, H.C.; Lee, M.H.; Oh, S.J.; Kim, J.C.; Lee, K.S. Clinical guidelines for interstitial cystitis and hypersensitive bladder updated in 2015. *Int. J. Urol.* **2016**, *23*, 542–549. [CrossRef] [PubMed]
5. Sant, G.R.; Kempuraj, D.; Marchand, J.E.; Theoharides, T.C. The mast cell in interstitial cystitis: Role in pathophysiology and pathogenesis. *Urology* **2007**, *69*, 34–40. [CrossRef] [PubMed]
6. Shie, J.H.; Kuo, H.C. Higher levels of cell apoptosis and abnormal E-cadherin expression in the urothelium are associated with inflammation in patients with interstitial cystitis/painful bladder syndrome. *BJU Int.* **2011**, *108*, 136–141. [CrossRef] [PubMed]
7. Southgate, J.; Varley, C.L.; Garthwaite, M.A.; Hinley, J.; Marsh, F.; Stahlschmidt, J.; Trejdosiewicz, L.K.; Eardley, I. Differentiation potential of urothelium from patients with benign bladder dysfunction. *BJU Int.* **2007**, *99*, 1506–1516. [CrossRef]
8. Zeng, Y.; Wu, X.X.; Homma, Y.; Yoshimura, N.; Iwaki, H.; Kageyama, S.; Yoshiki, T.; Kakehi, Y. Uroplakin III-delta4 messenger RNA as a promising marker to identify nonulcerative interstitial cystitis. *J. Urol.* **2007**, *178*, 1322–1327. [CrossRef]
9. Hauser, P.J.; Dozmorov, M.G.; Bane, B.L.; Slobodov, G.; Culkin, D.J.; Hurst, R.E. Abnormal expression of differentiation related proteins and proteoglycan core proteins in the urothelium of patients with interstitial cystitis. *J. Urol.* **2008**, *179*, 764–769. [CrossRef]
10. Kim, J.; Keay, S.K.; Dimitrakov, J.D.; Freeman, M.R. p53 mediates interstitial cystitis antiproliferative factor (APF)-induced growth inhibition of human urothelial cells. *FEBS Lett.* **2007**, *581*, 3795–3799. [CrossRef]
11. Parsons, C.L. The role of a leaky epithelium and potassium in the generation of bladder symptoms in interstitial cystitis/overactive bladder, urethral syndrome, prostatitis and gynaecological chronic pelvic pain. *BJU Int.* **2011**, *107*, 370–375. [CrossRef] [PubMed]
12. Lee, C.L.; Kuo, H.C. Long-term efficacy and safety of repeated intravescial onabotulinumtoxinA injections plus hydrodistention in the treatment of interstitial cystitis/ bladder pain syndrome. *Toxins* **2015**, *7*, 4283–4293. [CrossRef] [PubMed]

13. Shie, J.H.; Liu, H.T.; Wang, Y.S.; Kuo, H.C. Immunohistochemical evidence suggests repeated intravesical application of botulinum toxin A injections may improve treatment efficacy of interstitial cystitis/bladder pain syndrome. *BJU Int.* **2013**, *111*, 638–646. [CrossRef] [PubMed]
14. Keller, J.J.; Chen, Y.K.; Lin, H.C. Comorbidities of bladder pain syndrome/interstitial cystitis: A population-based study. *BJU Int.* **2012**, *110*, 903–909. [CrossRef] [PubMed]
15. Nickel, J.C.; Tripp, D.A.; International Interstitial Cystitis Study Group. Clinical and psychological parameters associated with pain pattern phenotypes in women with interstitial cystitis/bladder pain syndrome. *J. Urol.* **2015**, *193*, 138–144. [CrossRef]
16. Clemens, J.Q.; Elliott, M.N.; Suttorp, M.; Berry, S.H. Temporal ordering of interstitial cystitis/bladder pain syndrome and non-bladder conditions. *Urology* **2012**, *80*, 1227–1231. [CrossRef]
17. Fuoco, M.B.; Irvine-Bird, K.; Curtis Nickel, J. Multiple sensitivity phenotype in interstitial cystitis/bladder pain syndrome. *Can. Urol. Assoc. J.* **2014**, *8*, 758–761. [CrossRef]
18. Kuo, H.C.; Jiang, Y.H.; Tsai, Y.C.; Kuo, Y.C. Intravesical botulinum toxin-A injections reduce bladder pain of interstitial cystitis/bladder pain syndrome refractory to conventional treatment-A prospective, multicenter, randomized, double-blind, placebo-controlled clinical trial. *Urol. Sci.* **2016**, *35*, 609–614. [CrossRef]
19. Giannantoni, A.; Porena, M.; Costantini, E.; Zucchi, A.; Mearini, L.; Mearini, E. Botulinum A toxin intravesical injection in patients with painful bladder syndrome: 1-year followup. *J. Urol.* **2008**, *179*, 1031–1034. [CrossRef]
20. Kuo, H.C. Repeated onabotulinumtoxin-a injections provide better results than single injection in treatment of painful bladder syndrome. *Pain Physician* **2013**, *16*, E15–E23.
21. Smith, C.P.; Radziszewski, P.; Borkowski, A.; Somogyi, G.T.; Boone, T.B.; Chancellor, M.B. Botulinum toxin A has antinociceptive effects in treating interstitial cystitis. *Urology* **2004**, *64*, 871–875. [CrossRef] [PubMed]
22. Jhang, J.F.; Kuo, H.C. Novel treatment of chronic bladder pain syndrome and other pelvic pain disorders by onabotulinumtoxinA injection. *Toxins* **2015**, *7*, 2232–2250. [CrossRef] [PubMed]
23. Gamper, M.; Viereck, V.; Eberhard, J.; Binder, J.; Moll, C.; Welter, J.; Moser, R. Local immune response in bladder pain syndrome/interstitial cystitis ESSIC type 3C. *Int. Urogynecol. J.* **2013**, *24*, 2049–2057. [CrossRef] [PubMed]
24. Liu, H.T.; Shie, J.H.; Chen, S.H.; Wang, Y.S.; Kuo, H.C. Differences in mast cell infiltration, E-cadherin, and zonula occludens-1 expression between patients with overactive bladder and interstitial cystitis/bladder pain syndrome. *Urology* **2012**, *80*, 13–18. [CrossRef] [PubMed]
25. Schachar, J.S.; Evans, R.J.; Parks, G.E.; Zambon, J.; Badlani, G.; Walker, S.J. Histological evidence supports low anesthetic bladder capacity as a marker of a bladder-centric disease subtype in interstitial cystitis/bladder pain syndrome. *Int. Urogynecol. J.* **2019**, *30*, 1863–1870. [CrossRef]
26. Jhang, J.F.; Hsu, Y.H.; Kuo, H.C. Characteristics and electrocauterization of Hunner's lesions associated with bladder pain syndrome. *Urol. Sci.* **2013**, *24*, 51–55. [CrossRef]
27. Homma, Y. Interstitial cystitis, bladder pain syndrome, hypersensitive bladder, and interstitial cystitis/bladder pain syndrome—Clarification of definitions and relationships. *Int. J. Urol.* **2019**, *26* (Suppl. 1), 20–24. [CrossRef]
28. Chuang, Y.C.; Yoshimura, N.; Huang, C.C.; Chiang, P.H.; Chancellor, M.B. Intravesical botulinum toxin A administration produces analgesia against acetic acid induced bladder pain response in rats. *J. Urol.* **2004**, *172*, 1529–1532. [CrossRef]
29. Liu, H.T.; Kuo, H.C. Intravesical botulinum toxin A injections plus hydrodistension can reduce nerve growth factor production and control bladder pain in interstitial cystitis. *Urology* **2007**, *70*, 463–468. [CrossRef]
30. Hanno, P. Interstitial cystitis and related diseases. In *Campbell's Urology*, 7th ed.; Walsh, P.C., Retik, A.B., Vaughan, E.D., Wein, A.J., Eds.; WB Saunders Co.: Philadelphia, PA, USA, 1998; pp. 631–662.
31. Hanno, P.M.; Landis, J.R.; Matthews-Cook, Y.; Kusek, J.; Nyberg, L., Jr. The diagnosis of interstitial cystitis revisited: Lessons learned from the National Institutes of Health Interstitial Cystitis Database study. *J. Urol.* **1999**, *161*, 553–557. [CrossRef]
32. Lubeck, D.P.; Whitmore, K.; Sant, G.R.; Alvarez-Horine, S.; Lai, C. Psychometric validation of the OLeary-Sant interstitial cystitis symptom index in a clinical trial of pentosan polysulfate sodium. *Urology* **2001**, *57*, 62–66. [CrossRef]
33. Abrams, P.; Cardozo, L.; Fall, M.; Griffiths, D.; Rosier, P.; Ulmsten, U.; van Kerrebroeck, P.; Victor, A.; Wein, A.; Standardisation Sub-committee of the International Continence Society. The standardisation

of terminology of lower urinary tract function: Report from the Standardisation Sub-committee of the International Continence Society. *Neurourol. Urodyn.* **2002**, *21*, 167–178. [CrossRef] [PubMed]
34. Hsiao, S.M.; Lin, H.H.; Kuo, H.C. Videourodynamic Studies of Women with Voiding Dysfunction. *Sci. Rep.* **2017**, *7*, 6845. [CrossRef] [PubMed]
35. Parsons, C.L.; Housley, T.; Schmidt, J.D.; Lebow, D. Treatment of interstitial cystitis with intravesical heparin. *Br. J. Urol.* **1994**, *73*, 504–507. [CrossRef]

15

A Comparative Observational Study to Evaluate the Efficacy of Mid-Urethral Sling with Botulinum Toxin A Injection in Urinary Incontinence Patients

Yi-Huei Chang [1,2,†], Po-Jen Hsiao [1,2,3,†], Huang Chi-Ping [1,2], Hsi-Chin Wu [1,2,4], Po-Fan Hsieh [1,2,5,*] and Eric Chieh-Lung Chou [1,2,4,*]

1 Department of Urology, China Medical University Hospital, Taichung 40447, Taiwan; yihueichang1006@gmail.com (Y.-H.C.); pojenhsiao@gmail.com (P.-J.H.); Huangchiping@yahoo.com.tw (H.C.-P.); wuhc@mail.cmuh.org.tw (H.-C.W.)
2 School of Medicine, China Medical University, Taichung 40402, Taiwan
3 Department of Urology, China Medical University Hsinchu Hospital, Hsinchu 302056, Taiwan
4 Department of Urology, China Medical University Beigang Hospital, Beigang, Yunlin 651012, Taiwan
5 Graduate Institute of Biomedical Sciences, School of Medicine, China Medical University, Taichung 40402, Taiwan
* Correspondence: phdoublem@yahoo.com.tw (P.-F.H.); ericchou66@yahoo.com.tw (E.C.-L.C.)
† Yi-Huei Chang and Po-Jen Hsiao have equally contributed this study.

Abstract: This study aimed to evaluate and compare the efficacy and safety of mid-urethral sling (MUS) with botulinum toxin A (BoNT-A) versus MUS only in women with mixed urinary incontinence. This was a comparative observational study, and total of 73 patients were enrolled. A total of 38 and 35 patients received MUS only and MUS with BoNT-A injection, respectively. The efficacy outcome included change in Urinary Incontinence Outcome Scores (UIOS), change in Overactive Bladder Symptom Score (OABSS), and use of antimuscarinic agent or beta-3 agonist. Safety assessments included adverse events including urinary retention, increased postvoid residual volumes, and urinary tract infection. MUS with BoNT-A injection was insignificantly better than MUS only in urinary incontinence outcome (88% vs. 71%, respectively, $p = 0.085$) at week three. Among the 33 patients with detrusor overactivity (DO), patients who received BoNT-A had a higher cure rate of incontinence (88% vs. 41%, $p = 0.01$) and less required antimuscarinic agent or beta-3 agonist (31% vs. 94%, $p < 0.001$) compared to patients who did not receive BoNT-A injection. There was no significant difference in the incidences of adverse events between two groups. BoNT-A injection with MUS demonstrated efficacy and safety in the treatment of mixed urinary incontinence, specifically for women with DO.

Keywords: botulinum toxin A; mid-urethral sling; antimuscarinics; overactive bladder; urinary incontinence

Key Contribution: This study confirmed the efficacy and safety of BoNT-A injection along with MUS in women with mixed urinary incontinence.

---

1. Introduction

Urinary incontinence is a common disease observed in women, with an approximately 29–75% prevalence [1]. The common types of incontinence are stress urinary incontinence (SUI) and urge urinary incontinence (UUI). Management options for SUI include conservative treatment, pelvic floor training, and mid-urethral sling (MUS) operation. Treatments for UUI include behavioral modification and administration of antimuscarinic or beta-3 agonist agents. Furthermore, intravesical injection of botulinum toxin A (BoNT-A) is reserved for refractory patients. BoNT-A significantly decreases the number of UUI episodes and improves health-related quality of life in patients with overactive bladder (OAB) [2–5].

A high incidence of mixed urinary incontinence (MUI) is observed, or SUI and UUI coexist [6]. According to a previous study in women with MUI receiving MUS, approximately 53–79% of women experienced an improvement of UUI. However, 25–35% of women still experienced overactive bladder symptoms or de novo UUI [7].

We made a hypothesis that combining MUS and intravesical BoNT-A injection could have a therapeutic effect on MUI better than that of MUS alone. This study aimed to compare the efficacy and safety of MUS with or without intravesical BoNT-A injection in women who have MUI. The primary endpoints are changes in UUI episodes from baseline to week three. The secondary endpoints are add-ons in antimuscarinic agents or beta-3 agonists compared with baseline. Safety assessments included all common potential adverse events of MUS and BoNT-A intravesical injection, including urinary retention, increased postvoid residual volumes, and urinary tract infection (UTI).

2. Results

From July 2017 to June 2019, a total of 73 women with moderate to severe MUI were included in this observational study. The median age was 54.78 (range, 33 to 78) years. Of these, 38 patients underwent MUS only (group 1). Thirty-five patients received simultaneous MUS and intravesical injection of 80 units of BoNT-A (group 2). Detailed patient characteristics were shown in Table 1. Three months after the operation, 27 (71%) and 31 (88%) patients in group 1 and group 2 both scored 0 in the Urinary Incontinence Outcome Score (UIOS) [8] (p = 0.085, Table 2).

Table 1. Patient characteristics.

	MUS Only (n = 38)	MUS with BoNT-A (n = 35)	p Value
Age, median (years)	53.70 ± 11.10	55.30 ± 12.40	0.690
Body mass index, median (kg/m^2)	25.30 ± 2.40	26.20 ± 2.70	0.230
Parity, mean	2.60 ± 1.00	2.80 ± 0.8	0.390
OABSS, mean	8.47 ± 2.44	9.31 ± 2.37	0.084

MUS: Mid-urethral sling, BoNT-A: botulinum toxin A, OABSS: Overactive Bladder Symptom Score.

Table 2. Surgical outcomes of the study population.

	MUS Only (n = 38)	MUS with BoNT-A (n = 35)	p Value
Cure (UIOS = 0)	27 (71%)	31 (88%)	0.085
Need medication for OAB after operation	26 (68%)	9 (26%)	<0.001

UIOS: Urinary Incontinence Outcome Score, OAB: overactive bladder.

Seventeen of the 38 patients in group 1 had detrusor overactivity (DO), and 16 (94%) of them indicated that they wanted to receive treatment for OAB 3 weeks after surgery. On the contrary, 10 (48%) of the 21 patients without DO wanted to receive treatment for OAB. In group 2, 16 women had DO, and five patients wanted to receive medication treatment for OAB. In 19 patients without DO, only four patients wanted to receive medication treatment (Table 3).

Table 3. Surgical outcomes of patients with and without detrusor overactivity.

	MUS Only	MUS with BoNT-A	p Value
Patients with DO	17	16	1.000
Cure (UIOS = 0) after operation	7 (41%)	14 (88%)	0.010
Need medication after operation	16 (94%)	5 (31%)	<0.001
Patients without DO	21	19	1.000
Cure (UIOS = 0) after operation	20 (95%)	17 (89%)	0.596
Need medication after operation	10 (48%)	4 (21%)	0.105

DO: detrusor overactivity, UIOS: Urinary Incontinence Outcome Score.

The Overactive Bladder Symptom Scores (OABSS) in the MUS only group before and after 3 weeks of management were 8.5 and 6.1, which were not statistically different ($p = 0.084$). The OABSS in the MUS with BoNT-A group were 9.3 before surgery and 3.5 after 3 weeks of surgery, which showed significant improvement ($p < 0.001$, Table 4). Three months after surgery, patients with persistent bladder symptoms have been treated with oral medications, and the OABSS in groups 1 and 2 were 4.2 and 3.3, respectively.

Table 4. Evaluation of overactive bladder symptoms score at three weeks.

OABSS	Pre-Operation	Post-Operation
MUS only (n = 38)	8.5	6.1
MUS with BoNT-A (n = 35)	9.3	3.5
p value	0.084	<0.001

OABSS: Overactive Bladder Symptoms Score.

Based on further analysis of the data on week 12 after surgery, it was found that DO and OABSS ≥11 (area under the curve = 0.96, $p = 0.003$, 95% confidence interval, 0.893–1.000) were predictors of successful treatment when MUS was combined with BoNT-A injection (Table 5).

Table 5. Multiple linear regression analysis between successful treatment and factors.

Factors	Beta Coefficient	95% CI		p Value
		Lower Bound	Upper Bound	
OABSS	0.099	0.052	0.147	<0.001
DO	−0.505	−0.532	−0.113	0.004

DO: detrusor overactivity, OABSS: Overactive Bladder Symptoms Score.

The complication rates between the two groups were similar (Table 6). In the MUS with BoNT-A group, eight of the 35 patients complained of difficulty in urination. Six of them showed impaired detrusor contractility (bladder contractility index <100) in the urodynamic study before surgery [9]. These symptoms improved 12 weeks after the operation.

Table 6. Adverse events 3 weeks after operation.

Variable	MUS Only	MUS with BoNT-A	p Value
Urinary tract infection	5 (13%)	9 (26%)	0.237
Bladder perforation	0	0	N/A
Tape exposure	0	0	N/A
Acute urinary retention	0	0	N/A
Large PVR (>150 mL)	4 (11%)	7 (20%)	0.334
Difficulty in urination	6 (16%)	8 (23%)	0.556

PVR: post voiding residual urine volume.

3. Discussion

Urinary incontinence has a considerable impact on quality of life and significantly affects morbidity [10,11]. In women with urinary incontinence, approximately 50% and 30–40% have SUI and MUI, respectively [12]. Coexistence of SUI and UUI could increase the severity of leakage and significantly affect the patients' quality of life. Besides nonsurgical management, MUS for SUI is considered significantly effective in the treatment of storage symptoms [13,14]. On the contrary, conservative treatments for UUI mainly include behavioral modification, pelvic floor muscle training, and administration of oral medication [15]. New treatment modality should be considered considering that there is no single treatment applicable to treat both symptoms simultaneously.

Clinically, treatment decision will be determined according to the predominance of SUI or UUI. For example, if SUI is predominant, MUS surgery will be arranged, and patient may receive antimuscarinic agent after surgery [13,14]. However, some studies have pointed out that surgery for SUI is considered not beneficial or can even worsen the symptoms of OAB [16,17]. Moreover, approximately 6–8% of women treated with MUS will develop de novo OAB. On the contrary, if patient's symptom is UUI predominant, surgery is generally not recommended. Antimuscarinic agent and beta-3 agonist are administered to treat symptoms, but these patients often still experience persistent urinary leakage because of SUI. It is difficult for women to evaluate themselves whether SUI or UUI is more predominant. In some of these women, only SUI is treated; thus, they still experience UUI.

Intravesical injection of BoNT-A is also relatively effective for OAB-wet and has been approved by the Food and Drug Administration [18]. To the best of our knowledge, this is the first study to compare MUS with concomitant BoNT-A intravesical injection with MUS only to treat MUI. If two types of urinary incontinence can be treated simultaneously, it should be a good choice for patients. This study successfully expanded the clinical indication of BoNT-A in treating MUI.

Our results show that the continence rate of patients with moderate to severe MUI who received BoNT-A while undergoing MUS was slightly better than that of patients receiving MUS only (cure rate 88% vs. 71%, respectively), but the difference was statistically insignificant. More importantly, not only the symptoms of urinary leakage but also the symptoms of OAB improved in patients receiving both MUS and BoNT-A intravesical injection.

The possible complication of urinary retention is a great concern of patients with MUI receiving MUS and BoNT-A intravesical injection simultaneously. Sun et al. reported that the complication risks of 100 units of BoNT-A intravesical injection included UTI (35%) and urinary retention (8–10%) [18]. In our previous pilot study, five patients received 100 units of BoNT-A intravesical injection. All of them experienced difficulty in voiding and had postvoid residual urine greater than 150 mL. Moreover, three of these five patients required single catheterization after receiving MUS combined with 100 units of BoNT-A intravesical injection. Kuo et al. reported that the range of BoNT-A dosage from 50 U to 300 U showed significant improvement in OAB and urinary incontinence and in urodynamic measures, but receiving >100 units of BoNT-A ($p = 0.029$) was considered a predictor for the increasing incidence of adverse event such as straining to void [19]. Thus, we decreased the BoNT-A dosage to 80 units in this study, and patients did not experience urinary retention. Although 23% of the patients had transient difficulty in urination, these symptoms all improved 12 weeks after the operation.

We found that using a lower dose of 80 units of BoNT-A prevents urinary retention. Previous studies have pointed out that the lower BoNT-A dose has shorter efficacy [20]. Hence, proper explanation regarding the possible reinjection of BoNT-A in 3 months after surgery was provided to patients before surgery. We comprehensively discussed with the patients whether they needed to receive another BoNT-A intravesical injection or to undergo behavioral therapy combined with the administration of oral medication. Finally, 35% of patients decided to continuously receive BoNT-A intravesical injection.

There are several ways to treat urgency symptoms in MUI such as behavioral therapy, pelvic floor muscle training, and administration of oral medication [21]. Most MUI patients initially receive oral medications for their symptoms. However, these oral medications such as anticholinergic agents or beta-3 agonists have significant side effects. Side effects of anticholinergic agents include dry mouth, constipation, and cognitive problems in the elderly [22]. Although beta-3 agonists have relatively lesser side effects than anticholinergic agents, blood pressure may increase in some patients after receiving beta-3 agonists, and the long-term effects of beta-3 agonists on the elderly are still unclear [23,24]. In our study, only 26% continued to take the medication for OAB. Therefore, MUS combined with BoNT-A intravesical injection is considered beneficial in reducing the side effects of oral medications.

In our study, decreasing urination flow rate after surgery was associated with MUS or BoNT-A intravesical injection. However, none of the patients required urinary catheterization in our study. Moreover, adjusting the tension of the sling was not needed while we performed MUS surgery combined with BoNT-A intravesical injection, although BoNT-A may strongly reduce the contractility of the bladder. Previous studies pointed out that the mechanism of MUS was supported by a "tension-free" method instead of urethral obstruction [25].

In our study, all of the patients experienced MUI, but the proportion of DO that was observed during the urodynamic examination before surgery was 45%. According to the definition of the ICS [26], the diagnosis of UUI is based on the patient's symptoms. During the preoperative evaluation, the patient stated that it was difficult to distinguish whether SUI or UUI was predominant. For example, during certain movements, such as brisk walking or small jogging, increased abdominal pressure was accompanied by urgency to leak urine. In our study, we found that in patients who received both treatments, the symptoms still improve in patients without DO. However, patients with DO receiving MUS alone had higher risk of persistent UUI after surgery than patients receiving MUS combined with BoNT-A intravesical injection. We recommend that patients with MUI combined with DO should appropriately receive MUS and BoNT-A intravesical injection.

There were some limitations to this study. First, this was an observation study instead of a randomized controlled trial. According to the guideline of European Association of Urology and American Urological Association, both MUS and BoNT-A intravesical injection are standard treatments for urinary incontinence. In preoperative counseling we explained to every patient that BoNT-A intravesical injection carried 5% incidence of urinary retention and clean intermittent catheterization might be necessary [5]. Based on patients' autonomy, we let them choose whether to receive the BoNT-A intravesical injection or not. There was no significant difference in age, BMI, and OABSS between the two groups. Second, the case number was small. In addition, currently there is no objective and universally accepted tool to evaluate treatment outcomes of MUI. Nevertheless, the promising results shown in OABSS and UIOS improvement as well as freedom from OAB medications could support the rationale to conduct a prospective, large-scaled, randomized study to confirm the efficacy and safety of MUS combined with BoNT-A intravesical injection in treating MUI.

4. Conclusions

An 80-unit BoNT-A injection combined with MUS is not only effective but also safe in the treatment of MUI patients. DO and high OABSS are predictive factors for a satisfactory treatment outcome in patients.

5. Materials and Methods

This retrospective observational comparative study was done in a tertiary referral center. The inclusion criteria were women who had at least one episode of SUI and one episode of UUI in a 3-day voiding diary. Patients with urethral diverticulum, urinary fistula, previous urinary incontinence surgery, intravesical BoNT-A injection, or pelvic floor reconstruction, and history of neurogenic bladder were excluded. If they had previously taken medications for OAB, a 3-week washout period was required before surgery. This study was approved by the Ethic Committee of China Medical University Hospital, and the protocol number was DMR-94IRB-083(FR) (Approval date: 30 November 2016).

Preoperative evaluation including history assessment, physical examination, urinalysis, urodynamic study, and assessment of OABSS and UIOS were done at the outpatient clinic. The decision of MUS only or MUS with BoNT-A intravesical injection was made by the patient after a detailed explanation of the procedure and morbidities. All patients were reassessed at 1 week, 3 weeks, 3 months, and 6 months after surgery. According to the UIOS, cure, improvement, and failure scored 0, 1–4, and 5, respectively. In our study, a score ranging from 1–5 was defined as the absence of cure [8].

The patients in the MUS only group underwent a surgical procedure performed by a single surgeon (ECL Chou) using a transobturator MUS (Contasure-KIM®, Neomedic International, Leganés, Madrid, Spain). The patients in the MUS with BoNT-A group received transobturator MUS and 80-unit BoNT-A(BOTOX®, Allergan, Irvine, CA, USA) intravesical injection.

During a 3-week evaluation after surgery, patients in both groups were asked if they wanted to receive medication treatment for OAB to control the symptoms of urgency, frequent urination, and urgency incontinence. Six months after the operation, patients who had received BoNT-A intravesical injections were also evaluated if they wanted to repeatedly receive BoNT-A intravesical injection.

All comparisons of patients' categorical characteristics and outcomes were assessed using the Fisher's exact test. Mann-Whitney U test was used to compare the means of continuous variables such as OABSS in two groups. We compare continuous data before and after intervention by Wilcoxon signed rank test. The predictive factor of successful treatment was evaluated by mixed linear regression. All statistical assessments were performed by two-sided analysis, and significant differences were considered at a p-value < 0.05. The Statistical Package for the Social Sciences (SPSS) version 19.0 statistical software (SPSS Inc., Chicago, IL, USA) was used in all statistical analyses.

Author Contributions: Y.-H.C. and P.-J.H. drafted the manuscript. H.C.-P., H.-C.W., and P.-F.H. revised the manuscript. E.C.-L.C. supervised the drafting and revision of the manuscript. All authors have read and agreed to the published version of the manuscript.

Abbreviations

The following abbreviations are used in this manuscript:

MUS	mid-urethral sling
BoNT-A	botulinum toxin A
UIOS	Urinary Incontinence Outcome Scores
OABSS	Overactive Bladder Symptom Score
UUI	urge urinary incontinence
SUI	stress urinary incontinence
MUI	mixed urinary incontinence
OAB	overactive bladder
DO	detrusor overactivity

References

1. Luber, K.M. The Definition, Prevalence, and Risk Factors for Stress Urinary Incontinence. *Rev. Urol.* **2004**, *6*, S3–S9.
2. Chapple, C.R.; Sievert, K.-D.; MacDiarmid, S.; Khullar, V.; Radziszewski, P.; Nardo, C.; Thompson, C.; Zhou, J.; Haag-Molkenteller, C. OnabotulinumtoxinA 100 U Significantly Improves All Idiopathic Overactive Bladder Symptoms and Quality of Life in Patients with Overactive Bladder and Urinary Incontinence: A Randomised, Double-Blind, Placebo-Controlled Trial. *Eur. Urol.* **2013**, *64*, 249–256. [CrossRef] [PubMed]
3. Fowler, C.J.; Auerbach, S.; Ginsberg, D.A.; Hale, D.; Radziszewski, P.; Rechberger, T.; Patel, V.D.; Zhou, J.; Thompson, C.; Kowalski, J.W. OnabotulinumtoxinA Improves Health-Related Quality of Life in Patients With Urinary Incontinence Due to Idiopathic Overactive Bladder: A 36-Week, Double-Blind, Placebo-Controlled, Randomized, Dose-Ranging Trial. *Eur. Urol.* **2012**, *62*, 148–157. [CrossRef] [PubMed]

4. Sievert, K.-D.; Chapple, C.R.; Herschorn, S.; Joshi, M.; Zhou, J.; Nardo, C.; Nitti, V.W. OnabotulinumtoxinA 100U provides significant improvements in overactive bladder symptoms in patients with urinary incontinence regardless of the number of anticholinergic therapies used or reason for inadequate management of overactive bladder. *Int. J. Clin. Pr.* **2014**, *68*, 1246–1256. [CrossRef] [PubMed]
5. Nitti, V.W.; Dmochowski, R.R.; Herschorn, S.; Sand, P.; Thompson, C.; Nardo, C.; Yan, X.; Haag-Molkenteller, C. OnabotulinumtoxinA for the Treatment of Patients with Overactive Bladder and Urinary Incontinence: Results of a Phase 3, Randomized, Placebo Controlled Trial. *J. Urol.* **2013**, *189*, 2186–2193. [CrossRef] [PubMed]
6. Brubaker, L.; Lukacz, E.S.; Burgio, K.; Zimmern, P.; Norton, P.; Leng, W.; Johnson, H.; Kraus, S.; Stoddard, A. Mixed incontinence: Comparing definitions in non-surgical patients. *Neurourol. Urodyn.* **2011**, *30*, 47–51. [CrossRef]
7. Shin, J.H.; Choo, M.-S. De novo or resolved urgency and urgency urinary incontinence after midurethral sling operations: How can we properly counsel our patients? *Investig. Clin. Urol.* **2019**, *60*, 373–379. [CrossRef]
8. Groutz, A.; Blaivas, J.G.; Rosenthal, J.E. A simplified urinary incontinence score for the evaluation of treatment outcomes. *Neurourol. Urodyn.* **2000**, *19*, 127–135. [CrossRef]
9. Abrams, P. Bladder outlet obstruction index, bladder contractility index and bladder voiding efficiency: three simple indices to define bladder voiding function. *BJU Int.* **1999**, *84*, 14–15. [CrossRef]
10. Irwin, D.E.; Milsom, I.; Hunskaar, S.; Reilly, K.; Kopp, Z.; Herschorn, S.; Coyne, K.; Kelleher, C.; Hampel, C.; Artibani, W.; et al. Population-Based Survey of Urinary Incontinence, Overactive Bladder, and Other Lower Urinary Tract Symptoms in Five Countries: Results of the EPIC Study. *Eur. Urol.* **2006**, *50*, 1306–1315. [CrossRef]
11. Tennstedt, S.L.; Fitzgerald, M.P.; Nager, C.W.; Xu, Y.; Zimmern, P.; Kraus, S.; Goode, P.S.; Kusek, J.W.; Borello-France, D.; Mallett, V.; et al. Quality of life in women with stress urinary incontinence. *Int. Urogynecol. J. Pelvic Floor Dysfunct.* **2006**, *18*, 543–549. [CrossRef] [PubMed]
12. Ortiz, O.C. Stress urinary incontinence in the gynecological practice. *Int. J. Gynecol. Obstet.* **2004**, *86*, S6–S16. [CrossRef] [PubMed]
13. A Ford, A.; Rogerson, L.; Cody, J.D. Mid-urethral sling operations for stress urinary incontinence in women. *Cochrane Database Syst. Rev.* **2015**, *7*, CD006375. [CrossRef]
14. Nager, C.W. Midurethral slings: evidence-based medicine vs the medicolegal system. *Am. J. Obstet. Gynecol.* **2016**, *214*, 708. [CrossRef] [PubMed]
15. Gormley, E.A.; Lightner, D.J.; Faraday, M.; Vasavada, S.P. Diagnosis and Treatment of Overactive Bladder (Non-Neurogenic) in Adults: AUA/SUFU Guideline Amendment. *J. Urol.* **2015**, *193*, 1572–1580. [CrossRef] [PubMed]
16. Palva, K.; Nilsson, C.G. Prevalence of urinary urgency symptoms decreases by mid-urethral sling procedures for treatment of stress incontinence. *Int. Urogynecol. J.* **2011**, *22*, 1241–1247. [CrossRef] [PubMed]
17. Petri, E.; Ashok, K. Complications of synthetic slings used in female stress urinary incontinence and applicability of the new IUGA-ICS classification. *Eur. J. Obstet. Gynecol. Reprod. Boil.* **2012**, *165*, 347–351. [CrossRef]
18. Sun, Y.; Luo, D.; Tang, C.; Yang, L.; Shen, H. The safety and efficiency of onabotulinumtoxinA for the treatment of overactive bladder: A systematic review and meta-analysis. *Int. Urol. Nephrol.* **2015**, *47*, 1779–1788. [CrossRef]
19. Kuo, H.-C.; Liao, C.-H.; Chung, S.-D. Adverse Events of Intravesical Botulinum Toxin A Injections for Idiopathic Detrusor Overactivity: Risk Factors and Influence on Treatment Outcome. *Eur. Urol.* **2010**, *58*, 919–926. [CrossRef]
20. Dmochowski, R.R.; Chapple, C.R.; Nitti, V.W.; Chancellor, M.; Everaert, K.; Thompson, C.; Daniell, G.; Zhou, J.; Haag-Molkenteller, C. Efficacy and Safety of OnabotulinumtoxinA for Idiopathic Overactive Bladder: A Double-Blind, Placebo Controlled, Randomized, Dose Ranging Trial. *J. Urol.* **2010**, *184*, 2416–2422. [CrossRef]
21. Lukacz, E.S.; Santiago-Lastra, Y.; Albo, M.E.; Brubaker, L. Urinary Incontinence in Women. *JAMA* **2017**, *318*, 1592. [CrossRef] [PubMed]
22. Riemsma, R.; Hagen, S.; Kirschner-Hermanns, R.; Norton, C.; Wijk, H.; Andersson, K.-E.; Chapple, C.; Spinks, J.; Wagg, A.; Hutt, E.; et al. Can incontinence be cured? A systematic review of cure rates. *BMC Med.* **2017**, *15*, 63. [CrossRef] [PubMed]

23. Drake, M.J.; Chapple, C.R.; Esen, A.A.; Athanasiou, S.; Cambronero, J.; Mitcheson, D.; Herschorn, S.; Saleem, T.; Huang, M.; Siddiqui, E.; et al. Efficacy and Safety of Mirabegron Add-on Therapy to Solifenacin in Incontinent Overactive Bladder Patients with an Inadequate Response to Initial 4-Week Solifenacin Monotherapy: A Randomised Double-blind Multicentre Phase 3B Study (BESIDE). *Eur. Urol.* **2016**, *70*, 136–145. [CrossRef] [PubMed]
24. MacDiarmid, S.; Al-Shukri, S.; Barkin, J.; Fianu-Jonasson, A.; Grise, P.; Herschorn, S.; Saleem, T.; Huang, M.; Siddiqui, E.; Stölzel, M.; et al. Mirabegron as Add-On Treatment to Solifenacin in Patients with Incontinent Overactive Bladder and an Inadequate Response to Solifenacin Monotherapy. *J. Urol.* **2016**, *196*, 809–818. [CrossRef]
25. Cervigni, M.; Gambacciani, M. Female urinary stress incontinence. *Climacteric* **2015**, *18*, 30–36. [CrossRef]
26. Drake, M.J. Fundamentals of terminology in lower urinary tract function. *Neurourol. Urodyn.* **2018**, *37*, S13–S19. [CrossRef]

16

Using Botulinum Toxin A for Treatment of Interstitial Cystitis/Bladder Pain Syndrome—Possible Pathomechanisms and Practical Issues

Jia-Fong Jhang

Department of Urology, Hualien Tzu Chi Hospital, Buddhist Tzu Chi Medical Foundation, Tzu Chi University, Hualien 97047, Taiwan; alur1984@hotmail.com

Abstract: Treatment for patients with interstitial cystitis/bladder pain syndrome (IC/BPS) is always challenging for urologists. The main mechanism of the botulinum toxin A (BoNT-A) is inhibition of muscle contraction, but the indirect sensory modulation and anti-inflammatory effect in the bladder also play important roles in treating patients with IC/BPS. Although current guidelines consider BoNT-A injection to be a standard treatment, some practical issues remain debatable. Most clinical evidence of this treatment comes from retrospective uncontrolled studies, and only two randomized placebo-control studies with limited patient numbers have been published. Although 100 U BoNT-A is effective for most patients with IC/BPS, the potential efficacy of 200 U BoNT-A has not been evaluated. Both trigone and diffuse body BoNT-A injections are effective and safe for IC/BPS, although comparison studies are lacking. For IC/BPS patients with Hunner's lesion, the efficacy of BoNT-A injection remains controversial. Most patients with IC/BPS experience symptomatic relapse at six to nine months after a BoNT-A injection, although repeated injections exhibit a persistent therapeutic effect in long-term follow-up. Further randomized placebo-controlled studies with a larger number of patients are needed to support BoNT-A as standard treatment for patients with IC/BPS.

Keywords: interstitial cystitis; inflammation; treatment; Botulinum toxin

Key Contribution: This review summarized the mechanisms of using botulinum toxin for interstitial cystitis, and presented several clinical debatable practical issues which should be noticed by clinicians.

---

1. Introduction

Since the early 19th century, patients who exhibited chronic bladder pain, urinary frequency, and urgency without evidence of urinary tract infection or bladder stones have been diagnosed with interstitial cystitis (IC) [1]. As our understanding of IC has progressed over the past 200 years, its name and definition have changed many times.[1] Because patients with IC may not experience bladder inflammation, the term "interstitial cystitis/bladder pain syndrome" (IC/BPS) is considered to be more suitable and is widely used in current guidelines [2,3]. IC/BPS has attracted considerable attention among urologists. A recent epidemiology study revealed that the prevalence of IC/BPS is 4.2% for the high-sensitivity definition, whereas it is 1.9% for the high-specificity definition [4]. Although the prevalence has shown an increasing trend in recent years [4], the treatment of patients with IC/BPS remains challenging for urologists. Current guidelines recommend the use of oral medications, such as amitriptyline and cimetidine, as well as intravesical instillation therapy (i.e., heparin and hyaluronic acid) to treat patients with IC/BPS [2]. However, no single treatment is effective for all patients with IC/BPS, and symptomatic relapse after the abovementioned treatments is common among patients with IC/BPS. Thus, patients with IC/BPS need a more effective treatment with greater durability.

For complicated lower urinary-tract diseases (LUTDs), treatment options are sometimes limited. Over the past two decades, biotoxins (e.g., resiniferatoxin and capsaicin) have gradually been included as possible treatment modalities for complicated LUTDs [5,6]. Botulinum toxin (BoNT), which is produced by the bacterium *Clostridium botulinum* and related species, is regarded as the most potent poisonous neurotoxin worldwide [7]. In 1988, Dykstra et al. first used a BoNT type A (BoNT-A) injection to treat patients with spinal-cord injury and detrusor–sphincter dyssynergia [8]. Today, BoNT-A is widely used to treat various types of complicated LUTDs, and many clinical trials have proven its efficacy [9]. For patients with IC/BPS, the efficacy of traditional conservative treatments is typically insufficient [2]. In recent years, the treatment of IC/BPS has shown great progress with the use of the intravesical BoNT-A injection, and laboratory studies have demonstrated bladder improvement after BoNT-A injection [10]. This review summarizes the possible pathomechanisms of using BoNT-A for treatment of IC/BPS in the bladder and examines the practical issues and long-term efficacy of such treatment.

2. Methods

This is a non-systemic review. The PubMed search terms including "botulinum toxin" and "interstitial cystitis" were used to find published studies. The search results were used to summarize possible mechanisms and current evidence to analyze several practical issues with the use of BoNT-A in treating IC/BPS. The results were generated based on the author's knowledge and clinical experience in this field; hence, they were highly impacted by the author's bias in selecting and interpreting studies.

3. Results

3.1. Possible Pathomechanisms for BoNT-A in Treating IC/BPS

BoNT is well-known for its ability to inhibit acetylcholine release, which results in muscle paralysis [11]. However, current evidence shows that the possible pathomechanisms of using BoNT-A for treatment of IC/BPS involve additional pathways, including anti-inflammatory effects and sensory modulation in the urothelium [12].

3.1.1. Inhibition of Detrusor Muscle Activity

BoNT-A consists of a 50 kDa light chain and a 100 kDa heavy chain connected by a weak disulfide bond [13]. In presynaptic nerve endings, the C-terminal of the heavy chain binds to the synaptic vesicle protein 2 on the neuronal cell membrane, enabling BoNT-A to be internalized within the nerve terminal by endocytosis [14]. Although the heavy chain facilitates the entrance of BoNT-A into neurons, the light chain is the biologically active moiety of BoNT-A. Synaptosome-associated protein 25 facilitates intracellular vesicle docking and membrane fusion, and is involved in the exocytotic release of neurotransmitters during synaptic transmission [15]. The light chain of BoNT-A cleaves apart synaptosome-associated protein 25 in presynaptic neurons, thereby inhibiting the release of the acetylcholine neurotransmitter by disrupting vesicular fusion with the neuronal cell membrane, resulting in flaccid muscle paralysis [11]. A previous study showed that BoNT-A could attenuate bladder contractility. In a clinical study of intravesical injection of BoNT-A 200 U in patients with neurogenic detrusor overactivity, the maximum detrusor pressures during filling cystometry were significantly reduced at the four-week follow-up [16]. Recently, abnormal high tension or spasm in smooth muscle has been suggested to be a potential mechanism for the development of chronic visceral organ pain [17]. Tension-sensitive nerve endings in the smooth muscle of visceral organs may respond to luminal distension or stretching. Mechanotransduction of low-threshold afferent nerves is associated with transient receptor potential vanilloid receptor 1 (TRPV1) activation and resulting visceral pain [17]. Although electrophysiological evidence of this phenomenon in the human bladder is lacking, patients with IC/BPS commonly exhibit a tender bladder with "spasm-like" sensations [18]. Relaxation of bladder-muscle tension might be the mechanism by which BoNT-A treats bladder pain in patients with IC/BPS. Furthermore, although the core symptom of IC/BPS is bladder pain, most patients with IC/BPS also exhibit urinary frequency, urgency, and incontinence. Our previous study showed that detrusor overactivity could be detected in approximately 10% of patients with IC/BPS [19]. BoNT-A injection-induced inhibition of detrusor muscle overactivity could relieve frequency and urgency symptoms, thus improving the quality of life for patients with IC/BPS.

3.1.2. Sensory Modulation in the Urothelium

Generally, patients with botulism do not lose sensory nerve function. However, intravesical BoNT-A injection results in sensory modulation, both in pain reduction and urgency reduction in patients with IC/BPS or an overactive bladder [2,9]. Recent laboratory evidence revealed that BoNT-A injection indeed could alter the expression levels of sensory neurotransmitters and receptors in the bladder. Substance P and calcitonin gene-related peptide are small peptides that act as neurotransmitters in nociception [20,21]. In rats with cyclophosphamide-induced cystitis, the intravesical BoNT-A injection has been shown to significantly reduce the bladder expression levels of substance P and calcitonin gene-related peptide [22]. Glutamate is an excitatory neurotransmitter that plays a crucial role in central and peripheral pain pathways, along with its receptor [23]. BoNT-A injection induced significant downregulation of glutamate expression levels in human and rat skin [24,25]. In the bladder, adenosine 5′-triphosphate acts on the purinergic receptor, serving as the signal for the central nervous system to perceive bladder fullness [26]. In animal studies, BoNT-A intravesical injection was found to inhibit adenosine 5′-triphosphate release from rat bladder urothelium [27,28]. TRPV1 is a vanilloid receptor that is expressed in nociceptive afferent neurons, which can be activated by heat, protons, or vanilloid chemicals (e.g., capsaicin and resiniferatoxin) [29,30]. TRPV1 plays an important role in neural transmission in the pain pathway, and the upregulation of TRPV1 in certain diseases is accompanied by elevated pain [29,30]. In a clinical study of the use of intravesical BoNT-A injection in patients with an overactive bladder, a significant reduction of TRPV1-positive nerves was detected in bladder biopsy specimens [31]. Detrusor BoNT-A injections also led to significant reductions in the expression levels of the bladder muscarinic receptors M2 and M3, as well as the purinergic receptors P2X2 and P2X3, in patients with neurogenic detrusor overactivity [31,32]. Modulation of sensory neurotransmitters and their receptors in the bladder therefore constitutes an important mechanism by which BoNT-A can treat IC/BPS. In addition, the modulation of central nervous system sensory receptors in peripheral organs after BoNT-A injection has been observed in animal studies. The reduction of c-fos and calcitonin gene-related peptide expression levels in the dorsal horn of the spinal cord after pawl BoNT-A injection has been reported in association with the reduction of mechanical allodynia [33,34]. In a recent study, the injection of radiolabeled BoNT-A into the bladder caused retrograde transport to lumbosacral dorsal root ganglia [35]. Theoretically, intravesical injection of BoNT-A might change sensory receptor expression levels in the spinal cord, but further studies are needed to confirm this hypothesis. Although the Botulinum toxin does not directly block neurotransmitters released in the afferent nerve system, current clinical and laboratory evidence suggests that it indirectly modulates the sensory function in the bladder with pathological changes.

3.1.3. Anti-Inflammatory Effect in the Urothelium

Although some histopathology studies have reported contrary evidence, most experts and guidelines currently consider bladder inflammation to be present in patients with IC/BPS—bladder inflammation is presumed to play a central role in the pathogenesis of IC/BPS [2,36–38]. The infiltration of mast cells and lympho-plasmacytic cells is increased in the lamina propria and detrusor muscle of the bladder in patients with IC/BPS [37–39]. Immunohistochemical studies also have shown increased mast-cell activity and upregulation of pro-inflammatory cytokines in the bladders of patients with IC/BPS, including inducible nitric oxide synthase, interleukin-6 (IL-6), and IL-17A [40,41]. In urine and serum from patients with IC/BPS, inflammatory cytokines (e.g., IL-1β, IL-6, IL-8, tumor necrosis factor-α, and C-reactive protein) are reportedly elevated [42,43]. Although BoNT-A is well-known for its neurotransmitter-blocking effect, there is increasing evidence that BoNT-A can inhibit the release of inflammatory cytokines in different organs. In an in-vitro study, bladders were harvested from rats with acute or chronic cystitis, then incubated in organ baths containing BoNT-A or a vehicle [22]. Reduced substance-P release in the bladder was detected in models of both acute and chronic cystitis. In another in-vivo study, BoNT-A intravesical injection was shown to reduce histological inflammation in the bladders of rats with cyclophosphamide-induced cystitis [44]. Cyclooxygenase 2 and prostaglandin E2 receptor expression levels in the bladder also were reduced in the BoNT-A injection group [44]. In the human bladder, a single BoNT-A injection does not seem to reduce bladder inflammation in patients with neurogenic detrusor overactivity, but may improve bladder fibrosis [45]. In patients with IC/BPS, our previous study showed that repeated BoNT-A injections could significantly reduce the numbers of activated mast cells in the bladder, whereas a single injection could not [46]. The vascular endothelial growth-factor expression level and apoptotic cell count in the bladder were also reduced in patients with IC/BPS after repeated BoNT-A injections; however, these levels remained significantly higher than those of the controls [41]. Additionally, urothelial barrier-function impairment is a possible pathogenic mechanism in IC/BPS [47]. Improvement in urothelial barrier function might also be a possible mechanism by which BoNT-A is used for treatment of IC/BPS. Urothelial barrier-function recovery might contribute to improvement in suburothelial inflammation. Our previous study revealed that repeated BoNT-A injections could improve the expression levels of the urothelial barrier function protein, E-cadherin, and the tight junction protein, zonula occludens-1, in patients with neurogenic detrusor overactivity [48]. However, to the best of our knowledge, the effect of BoNT-A injection on the expression levels of urothelial barrier-function proteins in patients with IC/BPS has not yet been reported.

3.2. *The Practical Issues with the Use of BoNT-A in Treating IC/BPS*

Although BoNT-A is now widely used to treat IC/BPS, it still is a novel treatment that has only been included in guidelines since 2015 [2]. Clinical evidence is still relatively limited, and several technique details of BoNT-A injection to IC/BPS patients remain unclear. The following sections list the practical issues that should be noticed by clinicians, and summarize current evidence of the debatable issues.

3.2.1. Clinical Efficacy of BoNT-A in Treating IC/BPS

As noted previously, the treatment of patients with IC/BPS remains challenging for urologists. Because the pathogenesis of IC/BPS is not well-understood, it is rare for complete resolution of IC/BPS to occur after a single treatment [1]. Currently, most treatments for IC/BPS mainly target symptomatic relief, rather than resolution of disease; however, even satisfactory improvement of symptoms may not be achieved in all patients [49]. Researchers have used BoNT-A for treatment of patients with IC/BPS in clinical trials since 2004, and the initial results of various studies showed promising outcomes [50,51]. In 2004, Smith et al. first used submucosal injection of BoNT-A in the bladder trigone and floor, combined with cystoscopic hydrodistention. Among the 13 female patients in that study, the Interstitial Cystitis Problem and Symptom Index scores improved by 69% and 71% respectively; the pain, assessed by a visual analog scale, also decreased by 79%. In our pilot study, we used BoNT-A suburothelial injection into 20 sites alone to treat patients with IC/BPS for whom conventional treatments had failed [51]. The bladder visual analog scale pain score, functional bladder capacity, and daytime urinary frequency all showed mild but significant improvement at three months after treatment. More recently, many studies have shown the clinical efficacy of BoNT-A injection in treatment of IC/BPS. New double-blind, randomized controlled studies revealed that BoNT-A intravesical injection could relieve symptoms in patients with IC/BPS; these included reduced bladder pain and increased capacity [52–54]. BoNT-A injection is considered to be standard therapy in the American Urology Association (AUA) guidelines for IC/BPS [2], and is widely used among urologists. There are three types of BoNT-A available for treatment of patients with IC/BPS, including Botox®(onabotulinum toxin A, Allergan, Inc., CA), Dysport®(abobotulinum toxin A, Ipsen, Inc., UK), and LANTOX®(CBTX-A, Lanzhou Institute of

Biological Products, China) [50,51,55]. However, symptom relapse is common after BoNT-A injection in patients with IC/BPS, and most patients require repeated BoNT-A injections [56]. The use of BoNT-A for treatment of IC/BPS has several remaining practical issues that should be addressed.

3.2.2. Two Randomized, Double-Blinded, Placebo-Controlled Studies of the Use of BoNT-A Injection for Treatment of IC/BPS

Although there have been more than 50 clinical studies of the use of intravesical BoNT-A injection for treatment of patients with IC/BPS, clinicians should note that only two of those studies were randomized, double-blinded, and placebo-controlled [53,54,57]. In our first double-blinded study, we enrolled 60 patients with IC/BPS who were refractory to conventional treatments, and used normal saline intravesical injection as the placebo control [53]. At week 8, patients who received BoNT-A 100 U had significantly greater pain reduction than patients who received normal saline (-2.6 ± 2.8 vs. -0.9 ± 2.2, $P = 0.021$) [53]. The overall success rates (global response assessment ≥1) were also higher in the BoNT-A group (26/40, 63%) than in the normal saline group (3/20, 15%, $P = 0.028$). The adverse event rate was similar between the two groups. Pinto et al. published the second double-blinded study in 2018, in which 19 patients with IC/BPS were randomly assigned to intratrigonal injection of BoNT-A 100 U or normal saline [54]. At week 12, a significantly greater reduction of pain was observed in the BoNT-A group than in the normal saline group (-3.8 ± 2.5 vs. -1.6 ± 2.1, $p < 0.05$). O'Leary–Sant score reduction and quality of life improvement were also superior in the BoNT-A injection group. Notably, improvement of bladder symptoms was observed in the placebo group in both studies, which suggested that the placebo effect was strong in clinical treatment of patients with IC/BPS. The patient-inclusion criteria was also different between the two studies. Only a total of 79 patients with IC/BPS had been enrolled in randomized and placebo-controlled studies; [53,54] therefore, additional studies with high levels of evidence are necessary to confirm the therapeutic efficacy of BoNT-A injection. Recruiting more IC/BPS patients is necessary to analyze the therapeutic effect in the subgroup patients (e.g., classification with glomerulation grade).

3.2.3. Dose of BoNT-A Injection in IC/BPS

The dose of BoNT-A injection for treatment of patients with LUTDs is difficult to determine. Although mortality has not been reported following medical use of BoNT-A injection, the estimated lethal dose is 2800 U in humans [58]. Most urologists and studies have established doses based on previous experience, rather than on solid supporting evidence. Previous studies demonstrated a dose-response relationship in the use of BoNT-A to treat patients with detrusor overactivity, and showed that bladder-capacity improvement was also dose-dependent [59]. Moreover, residual bladder volume increased with an increasing BoNT-A dose [59]. For patients with neurogenic detrusor overactivity, the therapeutic effects of BoNT-A 200 U and BoNT-A 300 U were similar [60]. However, dose-comparison studies for patients with IC/BPS have not been reported. Initially, several studies reported satisfactory outcomes of BoNT-A 200 U for treatment of patients with IC/BPS [50,51,61–63], particularly those studies by the Giannantoni group in Italy [61,62]. Our initial experience with a very limited number of patients suggested that BoNT-A 200 U may have a better therapeutic effect than 100 U injection, but this was not found to be statistically significant [64]. However, the rates of dysuria and high residual-urine volume also seemed to be higher in the 200 U group. Most studies have used 100 U BoNT-A for patients with IC/BPS, and this dose is widely used in clinical practice. The American Urology Association guidelines suggest that the use of BoNT-A 100 U is an appropriate treatment and may substantially reduce morbidity compared to BoNT-A 200 U [2]. However, for refractory patients with IC/BPS who do not have satisfactory responses to BoNT-A 100 U, a 200 U injection might be a reasonable second-choice treatment option. The potential therapeutic effect of BoNT-A 200 U injection should be investigated in further dose-comparison studies.

3.2.4. Location of Bladder Injection: Trigone or Bladder Body

Most studies have used BoNT-A bladder-body injection to treat patients with bladder disease [65]. For the inhibition of bladder contractility and associated adverse effects, some researchers have used BoNT-A injection in the trigone and bladder floor, rather than the entire bladder body, for patients with IC/BPS [54,61,62,66]. The trigone has been regarded as the sensory input center in the bladder since the 1970s [67]. Neurophysiology analysis revealed that the trigone contains significantly higher levels of adrenergic and muscarinic nerve innervation relative to the bladder body [67]. A recent three-dimensional image reconstruction analysis of the nerve further demonstrated that bladder autonomic innervation is concentrated in the bladder trigone [68]. The injection of BoNT-A in the bladder trigone to block nociceptive neurotransmitters is a reasonable procedure, and has the potential to avoid inhibition of bladder contractility. However, the mechanisms of IC/BPS pathogenesis include abnormal bladder sensory input, as well as active inflammation in the bladder body. The anti-inflammatory effect of BoNT-A trigone injection may be inferior to that of diffuse bladder-body injection. Our previous study compared BoNT-A injection in the bladder body with that of injection in the trigone in patients with idiopathic detrusor overactivity [69]. There were no significant differences in treatment success rates or changes in urgency severity score, and the incidence of adverse events was similar between trigone and bladder-body injections. Another animal study used BoNT-A injection on one side of the bladder and found that synaptosome-associated protein 25 was cleaved on the opposite side of the bladder [70]. The findings of that study demonstrate that BoNT-A injection could spread across the guinea pig bladder; this phenomenon also may occur in the human bladder. Theoretically, trigone and bladder body BoNT-A injections might have similar therapeutic effects, but comparison studies are needed to confirm this hypothesis. For elderly IC/BPS patients with inadequate bladder contractility, the use of BoNT-A trigone injection appears to be reasonable.

3.2.5. Long-Term Therapeutic Effects of BoNT-A in IC/BPS

BoNT turnover in neurons is primarily mediated by the lysosomal/autophagic and ubiquitin-proteasome systems [71]. Most studies have shown persistent muscle paralysis in humans for four to six months following treatment with BoNT-A [72,73]. The persistence of the therapeutic effect after a single BoN-A injection in patients with LUTDs has varied among studies. In a study comparing the different types of BoNT-A injection for patients with neurogenic detrusor overactivity, approximately half of the patients (53.4%) exhibited continence at three months postinjection [74]. The mean interval of on-demand repeated injection was eight months, and no significant differences were found among types of BoNT-A injections. When assessing the therapeutic effect of a single BoNT-A injection in patients with IC/BPS, the longest follow-up duration in published studies is currently one year [52,62]. In 2008, Giannantoni et al. reported significant symptomatic relapse at five months after 200 U BoNT-A injection in the trigone and lateral wall, in terms of bladder pain, urinary frequency, and bladder capacity [62]. All patients exhibited recurrent pain at 12 months postinjection. In 2015, Akiyama et al. used 100 U BoNT-A trigone injections and reported similar results.[52] The response rates (global response assessment ≥+1: slightly improved) were 38.2% at six months postinjection and 20.6% at 12 months postinjection [52]. Although BoNT-A injection was effective for symptomatic relief in IC/BPS, remission was common and repeated injection was necessary for most patients.

Because symptomatic relapse is common, the persistence of therapeutic effects after repeated BoNT-A injection is an important issue. Evidence from cosmetic use of BoNT-A showed that treatment failure may occur after repeated injections [52,75]. The formation of neutralizing antibodies after repeated BoNT-A injections could include antibodies that target the functionally active part of BoNT-A, thereby leading to treatment failure [76]. In a human study, the formation of neutralizing antibodies after Botox®injection was observed in an estimated 5–15% of patients [77]. In cosmetic use, potential risk factors for development of neutralizing antibodies included a single injection of >200 U and repeated injection within one month [75]. For BoNT-A injection in patients with LUTDs, current evidence suggests that the therapeutic effect could persist after repeated injections. Kennelly et al.

performed a prospective study of 240 neurogenic detrusor overactivity patients who underwent up to six repeated BoNT-A injections within a four-year period [60]. Symptomatic improvement among injections did not reach statistical significance, particularly in terms of incontinence episodes and voided volume. For patients with IC/BPS, studies also showed that repeated BoNT-A injections could provide persistent symptomatic relief [78–80]. Notably, beginning in 2006, we performed a BoNT-A injection of 100 U every six months in patients with refractory IC/BPS until they wished to discontinue treatment [78]. Significant symptomatic improvement, including to bladder pain, O'Leary–Sant scores, and global response assessment, persisted after the fourth BoNT-A injection. Within a follow-up period of up to 79 months, patients who received repeated injections had a better success rate and longer therapeutic duration than those who received a single injection. The rate of adverse effects did not increase with the number of BoNT-A injections. Therefore, repeated BoNT-A injections may be both effective and safe for patients with IC/BPS.

However, one study detected serum BoNT-A antibodies in patients who received bladder BoNT-A injections, and the presence of such antibodies was associated with treatment failure [81]. Although repeated BoNT-A injections in the bladder are generally effective, the formation of neutralizing antibodies might cause treatment failure in some patients. Further study is necessary to investigate whether the neutralizing antibodies are present in the bladder after repeated BoNT-A injection.

3.2.6. BoNT-A Injection for IC/BPS with Hunner's Lesion

Hunner's lesion is a specific cystoscopic finding that is characterized by a circumscript, reddened mucosa with small vessels radiating toward a central scar [82]. Patients with IC/BPS and Hunner's lesion (HIC) typically experience significant sharp bladder pain and require cystoscopic bladder electrocauterization [1,82]. The efficacy of BoNT-A injection in HIC is controversial. Our study used diffuse bladder-body injection of BoNT-A in patients with HIC; notably, these patients showed no significant changes in any clinical or urodynamic variables [83]. Another study reported that the efficacy of BoNT-A injection in patients with HIC was not superior to treatment with hydrodistention alone [84]. In contrast, Pinto et al. compared the treatment outcomes of intratrigonal BoNT-A injection between patients with HIC and patients with IC/BPS without Hunner's lesion [85]. Both groups had equal responses to BoNT-A, as well as significant improvement that included lessening of bladder pain, urinary frequency, and O'Leary–Sant scores. In another study, complete remission of Hunner's lesion was observed in three of five patients with HIC after BoNT-A injection [86]. All of the abovementioned studies were limited to small numbers of patients (≤0 patients with HIC per study), and the results were conflicting among studies. In the past, the definition of Hunner's lesion might have differed among countries [82]; hence, the characteristics of patients with HIC included in previous studies may lack consistency. In the study by Pinto, the patients with HIC and patients with IC/BPS without Hunner's lesion had similar symptom severity at baseline; in contrast, the patients with HIC in our study had much more severe baseline symptoms. From our perspective, BoNT-A injection alone is insufficient for satisfactory symptomatic relief in patients with severe HIC. Further studies with larger numbers of patients and clear definitions of Hunner's lesion are necessary.

4. Conclusions

Intravesical BoNT-A injection provides a promising option in treating IC/BPS. Randomized placebo-controlled trials have revealed that intravesical BoNT-A injection is effective for relief of pain and urinary symptoms. The mechanisms by which BoNT-A is effective for treatment of IC/BPS include inhibition of detrusor muscle activity, as well as directly sensory modulation and inflammation control in the urothelium. Although current guidelines consider BoNT-A injection to be the standard treatment, some practical issues remain. Most clinical evidence comes from retrospective uncontrolled studies, and there are only two randomized, placebo-controlled studies with limited patients numbers to support BoNT-A efficacy in IC/BPS. Most patients with IC/BPS experience symptom relapse at six to nine months after BoNT-A injection, although repeated BoNT-A injections have persistent therapeutic effects. The optimal BoNT-A injection dose and site have not been well-investigated in comparison studies. For the IC/BPS patients with Hunner's lesion, clinical efficacy is still unclear. Further high-level evidence studies with greater numbers of patients are necessary to support using BoNT-A injection as a standard treatment for patients with IC/BPS.

References

1. Meijlink, J.M. Interstitial cystitis and the painful bladder: A brief history of nomenclature, definitions and criteria. *Int. J. Urol.* **2014**, *21* (Suppl. 1), 4–12. [CrossRef] [PubMed]
2. Hanno, P.M.; Erickson, D.; Moldwin, R.; Faraday, M.M.; American Urological, A. Diagnosis and treatment of interstitial cystitis/bladder pain syndrome: AUA guideline amendment. *J. Urol.* **2015**, *193*, 1545–1553. [CrossRef]
3. van de Merwe, J.P.; Nordling, J.; Bouchelouche, P.; Bouchelouche, K.; Cervigni, M.; Daha, L.K.; Elneil, S.; Fall, M.; Hohlbrugger, G.; Irwin, P.; et al. Diagnostic criteria, classification, and nomenclature for painful bladder syndrome/interstitial cystitis: An ESSIC proposal. *Eur. Urol.* **2008**, *53*, 60–67. [CrossRef] [PubMed]
4. Suskind, A.M.; Berry, S.H.; Ewing, B.A.; Elliott, M.N.; Suttorp, M.J.; Clemens, J.Q. The prevalence and overlap of interstitial cystitis/bladder pain syndrome and chronic prostatitis/chronic pelvic pain syndrome in men: Results of the RAND Interstitial Cystitis Epidemiology male study. *J. Urol.* **2013**, *189*, 141–145. [CrossRef] [PubMed]
5. Kuo, H.C. Reversibility of the inhibitory effect of intravesical capsaicin on the micturition reflex in rats. *J. Formos. Med. Assoc.* **1997**, *96*, 819–824. [PubMed]
6. Kuo, H.C. Multiple intravesical instillation of low-dose resiniferatoxin is effective in the treatment of detrusor overactivity refractory to anticholinergics. *BJU Int.* **2005**, *95*, 1023–1027. [CrossRef] [PubMed]
7. Montecucco, C.; Molgo, J. Botulinal neurotoxins: Revival of an old killer. *Curr. Opin. Pharmacol.* **2005**, *5*, 274–279. [CrossRef] [PubMed]
8. Dykstra, D.D.; Sidi, A.A.; Scott, A.B.; Pagel, J.M.; Goldish, G.D. Effects of botulinum A toxin on detrusor-sphincter dyssynergia in spinal cord injury patients. *J. Urol.* **1988**, *139*, 919–922. [CrossRef]
9. Jhang, J.F.; Kuo, H.C. Novel Applications of OnabotulinumtoxinA in Lower Urinary Tract Dysfunction. *Toxins* **2018**, *10*, 260. [CrossRef]
10. Jhang, J.F.; Kuo, H.C. Botulinum Toxin A and Lower Urinary Tract Dysfunction: Pathophysiology and Mechanisms of Action. *Toxins* **2016**, *8*, 120. [CrossRef]
11. Meunier, F.A.; Schiavo, G.; Molgo, J. Botulinum neurotoxins: From paralysis to recovery of functional neuromuscular transmission. *J. Physiol. Paris* **2002**, *96*, 105–113. [CrossRef]
12. Chiu, B.; Tai, H.C.; Chung, S.D.; Birder, L.A. Botulinum Toxin A for Bladder Pain Syndrome/Interstitial Cystitis. *Toxins* **2016**, *8*, 201. [CrossRef] [PubMed]
13. Dolly, J.O.; O'Connell, M.A. Neurotherapeutics to inhibit exocytosis from sensory neurons for the control of chronic pain. *Curr. Opin. Pharmacol.* **2012**, *12*, 100–108. [CrossRef] [PubMed]
14. Rummel, A. The long journey of botulinum neurotoxins into the synapse. *Toxicon* **2015**, *107 Pt A*, 9–24. [CrossRef]
15. Antonucci, F.; Corradini, I.; Fossati, G.; Tomasoni, R.; Menna, E.; Matteoli, M. SNAP-25, a Known Presynaptic Protein with Emerging Postsynaptic Functions. *Front. Synaptic Neurosci.* **2016**, *8*, 159. [CrossRef] [PubMed]
16. Sahai, A.; Sangster, P.; Kalsi, V.; Khan, M.S.; Fowler, C.J.; Dasgupta, P. Assessment of urodynamic and detrusor contractility variables in patients with overactive bladder syndrome treated with botulinum toxin-A: Is incomplete bladder emptying predictable? *BJU Int.* **2009**, *103*, 630–634. [CrossRef]
17. Sengupta, J.N. Visceral pain: The neurophysiological mechanism. *Handb. Exp. Pharmacol.* **2009**, *194*, 31–74.
18. Macdiarmid, S.A.; Sand, P.K. Diagnosis of interstitial cystitis/painful bladder syndrome in patients with overactive bladder symptoms. *Rev. Urol.* **2007**, *9*, 9–16.
19. Kuo, Y.C.; Kuo, H.C. Videourodynamic characteristics of interstitial cystitis/bladder pain syndrome-The role of bladder outlet dysfunction in the pathophysiology. *Neurourol. Urodyn.* **2018**, *37*, 1971–1977. [CrossRef]

20. De Felipe, C.; Herrero, J.F.; O'Brien, J.A.; Palmer, J.A.; Doyle, C.A.; Smith, A.J.; Laird, J.M.; Belmonte, C.; Cervero, F.; Hunt, S.P. Altered nociception, analgesia and aggression in mice lacking the receptor for substance P. *Nature* **1998**, *392*, 394–397. [CrossRef]
21. Brain, S.D.; Williams, T.J.; Tippins, J.R.; Morris, H.R.; MacIntyre, I. Calcitonin gene-related peptide is a potent vasodilator. *Nature* **1985**, *313*, 54–56. [CrossRef] [PubMed]
22. Lucioni, A.; Bales, G.T.; Lotan, T.L.; McGehee, D.S.; Cook, S.P.; Rapp, D.E. Botulinum toxin type A inhibits sensory neuropeptide release in rat bladder models of acute injury and chronic inflammation. *BJU Int.* **2008**, *101*, 366–370. [CrossRef] [PubMed]
23. Bleakman, D.; Alt, A.; Nisenbaum, E.S. Glutamate receptors and pain. *Semin. Cell Dev. Biol.* **2006**, *17*, 592–604. [CrossRef]
24. Aoki, K.R. Review of a proposed mechanism for the antinociceptive action of botulinum toxin type A. *Neurotoxicology* **2005**, *26*, 785–793. [CrossRef] [PubMed]
25. Bittencourt da Silva, L.; Karshenas, A.; Bach, F.W.; Rasmussen, S.; Arendt-Nielsen, L.; Gazerani, P. Blockade of glutamate release by botulinum neurotoxin type A in humans: A dermal microdialysis study. *Pain Res. Manag.* **2014**, *19*, 126–132. [CrossRef]
26. Burnstock, G. Purinergic signalling in the urinary tract in health and disease. *Purinergic Signal.* **2014**, *10*, 103–155.
27. Hanna-Mitchell, A.T.; Wolf-Johnston, A.S.; Barrick, S.R.; Kanai, A.J.; Chancellor, M.B.; de Groat, W.C.; Birder, L.A. Effect of botulinum toxin A on urothelial-release of ATP and expression of SNARE targets within the urothelium. *Neurourol. Urodyn.* **2015**, *34*, 79–84. [CrossRef]
28. Khera, M.; Somogyi, G.T.; Kiss, S.; Boone, T.B.; Smith, C.P. Botulinum toxin A inhibits ATP release from bladder urothelium after chronic spinal cord injury. *Neurochem. Int.* **2004**, *45*, 987–993. [CrossRef]
29. Adcock, J.J. TRPV1 receptors in sensitisation of cough and pain reflexes. *Pulm. Pharmacol. Ther.* **2009**, *22*, 65–70. [CrossRef]
30. Min, J.W.; Liu, W.H.; He, X.H.; Peng, B.W. Different types of toxins targeting TRPV1 in pain. *Toxicon* **2013**, *71*, 66–75. [CrossRef]
31. Apostolidis, A.; Popat, R.; Yiangou, Y.; Cockayne, D.; Ford, A.; Davis, J.; Dasgupta, P.; Fowler, C.; Anand, P. Decreased sensory receptors P2X3 and TRPV1 in suburothelial nerve fibers following intradetrusor injections of botulinum toxin for human detrusor overactivity. *J. Urol.* **2005**, *174*, 977–982. [CrossRef] [PubMed]
32. Schulte-Baukloh, H.; Priefert, J.; Knispel, H.H.; Lawrence, G.W.; Miller, K.; Neuhaus, J. Botulinum toxin A detrusor injections reduce postsynaptic muscular M2, M3, P2X2, and P2X3 receptors in children and adolescents who have neurogenic detrusor overactivity: A single-blind study. *Urology* **2013**, *81*, 1052–1057. [CrossRef] [PubMed]
33. Drinovac, V.; Bach-Rojecky, L.; Babic, A.; Lackovic, Z. Antinociceptive effect of botulinum toxin type A on experimental abdominal pain. *Eur. J. Pharmacol.* **2014**, *745*, 190–195. [CrossRef] [PubMed]
34. Lee, W.H.; Shin, T.J.; Kim, H.J.; Lee, J.-K.; Suh, H.-W.; Lee, S.C.; Seo, K. Intrathecal administration of botulinum neurotoxin type A attenuates formalin-induced nociceptive responses in mice. *Anesth. Analg.* **2011**, *112*, 228–235. [CrossRef]
35. Papagiannopoulou, D.; Vardouli, L.; Dimitriadis, F.; Apostolidis, A. Retrograde transport of radiolabelled botulinum neurotoxin type A to the CNS after intradetrusor injection in rats. *BJU Int.* **2016**, *117*, 697–704. [CrossRef]
36. Birder, L.A. Pathophysiology of interstitial cystitis. *Int. J. Urol.* **2019**, *26* (Suppl. 1), 12–15. [CrossRef]
37. Kim, H.J. Update on the Pathology and Diagnosis of Interstitial Cystitis/Bladder Pain Syndrome: A Review. *Int. Neurourol. J.* **2016**, *20*, 13–17. [CrossRef]
38. Lynes, W.L.; Flynn, S.D.; Shortliffe, L.D.; Stamey, T.A. The histology of interstitial cystitis. *Am. J. Surg. Pathol.* **1990**, *14*, 969–976. [CrossRef]
39. Maeda, D.; Akiyama, Y.; Morikawa, T.; Kunita, A.; Ota, Y.; Katoh, H.; Niimi, A.; Nomiya, A.; Ishikawa, S.; Goto, A.; et al. Hunner-Type (Classic) Interstitial Cystitis: A Distinct Inflammatory Disorder Characterized by Pancystitis, with Frequent Expansion of Clonal B-Cells and Epithelial Denudation. *PLoS ONE* **2015**, *10*, e0143316. [CrossRef]
40. Logadottir, Y.; Delbro, D.; Lindholm, C.; Fall, M.; Peeker, R. Inflammation characteristics in bladder pain syndrome ESSIC type 3C/classic interstitial cystitis. *Int. J. Urol.* **2014**, *21* (Suppl. 1), 75–78. [CrossRef]

41. Peng, C.H.; Jhang, J.F.; Shie, J.H.; Kuo, H.C. Down regulation of vascular endothelial growth factor is associated with decreased inflammation after intravesical OnabotulinumtoxinA injections combined with hydrodistention for patients with interstitial cystitis–clinical results and immunohistochemistry analysis. *Urology* **2013**, *82*, 1452.e1–1452.e6. [PubMed]
42. Jiang, Y.H.; Peng, C.H.; Liu, H.T.; Kuo, H.C. Increased pro-inflammatory cytokines, C-reactive protein and nerve growth factor expressions in serum of patients with interstitial cystitis/bladder pain syndrome. *PLoS ONE* **2013**, *8*, e76779. [CrossRef] [PubMed]
43. Peters, K.M.; Diokno, A.C.; Steinert, B.W. Preliminary study on urinary cytokine levels in interstitial cystitis: Does intravesical bacille Calmette-Guerin treat interstitial cystitis by altering the immune profile in the bladder? *Urology* **1999**, *54*, 450–453. [CrossRef]
44. Chuang, Y.C.; Yoshimura, N.; Huang, C.C.; Wu, M.; Chiang, P.H.; Chancellor, M.B. Intravesical botulinum toxin A administration inhibits COX-2 and EP4 expression and suppresses bladder hyperactivity in cyclophosphamide-induced cystitis in rats. *Eur. Urol.* **2009**, *56*, 159–166. [CrossRef] [PubMed]
45. Comperat, E.; Reitz, A.; Delcourt, A.; Capron, F.; Denys, P.; Chartier-Kastler, E. Histologic features in the urinary bladder wall affected from neurogenic overactivity—A comparison of inflammation, oedema and fibrosis with and without injection of botulinum toxin type A. *Eur. Urol.* **2006**, *50*, 1058–1064. [CrossRef]
46. Shie, J.H.; Liu, H.T.; Wang, Y.S.; Kuo, H.C. Immunohistochemical evidence suggests repeated intravesical application of botulinum toxin A injections may improve treatment efficacy of interstitial cystitis/bladder pain syndrome. *BJU Int.* **2013**, *111*, 638–646. [CrossRef]
47. Parsons, C.L. The role of the urinary epithelium in the pathogenesis of interstitial cystitis/prostatitis/urethritis. *Urology* **2007**, *69* (Suppl. 4), 9–16. [CrossRef]
48. Chen, S.F.; Chang, C.H.; Kuo, H.C. Clinical Efficacy and Changes of Urothelial Dysfunction after Repeated Detrusor Botulinum Toxin A Injections in Chronic Spinal Cord-Injured Bladder. *Toxins* **2016**, *8*, 164. [CrossRef]
49. Yeh, H.L.; Jhang, J.F.; Kuo, Y.C.; Kuo, H.C. Long-term outcome and symptom improvement in patients with interstitial cystitis/bladder pain syndrome with or without regular follow-up and treatment. *Neurourol. Urodyn.* **2019**, *38*, 1985–1993. [CrossRef]
50. Smith, C.P.; Radziszewski, P.; Borkowski, A.; Somogyi, G.T.; Boone, T.B.; Chancellor, M.B. Botulinum toxin a has antinociceptive effects in treating interstitial cystitis. *Urology* **2004**, *64*, 871–875. [CrossRef]
51. Kuo, H.C. Preliminary results of suburothelial injection of botulinum a toxin in the treatment of chronic interstitial cystitis. *Urol. Int.* **2005**, *75*, 170–174. [CrossRef] [PubMed]
52. Akiyama, Y.; Nomiya, A.; Niimi, A.; Yamada, Y.; Fujimura, T.; Nakagawa, T.; Fukuhara, H.; Kume, H.; Igawa, Y.; Homma, Y. Botulinum toxin type A injection for refractory interstitial cystitis: A randomized comparative study and predictors of treatment response. *Int. J. Urol.* **2015**, *22*, 835–841. [CrossRef] [PubMed]
53. Kuo, H.C.; Jiang, Y.H.; Tsai, Y.C.; Kuo, Y.C. Intravesical botulinum toxin—A injections reduce bladder pain of interstitial cystitis/bladder pain syndrome refractory to conventional treatment—A prospective, multicenter, randomized, double-blind, placebo-controlled clinical trial. *Neurourol. Urodyn.* **2016**, *35*, 609–614. [CrossRef] [PubMed]
54. Pinto, R.A.; Costa, D.; Morgado, A.; Pereira, P.; Charrua, A.; Silva, J.; Cruz, F. Intratrigonal OnabotulinumtoxinA Improves Bladder Symptoms and Quality of Life in Patients with Bladder Pain Syndrome/Interstitial Cystitis: A Pilot, Single Center, Randomized, Double-Blind, Placebo Controlled Trial. *J. Urol.* **2018**, *199*, 998–1003. [CrossRef]
55. Krivoborodov, G.G.; Shumilo, D.V.; Vasil'ev, A.V. [First experience of using lantox (botulinum toxin A) in chronic pelvic pain syndrome combined with bladder emptying dysfunction]. *Urologiia* **2010**, 60–62. [PubMed]
56. Gao, Y.; Liao, L. Intravesical injection of botulinum toxin A for treatment of interstitial cystitis/bladder pain syndrome: 10 years of experience at a single center in China. *Int. Urogynecol. J.* **2015**, *26*, 1021–1026. [CrossRef]
57. Zhang, W.; Deng, X.; Liu, C.; Wang, X. Intravesical treatment for interstitial cystitis/painful bladder syndrome: A network meta-analysis. *Int. Urogynecol. J.* **2017**, *28*, 515–525. [CrossRef]
58. Binder, W.J.; Brin, M.F.; Blitzer, A.; Pogoda, J.M. Botulinum toxin type A (BOTOX) for treatment of migraine. *Dis. Mon.* **2002**, *48*, 323–335. [CrossRef]

59. Rovner, E.; Kennelly, M.; Schulte-Baukloh, H.; Zhou, J.; Haag-Molkenteller, C.; Dasgupta, P. Urodynamic results and clinical outcomes with intradetrusor injections of onabotulinumtoxinA in a randomized, placebo-controlled dose-finding study in idiopathic overactive bladder. *Neurourol. Urodyn.* **2011**, *30*, 556–562. [CrossRef]
60. Kennelly, M.; Dmochowski, R.; Schulte-Baukloh, H.; Ethans, K.; Del Popolo, G.; Moore, C.; Jenkins, B.; Guard, S.; Zheng, Y.; Karsenty, G.; et al. Efficacy and safety of onabotulinumtoxinA therapy are sustained over 4 years of treatment in patients with neurogenic detrusor overactivity: Final results of a long-term extension study. *Neurourol. Urodyn.* **2017**, *36*, 368–375. [CrossRef]
61. Giannantoni, A.; Costantini, E.; Di Stasi, S.M.; Tascini, M.C.; Bini, V.; Porena, M. Botulinum A toxin intravesical injections in the treatment of painful bladder syndrome: A pilot study. *Eur. Urol.* **2006**, *49*, 704–709. [CrossRef] [PubMed]
62. Giannantoni, A.; Porena, M.; Costantini, E.; Zucchi, A.; Mearini, L.; Mearini, E. Botulinum A toxin intravesical injection in patients with painful bladder syndrome: 1-year followup. *J. Urol.* **2008**, *179*, 1031–1034. [CrossRef] [PubMed]
63. Smith, C.P.; Nishiguchi, J.; O'Leary, M.; Yoshimura, N.; Chancellor, M.B. Single-institution experience in 110 patients with botulinum toxin A injection into bladder or urethra. *Urology* **2005**, *65*, 37–41. [CrossRef] [PubMed]
64. Kuo, H.C.; Chancellor, M.B. Comparison of intravesical botulinum toxin type A injections plus hydrodistention with hydrodistention alone for the treatment of refractory interstitial cystitis/painful bladder syndrome. *BJU Int.* **2009**, *104*, 657–661. [CrossRef] [PubMed]
65. Groen, J.; Pannek, J.; Castro Diaz, D.; Del Popolo, G.; Gross, T.; Hamid, R.; Karsenty, G.; Kessler, T.M.; Schneider, M.; Hoen, L.T.; et al. Summary of European Association of Urology (EAU) Guidelines on Neuro-Urology. *Eur. Urol.* **2016**, *69*, 324–333. [CrossRef] [PubMed]
66. Pinto, R.; Lopes, T.; Frias, B.; Silva, A.; Silva, J.A.; Silva, C.M.; Cruz, C.D.; Cruz, F.; Dinis, P. Trigonal injection of botulinum toxin A in patients with refractory bladder pain syndrome/interstitial cystitis. *Eur. Urol.* **2010**, *58*, 360–365. [CrossRef] [PubMed]
67. Gosling, J.A.; Dixon, J.S. Sensory nerves in the mammalian urinary tract. An evaluation using light and electron microscopy. *J. Anat.* **1974**, *117 Pt 1*, 133–144.
68. Spradling, K.; Khoyilar, C.; Abedi, G.; Okhunov, Z.; Wikenheiser, J.; Yoon, R.; Huang, J.; Youssef, R.F.; Ghoniem, G.; Landman, J. Redefining the Autonomic Nerve Distribution of the Bladder Using 3-Dimensional Image Reconstruction. *J. Urol.* **2015**, *194*, 1661–1667. [CrossRef]
69. Kuo, H.C. Bladder base/trigone injection is safe and as effective as bladder body injection of onabotulinumtoxinA for idiopathic detrusor overactivity refractory to antimuscarinics. *Neurourol. Urodyn.* **2011**, *30*, 1242–1248. [CrossRef]
70. Coelho, A.; Cruz, F.; Cruz, C.D.; Avelino, A. Spread of onabotulinumtoxinA after bladder injection. Experimental study using the distribution of cleaved SNAP-25 as the marker of the toxin action. *Eur. Urol.* **2012**, *61*, 1178–1184. [CrossRef]
71. Shoemaker, C.B.; Oyler, G.A. Persistence of Botulinum neurotoxin inactivation of nerve function. *Curr. Top. Microbiol. Immunol.* **2013**, *364*, 179–196. [PubMed]
72. Eleopra, R.; Tugnoli, V.; Rossetto, O.; De Grandis, D.; Montecucco, C. Different time courses of recovery after poisoning with botulinum neurotoxin serotypes A and E in humans. *Neurosci. Lett.* **1998**, *256*, 135–138. [CrossRef]
73. Sloop, R.R.; Cole, B.A.; Escutin, R.O. Human response to botulinum toxin injection: Type B compared with type A. *Neurology* **1997**, *49*, 189–194. [CrossRef] [PubMed]
74. Lombardi, G.; Musco, S.; Bacci, G.; Celso, M.; Bellio, V.; Del Popolo, G. Long-term response of different Botulinum toxins in refractory neurogenic detrusor overactivity due to spinal cord injury. *Int. Braz. J. Urol.* **2017**, *43*, 721–729. [CrossRef] [PubMed]
75. Nigam, P.K.; Nigam, A. Botulinum toxin. *Indian J. Dermatol.* **2010**, *55*, 8–14. [CrossRef] [PubMed]
76. Fabbri, M.; Leodori, G.; Fernandes, R.M.; Bhidayasiri, R.; Marti, M.J.; Colosimo, C.; Ferreira, J.J. Neutralizing Antibody and Botulinum Toxin Therapy: A Systematic Review and Meta-analysis. *Neurotox. Res.* **2016**, *29*, 105–117. [CrossRef] [PubMed]
77. Goschel, H.; Wohlfarth, K.; Frevert, J.; Dengler, R.; Bigalke, H. Botulinum A toxin therapy: Neutralizing and nonneutralizing antibodies–therapeutic consequences. *Exp. Neurol.* **1997**, *147*, 96–102. [CrossRef]

78. Lee, C.L.; Kuo, H.C. Long-Term Efficacy and Safety of Repeated Intravescial OnabotulinumtoxinA Injections Plus Hydrodistention in the Treatment of Interstitial Cystitis/Bladder Pain Syndrome. *Toxins* **2015**, *7*, 4283–4293. [CrossRef]
79. Pinto, R.; Lopes, T.; Silva, J.; Silva, C.; Dinis, P.; Cruz, F. Persistent therapeutic effect of repeated injections of onabotulinum toxin a in refractory bladder pain syndrome/interstitial cystitis. *J. Urol.* **2013**, *189*, 548–553. [CrossRef]
80. Kuo, H.C. Repeated onabotulinumtoxin-a injections provide better results than single injection in treatment of painful bladder syndrome. *Pain Physician* **2013**, *16*, E15–E23.
81. Schulte-Baukloh, H.; Bigalke, H.; Miller, K.; Heine, G.; Pape, D.; Lehmann, J.; Knispel, H.H. Botulinum neurotoxin type A in urology: Antibodies as a cause of therapy failure. *Int. J. Urol.* **2008**, *15*, 407–415. [CrossRef] [PubMed]
82. Doggweiler, R.; Whitmore, K.E.; Meijlink, J.M.; Drake, M.J.; Frawley, H.; Nordling, J.; Hanno, P.; Fraser, M.O.; Homma, Y.; Garrido, G.; et al. A standard for terminology in chronic pelvic pain syndromes: A report from the chronic pelvic pain working group of the international continence society. *Neurourol. Urodyn.* **2017**, *36*, 984–1008. [CrossRef] [PubMed]
83. Lee, C.L.; Kuo, H.C. Intravesical botulinum toxin a injections do not benefit patients with ulcer type interstitial cystitis. *Pain Physician* **2013**, *16*, 109–116. [PubMed]
84. Kasyan, G.; Pushkar, D. 822 Randomized Controlled Trial for Efficacy of Botulinum Toxin Type A in Treatment of Patients Suffering Bladder Pain Syndrome/Interstitial Cystitis with Hunners' Lesions Preliminary Results. *J. Urol.* **2012**, *187*, e335–e336. [CrossRef]
85. Pinto, R.; Lopes, T.; Costa, D.; Barros, S.; Silva, J.; Silva, C.; Cruz, C.D.; Dinis, P.; Cruz, F. Ulcerative and nonulcerative forms of bladder pain syndrome/interstitial cystitis do not differ in symptom intensity or response to onabotulinum toxin A. *Urology* **2014**, *83*, 1030–1034. [CrossRef]
86. Al Mousa, R.; Alsowayan, Y.; Alfadagh, A.; Almuhrij, A. [7] Efficacy, complications and tolerability of repeated intravesical onabotulinumtoxinA injections in interstitial cystitis/bladder pain syndrome. *Arab J. Urol.* **2018**, *16* (Suppl. 1), S5. [CrossRef]

17

Therapeutic Effect of Botulinum Toxin A on Sensory Bladder Disorders—From Bench to Bedside

Yuan-Hong Jiang [1,2], Wan-Ru Yu [3] and Hann-Chorng Kuo [1,2,*]

1 Department of Urology, Hualien Tzu Chi Hospital, Buddhist Tzu Chi Medical Foundation, Hualien 970, Taiwan; redeemer1019@yahoo.com.tw
2 Department of Urology, Buddhist Tzu Chi University, Hualien 970, Taiwan
3 Department of Nursing, Hualien Tzu Chi General Hospital, Tzu Chi Medical Foundation, Tzu Chi University, Hualien 970, Taiwan; wanzu666@gmail.com
* Correspondence: hck@tzuchi.com.tw

Abstract: Bladder oversensitivity arises from several different conditions involving the bladder, bladder outlet, systemic or central nervous system diseases. Increase of the bladder sensation results from activation of the sensory receptors in the urothelial cells or suburothelial tissues. Medical treatment targeting the overactive bladder (OAB) or interstitial cystitis (IC) might relieve oversensitive bladder symptoms (frequency, urgency and pain) in a portion of patients, but a certain percentage of patients still need active management. Botulinum toxin A (BoNT-A) has been demonstrated to have anti-inflammatory and antinociceptive effects in bladder sensory disorders and has been shown effective in the reduction of bladder oversensitivity and the increase of functional bladder capacity. For patients with OAB, urgency and urinary incontinence improved, while in patients with IC, bladder pain could be relieved in association with reduction of bladder oversensitivity after BoNT-A intravesical injection. Histological evidence has confirmed the therapeutic mechanism and clinical efficacy of intravesical BoNT-A injection on patients with OAB or IC. Bladder oversensitivity can also be relieved with the instillation of liposome encapsulated BoNT-A or low energy show waves (LESWs), which enable the BoNT-A molecule to penetrate into the urothelium and suburothelial space without affecting the detrusor contractility. Liposome encapsulated BoNT-A or combined LESWs and BoNT-A instillation might be future treatment alternatives for bladder oversensitivity in sensory bladder disorders.

Keywords: bladder; sensation; therapy; pathophysiology

Key Contribution: This study reviews the main pathophysiology and pharmacological mechanisms of botulinum toxin action on the treatment of sensory bladder disorders.

---

1. Introduction

Bladder sensation arises from the urothelial cell and detrusor muscle stretching by signal transduction from peripheral receptors to the cerebral cortex. Many factors may contribute and effect the sensory transduction pathways, resulting in increased bladder sensation with or without associated symptoms such as urgency, urgency incontinence or bladder pain. The factors which will increase bladder sensation include aging, the urinary bladder, bladder outlet conditions, or systemic diseases. Currently, there is no definite definition nor specific medication targeting bladder oversensitivity. Bladder oversensitivity is usually existent with other lower urinary tract disorders (LUTD) such as bacterial cystitis, ketamine cystitis, interstitial cystitis (IC), bladder outlet obstruction (BOO), overactive bladder syndrome (OAB), idiopathic detrusor overactivity (DO), neurogenic DO (NDO); or systemic diseases such as diabetes mellitus, end-stage renal disease, or congestive heart failure [1].

Antimuscarinics or beta-3 adrenoceptor agonists have therapeutic effects on OAB and DO and also have some effect on reducing bladder oversensitivity. [2,3] Treatment of bladder oversensitivity should begin with treating the underlying causative diseases such as BOO, acute or chronic bladder inflammatory diseases, diabetes mellitus, or other systemic diseases. Previous studies of botulinum toxin A (BoNT-A) treatments for OAB, DO and IC have shown significant improvement of bladder oversensation and increased bladder capacity, in addition to the main target of urinary urgency or bladder pain. If medical treatment fails, intravesical BoNT-A might play a second- or third-line therapeutic alternative for bladder oversensitivity. This article reviews the pathophysiology, therapeutic mechanisms and treatment effects of BoNT-A on the improvement of the increased bladder sensation in bladder disorders, specifically focused on OAB, DO, IC and bladder oversensitivity. This review study searched relevant articles identified by a literature search using MEDLINE/PubMed. Key words included OAB, bladder oversensitivity, DO, IC, bladder sensation, botulinum toxin A, BOTOX, and BTX-A. References of retrieved articles were also hand searched to find additional articles related to the topic of this review. All trials examining the use of BoNT-A injections into the urinary bladder for the treatment of OAB, DO, IC and bladder oversensitivity, and the studies reporting the treatment outcome such as urodynamic parameters, urinary incontinence improvement, and adverse events were included in this review.

2. Lower Urinary Tract Disorder and Bladder Oversensitivity

Lower urinary tract symptoms (LUTS) are highly prevalent and greatly impact the health-related quality of life and cause social economic burden, especially in elderly men and women [4–6]. The etiology of LUTS could be bladder outlet dysfunction or bladder dysfunction, including bladder oversensitivity and DO, or a combination of both bladder and bladder outlet dysfunctions. [7] Recent studies revealed the prevalence of OAB is high in Europe and the United States, as well as in Asian countries. [8,9] As most men with clinical OAB do not have urinary incontinence, they are frequently mis-diagnosed with bladder outlet obstruction (BOO) [10].

The bladder epithelium, known as urothelium, provides a passive barrier to prevent absorption of urine and its contents. Recent evidence suggests the urothelium might be a responsive organ with sensory and transducer functions. [11] The urothelial cells and suburothelial afferent nerves exhibit a number of common properties, including sensory receptors and ion channels. The local or systemic conditions which alter the afferent nerves or urothelial cells might contribute to the abnormal sensory of the urinary bladder. [11] Patients with several lower urinary tract disorders such as BOO, IC, ketamine cystitis, spinal cord injured (SCI), neurogenic bladder dysfunction, or systemic diseases such as diabetes mellitus, end-stage renal disease, or congestive heart failure may also have symptoms of OAB or bladder oversensitivity [12].

3. Pathophysiology of Bladder Oversensitivity

The pathophysiology of OAB and bladder oversensitivity is multifactorial. Occult neurogenic bladder, undetected BOO, provoked DO due to urethral incompetence, aging or diseases, chronic bladder ischemia, chronic bladder inflammation, central nervous system (CNS) sensitization, and autonomic dysfunction are possible etiologies of refractory OAB. [1] The bladder urothelium and afferent nerves express transient receptor potential vanilloid receptor 1 (TRPV1), the purinergic receptor P2X3, the sensory neuropeptides substance P, and calcitonin gene-related peptide (CGRP). [13–15] These receptors are believed to be involved in the afferent pathways that control bladder sensation and urinary volume reflexes [16].

Bladder sensation can be transmitted by the myelinated A-δnerves and unmyelinated C-fibers. In mammalian bladders after SCI, the unmyelinated afferent C-fibers are found to become predominant and mediate the voiding reflex. [17] Intravesical vanilloid treatment using capsaicin or resiniferatoxin had been found effective in SCI patients with NDO or idiopathic DO through acting on TRPV1 [18,19]. After intravesical instillation of resiniferatoxin, urinary frequency significantly decreased and maximal cystometric capacity increased, and patients with NDO became dry days after treatment. [20] In addition, many C-fibers in the bladder urothelium contain sensory neuropeptides which can modulate the micturition reflex and cause DO [21]. Since TRPV1 receptors are found on the afferent nerves and co-localized with P2X3 receptors and other sensory nerves expressing substance P and CGRP, desensitization of the TRPV1 by vanilloid treatment can also decrease bladder oversensitivity and DO [22–24].

The urothelium functions as a sensory organ which receives information from the urinary bladder content and responds to mechanical, thermal or chemical stimuli by releasing adenosine triphosphate (ATP), nitric oxide and acetylcholine (Ach). Changes in the external environment or direct insult on the urothelium produced by different bladder disorders may convey these signals to nerves, detrusor muscles, and transmit to the CNS, resulting in bladder oversensitivity or detrusor contractions. [25] The suburothelial sensory nerves of the urinary bladder are abundant with vesicles containing Ach and ATP, suggesting the bladder lamina propria also play an important role in the transmission of bladder filling and fullness in response to bladder stretch by activating $P2X_3$ receptors [26–28]. When the urinary bladder is infected or under traumatic conditions, the production of ATP, CGRP and substance P acts on afferent nerves in an autocrine fashion to increase afferent nerve activity [29]. Recent studies also found a suburothelial nexus of myofibroblasts or interstitial cells which might be involved in the micturition reflexes [30]. These cells are closely linked by gap junctions and have a response to ATP in a mode similar to the activated ATP-gated P2Y receptors [31,32]. The Ach and ATP released from urothelial cells on bladder filling were noted in patients with aging, which also implies the main pathological mechanism of OAB and bladder oversensitivity in older people [33]. In addition, increase of stretch-activated ATP release was found in the cultured human urothelial cells from patients with IC and SCI, suggesting the involvement of these neurotransmitters in DO and bladder oversensitivity [34].

Bladder inflammation is commonly found in patients with OAB, IC, and systemic diseases and lower urinary tract disorders, resulting in bladder storage symptoms such as urgency and frequency [12]. In previous studies of IC, chronic inflammation leads to increase of urothelial cell apoptosis, lower adhesive protein E-cadherin and lower tight junction protein zonula occludens-1 expression [35]. The chronic inflammation in the IC bladders also inhibits the basal cell proliferation, causing defective apical cell maturation and impaired barrier function [36]. Further study of apoptotic markers such as Bad, Bax, and caspase 3 all increased in the IC bladder tissues, and the inflammatory signals such as p38 mitogen-activated protein kinase and tumor necrosis factor alpha were upregulated [37]. Chronic inflammation is also found in a large proportion of patients with OAB [38]. Chronic neural plasticity due to chronic inflammation and activation of sensory receptors may change the sensory afferent activity via influencing antinociceptive activity, resulting in bladder oversensitivity or DO. The urinary nerve growth factor (NGF) levels in patients with OAB, IC, or other types of bladder oversensitivity have been found to elevate, suggesting these different lower urinary tract disorders might share common pathways in increasing bladder sensation [39–41].

Based on the above evidence, the pathophysiology of bladder oversensitivity or IC syndrome might be sequentially developed by: (1) urothelial injury caused by bacterial cystitis, foreign body, instrumentation, or surgical trauma; (2) suburothelial inflammation developed after urothelial trauma, toxin or autoimmune response; (3) acute inflammatory cell infiltrations in the bladder wall after the acute injury; (4) chronic inflammatory reaction and scar formation in the bladder wall; (5) increased inflammatory reaction leading to neuroplasticity in the dorsal horn ganglia and corresponding sacral cord, resulting in lowering bladder sensation threshold and oversensitivity [42]. The insult of the bladder wall initiates an acute inflammatory process. The sensory impulse from the bladder wall also ascends to the corresponding cortical gyrus and produces frequency symptoms. Therefore, patients might have an early inflammatory reaction and characteristic IC symptoms, such as urgency, frequency and bladder pain. If the urothelial insult ceases, the urothelial cell regeneration will rebuild the defense mechanism and solves the inflammatory reaction to relieve bladder symptoms after treatment. However, if the urothelial insult continues, the inflammatory reaction might exacerbate not only at the bladder wall but also at the spinal cord or cortical gyrus, causing permanent inflammation printing [43].

Similar pathogenesis might also occur in OAB, in which bladder condition may progress from early stage (bladder oversensitivity) to late stage (urgency urinary incontinence) bladder conditions [44].

4. Therapeutic Mechanism of Botulinum Toxin A on Bladder Oversensitivity

BoNT-A has both motor and sensory effects in treating patients with DO or OAB. BoNT-A can inhibit the release of ACh and other neuropeptides from nerve terminals by cleaving the synaptosomal associated protein 25 kDa (SNAP-25), causing paralysis of the affected neuromuscular junctions [45]. In human bladders, Coelho et al. revealed that synaptic vesicle protein 2 (SV2) and SNAP-25 immunoreactive fibers were distributed throughout the suburothelium and muscle layer. Extensive co-localization of both proteins was noted in nerve fibers. SV2 is expressed more in parasympathetic fibers than in sympathetic or sensory fibers [46]. In nerve terminals, synaptic vesicles fuse with the presynaptic membrane where they release the neurotransmitter into the neuromuscular or neuroglandular junction. Intravesical BoNT-A injection relieves OAB symptoms as it enters bladder neurons binding to SV2, causing cleavage of SNAP-25 and preventing exocytosis of the neurotransmitter-containing vesicle at the nerve terminal [47,48]. Further studies revealed that after a single BoNT-A injection, cleaved SNAP-25 immunoreactive fibers were abundant throughout the guinea pig bladder tissue in the mucosa and muscular layer, significantly affecting the parasympathetic fibers. [49] However, because of the tight barrier function of the urothelium, intravesical instillation of BoNT-A cannot cleave SNAP-25 in nerve fibers. The bladder urothelium also expresses intracellular targets SNARE (Soluble *N*-ethylmaleimide-sensitive fusion Attachment protein REceptor) and binding receptor SV2 for BoNT-A uptake. BoNT-A has been shown to suppress the hypotonic-evoked ATP release from the cultured rat urothelial cells. BoNT-A injection can suppress sensory mechanisms and micturition reflexes after affecting the urothelial function of transmitter release [50].

Reduction of the expressions of TRPV1 and P2X3 on the suburothelial sensory afferents had been found in patients with DO treated with detrusor BoNT-A injections. [51] Patients also experience improvement of urinary frequency and reduction of the urgency severity after BoNT-A injection [52,53]. However, not all patients have similar sensory and motor therapeutic effects after BoNT-A injection. The reported success rates are between 60%-80% in patients with OAB [52–59]. Reduction of the urgency severity has been noted to be associated with long-term therapeutic efficacy after BoNT-A injections in patients with idiopathic DO [60]. Patients with both sensory and motor effects after BoNT-A injection showed a significantly better long-term therapeutic effect than the patients with motor or sensory effects alone. [60] Change of bladder capacity and increase of bladder fullness sensation after BoNT-A injections are also noted in these clinical trials. The improvement of bladder oversensitivity is likely to result from reduction of P2X3 and TRPV1 receptor expressions on the suburothelial afferent nerves [51].

In addition, BoNT-A injections for OAB and IC can effectively improve bladder sensory symptoms of frequency urgency and bladder pain in association with reduction of urinary NGF levels [61–64]. Recent studies also demonstrated that BoNT-A injection can inhibit cyclooxygenase-2 (COX-2) and prostaglandin E2 receptor 4 (EP4) expressions in the bladder tissue and block cyclophosphamide-induced bladder inflammation and overactivity. The increase of intercontractile intervals after BoNT-A injection indicates that BoNT-A can effectively improve both sensory and motor functions [65]. BoNT-A might also have a neuromodulatory or anti-inflammatory effect on the bladder wall in patients with OAB or IC, resulting in long-term sensory effect, possibly through CNS desensitization.

5. Clinical Effects of Botulinum Toxin A on Bladder Oversensitivity in OAB

The pathophysiology of OAB might be urotheliogenic or myogenic or could be due to neurogenic inflammation or BOO. As the pathophysiology of OAB might not clearly be determined before treatment, antimuscarinic agents or beta-3 adrenoceptor agonists usually cannot effectively treat all patients [66,67]. Recent investigation hypothesized that OAB might be a sensory disorder due to conditions activating the afferent nerve activities and resulting from the mild OAB subtype (hypersensitive bladder, frequency without urgency) to the moderate subtype (OAB dry, with urgency but no urgency incontinence) or severe subtype (OAB wet, with urgency urinary incontinence). [44] In a long-term, large-scale study, Wennberg et al. found the incidence of urgency incontinence and OAB increased over a 16-year span, with a certain percentage of patients having symptoms progress or regress [68].

Histological study revealed that chronic inflammation exists in half of the OAB bladders [38]. OAB had also been postulated as a subtype of neurogenic inflammation with vascular and non-vascular inflammatory responses through activation of bladder sensory afferents and release of sensory neuropeptides such as substance P and CGRP [69]. The inflammation might involve locally over-expressed suburothelial receptors such as TRPV1 and P2X3, or central inflammatory responses in the dorsal root ganglia [23,70]. Bladder inflammation leads to afferent nerve activation and results in long-term neuroplasticity which lowers the threshold of nociceptive and mechanoceptive afferent fibers, causing bladder oversensitivity. [71] The dynamic changes of OAB presentation with time might be due to different bladder conditions affecting afferent nerve activities [72].

Although many factors could cause OAB, the downstream pathophysiology of bladder oversensitivity and DO is similar. Through BoNT-A injection, the release of neuropeptides and neurotransmitters such ACh, ATP, substance P, or CGRP can be effectively reduced, causing impairment of sensory afferents and paralysis of the detrusor muscles. Treatment of OAB by intravesical BoNT-A injection has achieved satisfactory results in recent decades [52,58,73–77]. Currently, BoNT-A has been widely used in treatment of urinary urgency and incontinence in OAB patients' refractory to oral medical treatment, and relief of frequency and bladder pain in patients with IC. The application of BoNT-A in OAB has been approved by the U.S. and European FDA and is listed as the third-line treatment in the AUA and EAU guidelines for OAB and urinary incontinence [78,79].

The dose of BoNT-A for OAB has been changed from 200 U or 300 U initially to the currently used 100 U [73]. A recent phase 3 clinical trial confirmed that the therapeutic results are similar between doses of 100 U and greater than 100 U [74,75]. BoNT-A at the dose of greater than 100 U increased the risk of adverse events of acute urinary retention and large post-void residual (PVR), as well as the incidence of urinary tract infection (UTI) [77,80]. Injecting BoNT-A at the trigone or bladder base for patients with OAB could effectively decrease the risk of acute urinary retention or large PVR without affecting the therapeutic effects of reduction of urgency and urgency incontinence [81]. The increased bladder sensation in OAB patients can effectively be decreased and bladder capacity increased after effective BoNT-A injection. Table 1 shows some representative study results on the improvement of bladder oversensitivity, reduction of frequency and urgency episodes, and increase of bladder capacity in OAB patients after different doses of BoNT-A injections.

Table 1. The therapeutic effects of botulinum toxin A on the increase of bladder capacity in patients with overactive bladder syndrome.

Authors	Patients and OAB Subtype	Dose of BoNT-A	Change of Bladder Capacity after BoNT-A Treatment at 3 M	Reference
Kuo HC 2004	30 IDO + NDO	200(D)	223 ± 101 to 247 ± 96.3 mL	[54]
Schulte-Baukloh H 2005	44 OAB	200–300(D)	228 ± 19.2 to 305 ± 19.0 mL	[82]
Kuo HC 2005	20 IDO	200 (SU)	224 ± 125 to 315 ± 136 mL	[53]
Rajkumar GN 2005	15 IDO	300 (D)	MCC increased in 10 patients FDV increased in 12 patients	[58]
Smith CP 2005	110 IDO + NDO	100–300 (D)	153 ± 55 to 246 ± 64 mL	[83]
Popat R 2005	31 IDO	200 (D)	194 ± 24 to 327 ± 36.1 mL	[57]
Schmid DM 2006	100 OAB	100 (D)	246 to 381 mL	[84]
Kuo HC 2007	23 IDO + NDO	100 (SU)	185 ± 83 to 252 ± 159 mL	[85]
	25 IDO + NDO	150 (SU)	223 ± 133 to 303 ± 175 mL	
	27 IDO + NDO	200 (SU)	215 ± 124 to 315 ± 136 mL	
Sahai A 2007	16 IDO	200 (D)	MCC increased by 95.7 mL	[55]
Karsenty G 2007	12 OAB	200 (base)	MCC increased 162 to 370 mL	[86]
Kuo HC 2007	15 IDO	100 (SU)	243 ± 133 to 368 ± 132 mL	[87]
	15 IDO	100 (D)	260 ± 105 to 330 ± 116 mL	
	15 IDO	100 (base)	283 ± 167 to 318 ± 138 mL	

Table 1. *Cont.*

Authors	Patients and OAB Subtype	Dose of BoNT-A	Change of Bladder Capacity after BoNT-A Treatment at 3 M	Reference
Rovner E 2011	57 OAB	50 (D)	MCC increased 50 ± 120 mL	[76]
	54 OAB	100 (D)	MCC increased 71 ± 129 mL	
	49 OAB	150 (D)	MCC increased 102 ± 127 mL	
	53 OAB	200 (D)	MCC increased 9 ± 1129 mL	
	53 OAB	300 (D)	MCC increased 131 ± 130 mL	
Tincello DG 2012	122 OAB women	200 (D)	Daily frequency 10.3 to 8.0	[88]
Fowler CJ 2012	57 OAB	50 (D)	UUI decreased 20.7/week	[89]
	54 OAB	100 (D)	UUI increased 18.4/week	
	49 OAB	150 (D)	UUI increased 23.0/week	
	53 OAB	200 (D)	UUI increased 19.6/week	
	56 OAB	300 (D)	UUI increased 19.4/week	
Denys P 2012	23 OAB	50 (D)	MCC increased by 38.4 ± 94.8 mL	[90]
	23 OAB	100 (D)	MCC increased by 85.5 ± 135.1 mL	
	30 OAB	150 (D)	MCC increased by 91.3 ± 125.2 mL	
Liao CH 2013	61 IDO frail	100 (SU)	247 ± 105 to 309 ± 133 mL	[91]
	63 IDO elderly	100 (SU)	266 ±124 to 309 ± 154 mL	
	42 IDO <65 yr	100 (SU)	254 ± 113 to 342 ± 103 mL	
Chapple C 2013	277 OAB	100 (D)	Frequency decreased by 19.7% Urgency decreased by 41.1%	[75]
Nitti V 2013	267 OAB	100 (D)	Vol voided increased 41.1 mL (37.7%)	[74]
Mangera A 2014	IDO		MCC Improved by 58%	[92]
Wang CC 2016	21 DHIC	100 (SU)	Vol + PVR 255 to 365 mL	[93]
	21 OAB	100 (SU)	Vol + PVR 198 to 286 mL	
Onem K 2018	80 OAB	100 (D)	280 ± 134 to 330 ± 124 mL	[94]

OAB: overactive bladder, IDO: idiopathic detrusor overactivity, NDO: neurogenic detrusor overactivty, DHIC: detrusor overactivity and inadequate contractility, SU: suburethelial injection, D: detrusor injection, MCC: maximal cystometric capacity, FDV: first desire volume, MBC: maximal bladder capacity, Vol: voided volume, PVR: post-void residual.

6. Clinical Effects of Botulinum Toxin A on Bladder Oversensitivity in IC Patients

As BoNT-A injections can inhibit the release of ACh at the presynaptic neuromuscular junction and reduce the expressions of TRPV1, P2X3, CGRP and substance P in the urothelial cells and sensory fibers, this treatment has been enthusiastically applied in the treatment of IC [95]. Intravesical BoNTA injection can reduce bladder pain response and inhibit CGRP release from bladder afferent nerves in rat models [96]. The effect of BoNT-A on pain response to irritants might not only reduce bladder oversensitivity but also result in desensitization of the CNS in dorsal horn ganglia after long-term neuroplasticity [97].

An initial pilot trial was performed by Smith et al. who treated 13 IC patients with 100 U to 200 U of Dysport or BoNT-A into the trigone and bladder base and found subjective improvement in 69% of patients after treatment. They concluded that BoNT-A might have an antinociceptive effect on bladder afferent nerves [98]. Kuo et al. injected BoNT-A suburothelially to treat 10 women with IC and seven had symptom improvement. The cystometric bladder capacity significantly increased from 210 ± 63.8 mL to 287 ± 115 mL ($p = 0.05$), however, patients who responded to treatment also had dysuria after BoNT-A injection [95]. The therapeutic effect of BoNT-A on IC patients was further confirmed by Giannantoni et al., who treated 14 patients with 200 U of BoNT-A at 20 sites of the trigone and bladder base. After treatment, 12 patients (85.7%) had subjective improvement at one and three months, where urinary frequency and bladder pain decreased and functional capacity increased significantly [99]. However, the therapeutic efficacy decreased to none at the one-year follow-up [100]. Nevertheless, intravesical BoNT-A injection could reduce bladder pain, urinary frequency, and improve psychosocial functioning. Table 2 shows some representative study results of the changes of bladder capacity and improvement of bladder oversensitivity that are significant in IC bladders after different doses of BoNT-A injections. Due to significant therapeutic efficacy the application of BoNT-A on IC, it has also been recommended as the third-line for IC refractory to lifestyle modulation and medication for pain and urothelial glycosaminoglycan replenishment [101].

Table 2. The therapeutic effects of botulinum toxin A on the increase of bladder capacity and decrease of bladder oversensitivity in patients with interstitial cystitis.

Authors	Patients and IC Subtype	Dose of BoNT-A	Change of Bladder Capacity after BoNT-A Treatment at 3 M	Reference
Smith CP 2004	13 IC	100–200	159 ± 39.9 to 250 ± 46.10 mL	[98]
Kuo HC 2005	10 non-ulcer	100 (SU)	210 ± 63.8 to 287 ± 115 mL	[96]
Giannantoni A 2006	14 IC	200 (D)	262 ± 34.8 to 342 ± 52.4 mL	[99]
Giannantoni A 2008	15 IC	200 (D)	256.4 ± 33.5 to 352.5 ± 50 mL	[100]
Kuo HC 2009	29 non-ulcer	100 (SU)	309 ± 135 to 388 ± 127 mL	[102]
	15 non-ulcer	200 (SU)	251 ± 86.7 to 407 ± 179 mL	
Giannantoni A 2010	13 IC	200 (D)	211.3 ± 48.9 to 341.4 ± 60.6 mL	[103]
Pinto R 2010	26 IC	100 (T)	106 ± 42 to 279 ± 82 mL	[104]
Chung SD 2012	67 IC	100 (SU)	261 ± 108 to 278 ± 144 mL	[105]
Kuo HC 2013	23 IC	100 x 3	277.2 ± 95.2 to 370.5 ± 173 mL	[106]
Kuo HC 2013	81 IC	100 x 3	270 ± 112 to 321 ± 160 mL	[107]
Lee CL 2013	30 non-ulcer	100 (SU)	305–316 to 379–395 mL	[108]
	10 ulcer IC	100 (SU)	142 to 110 mL	
Pinto R 2014	10 ulcer	100 (T)	Frequency 11.2 ± 2.4 to 7.9 ± 1	[109]
	14 non-ulcer	100 (T)	Frequency 10.3 ± 1.9 to 7.9 ± 0.9	
Wang J 2016	Non-ulcer	100–300	MBC increased by 50.5 mL	[110]
Kuo HC 2016	40 non-ulcer	100 (SU)	264.1 ± 120.1 to 332.0 ± 157.5 mL	[111]
Pinto R 2018	19 non-ulcer	100 (T)	Frequency 14.4 ± 6.3 to 9.5 ± 5.5	[112]

SU: suburothelial injection, D: detrusor injection, T: trigonal injection, MBC: maximal bladder capacity, IC: interstitial cystitis, BoNT-A botulinum toxin A.

The dose of BoNT-A for IC has not been well determined. Pinto et al. used 100 U of BoNT-A to treat IC women by 10 trigonal injections and found subjective improvement in all patients at one- and three-month follow-up and the therapeutic efficacy remained for nine months in more than 50% of patients [104]. The therapeutic efficacy of 100 U of BoNT-A on IC patients was demonstrated in a large cohort. Significant improvement of interstitial cystitis symptom index (ICSI) and interstitial cystitis problem index (ICPI, 23.6 ± 5.9 versus 15.2 ± 8.5, $p = 0.000$), VAS (5.3 ± 2.2 versus 3.3 ± 2.4, $p = 0.000$), functional bladder capacity (136 ± 77.6 versus 180 ± 78.2, $p = 0.000$) and global response assessment (0.3 ± 0.8 versus 1.4 ± 1.0, $p = 0.000$) were shown at six months after 100 U of BoNT-A injection. BoNT-A injection has been proven to be a safe and effective procedure for relief of bladder pain and increase of bladder capacity in IC patients [105].

Kuo et al. conducted a randomized controlled trial (RCT) to compare the clinical effectiveness of 100 U or 200 U of BoNT-A intravesical injections followed by cystoscopic hydrodistention and hydrodistention alone in 67 IC patients. Among three groups, IC symptom score significantly decreased in all, but bladder pain VAS reduction and functional and cystometric bladder capacity increases were only noted in the BoNT-A groups at three months [102]. Recently, Pinto et al. compared the efficacy and safety of trigonal injections of onabotulinumtoxinA and saline in patients with IC. They found significant reduction of bladder pain in the BoNT-A group than the saline group at week 12. BoNT-A significantly improved IC symptom score and quality of life at all timepoints and the PVR did not increase at the endpoint, indicating that BoNT-A trigonal injection had safe and effective treatment outcomes without PVR increase [112].

In the histopathological investigations, Kuo et al. also investigated bladder tissue NGF mRNA at baseline and after BoNT-A treatment and found the NGF levels significantly increased in IC patients at baseline and decreased to normal in responders after BoNT-A treatment [61]. Shie et al. found that mast cell activity and apoptotic cell count did not decrease significantly; Bax and p-p38 but not tryptase content decreased significantly after a single BoNT-A injection [106]. After three repeated BoNT-A injections every six months, significant decrease of tryptase, Bax, p-p38 contents and apoptotic cell counts were noted, and SNAP-25 content in the bladder also decreased after BoNT-A injections. The immunohistochemistric improvements are also associated with clinical symptomatic improvements. This evidence further confirms that chronic inflammation and apoptotic signaling molecules in the IC bladder wall can be reduced significantly after repeated BoNT-A injections in IC bladders [42]. Repeat BoNT-A injections are needed to achieve a better and more durable success in the treatment of IC [107]. Repeated BoNT-A injections plus hydrodistention provides bladder pain relief and bladder capacity increase in responders. Through reduction of bladder suburothelial inflammation, the defective urothelial repair and improvement of cell differentiation ensue, leading to a healthy urothelium and thereby improving the clinical symptoms of IC [36].

7. Adverse Events after BoNT-A Injection for Sensory Bladder Disorders

Intravesical injection of BoNT-A has been demonstrated to be effective in treatment of NDO, IDO, OAB and IC, however, the high rates of treatment-related adverse events (AEs) still need attention. The most common AEs are large PVR, difficulty in urination, UTI and acute urinary retention [80]. For the male gender with IDO, a baseline PVR more than 100 mL with medical comorbidity and BoNT-A dose greater than 100 U are risk factors for AEs to increase after treatment [80]. The odds of increased PVR after BoNT-A injection were a nine-fold increase in comparison with placebo [92]. At the first treatment, the incidence of needing clean intermittent catheterization (CIC) was 35% and bacteriuria was 21% [113]. Poor efficiency, UTI and CIC-related issues are the most common causes of discontinuation of BoNT-A injections for DO over a seven-year span [114]. Large PVR after BoNT-A injection was significantly more in the frail elderly than elderly without frailty and younger patients; in frail elderly patients (60.7% v 39.7% v 35.7%, $p = 0.018$), the long-term success rate was significantly lower [82]. The incidence of AEs is closely related with the injected BoNT-A dose [77].

Regarding the AEs after BoNT-A injection for treatment of bladder and frequency in patients with IC, difficulty in urination and large PVR are the most common AEs [115]. The incidence of AEs in IC or OAB patients after BoNT-A injection is also related to the dose of BoNT-A. Injecting 100 U of onabotulinumtoxinA has less AEs than 200 U, while injecting 100 U of BoNT-A into the trigone showed no acute urinary retention and minimal AEs in both IC and OAB patients [102,104,112]. Interestingly, compared with IC, OAB patients suffered more frequently from AEs of hematuria, UTI, and large PVR (>200 mL) after BoNT-A injection, but less frequently from events of straining to void. OAB women had higher PVR volume and lower voiding efficiency than those in IC after BoNT-A injections, implying the bladder contractility of OAB patients are more susceptible to BoNT-A than IC patients [115]. However, in a randomized, double blind, placebo-controlled trial examining the effects of BoNT-A in patients with bladder oversensitivity, the significant increase in maximal cystometric capacity did not translate to clinical benefit in the majority of patients. Patients with bladder oversensitivity without DO had storage symptoms remain unchanged following BoNT-A injection and CIC was needed in three patients without clinical improvement [116].

8. Perspectives of Botulinum Toxin A on Sensory Bladder Disorders

Intravesical BoNT-A injection for OAB and IC have been demonstrated to be effective and well tolerated. However, large PVR and difficulty with urination remain problems to be solved [80]. Patients with OAB can benefit from BoNT-A for urgency and urgency incontinence relief, and patients with IC can have bladder pain relief after BoNT-A injection. However, for patients with bladder oversensitivity who do not have urgency or bladder pain, the adverse events that occurr after BoNT-A might not be acceptable [116].

Liposome instillation into the inflammatory bladder models have been shown effective to treat bladder hyperactivity in rat models [117]. As BoNT-A has a large molecular weight of 150 kDa, this neurotoxin cannot be delivered across the bladder urothelial cell membrane without an injection. Liposome encapsulated BoNT-A has also been demonstrated effective in improving the acetic acid-induced bladder hyperactivity in rat models [118]. The rats that received liposome encapsulated BoNT-A (Lipotoxin) showed significant decrease of response to acetic acid pretreatment without compromising the voiding function. Lipotoxin treatment also showed cleavage of SNAP-25, inhibition of CGRP from afferent nerves and blockage of hyperactivity induced by acetic acid. This evidence supports the idea that liposome can effectively carry BoNT-A across the urothelial barrier and has effects on bladder inflammation.

In a proof-of-concept clinical trial, Kuo et al. found that the BoNT-A binding protein SV2 could be demonstrated in the apical cells, urothelial cells and suburothelial tissues of the normal and OAB patients by immunohistochemistric or western blotting studies [119]. The changes of three-day urinary frequency (−6.50, IQR −18.3 to −0.25) and urgency (−12.0, IQR −20.3 to −2.75) significantly improved in the Lipotoxin group but not in the control group at one month post intravesical instillation of Lipotoxin containing 80 mg of liposome and 200 U of BoNT-A or normal saline [119]. A multicentric double-blind randomized trial using the same regimens also demonstrated that a single intravesical instillation of Lipotoxin could significantly decrease OAB symptoms and three-day frequency episodes (−4.64 for Lipotoxin and −0.19 for placebo, $p = 0.0252$) without adverse events of dysuria, large PVR or urinary tract infection [120].

Another recent study using Lipotoxin (containing 80 mg of liposome and 200 U of BoNT-A) for treatment of IC refractory to conventional medication revealed that a single Lipotoxin instillation was associated with a significant decrease in O'Leary-Sant symptom score (mean 7.38 ± 8.75), ICSI (4.00 ± 4.28), ICPI (3.35 ± 5.11) and VAS (1.64 ± 2.52); and an increase in the GRA score (1.35 ± 1.28). However, patients allocated to receive normal saline or BoNT-A in saline also had similar results [121]. Although the results of this study were negative, the effect of Lipotoxin on urinary frequency is similar to the results from Lipotoxin on OAB patients [120]. As patients with OAB or IC have symptom improvement, no difficulty with urination or large PVR after Lipotoxin intravesical instillation, this suggests that the penetration depth of BoNT-A carried by liposome is not as deep as that of a detrusor injection. The effect of BoNT-A in liposome might be limited to the urothelium. It seems rational to treat patients with bladder oversensitivity by liposome encapsulated BoNT-A rather than detrusor injection. However, the therapeutic duration of Lipotoxin instillation is short and the study was carried out in a small number of patients, indicating that the amount of BoNT-A protein diffused into the bladder urothelium was small. A large, randomized control trial is needed to clarify the effect of Lipotoxin on bladder oversensitivity.

Recently, low energy shock wave (LESW) has been enthusiastically applied in treatment of lower urinary tract disorders in animal models for bladder inflammation and overactivity [122,123]. LESWs suppressed cyclophosphamide-induced bladder pain, inflammation, and overactivity involved with the activation of IL6, NGF, and COX2 expression, indicating that it is a potential candidate for relieving bladder inflammatory conditions and overactivity [123]. LESWs also increased urothelial permeability, facilitated intravesical BoNT-A delivery and blocked acetic acid-induced hyperactive bladder [124]. In a preliminary clinical study including 15 patients with refractory OAB, Nageib et al. used intravesical instillation of 100 U of BoNT-A followed by LESWs (3000 shocks over 10 min) of exposure to the supra-pubic area. They found significant improvements in all OABSS domains and a total score at one and two months after treatment without an increase of PVR. [125] In the future, BoNT-A might be delivered via LESW to treat bladder oversensitivity without a need of intravesical injection.

9. Conclusions

The underlying pathophysiology of bladder oversensitivity in lower urinary tract disorders has not been well elucidated. However, chronic inflammation resulting in activation of the suburothelial sensory fibers, over-expression of the sensory receptors, and increased production of inflammatory proteins are likely to develop in patients with OAB, IC or bladder oversensitivity. Intravesical BoNT-A injection at the dose of 100 U can effectively reduce bladder inflammation, decrease the hyperactivity of sensory afferent nerves, restore normal urothelial barrier function, and desensitize the inflammatory printings in the central nervous system. The bladder oversensitive symptoms of OAB and IC can be improved after BoNT-A injections. However, large PVR and dysuria might develop after intravesical BoNT-A injection, especially in the elderly patients with low detrusor contractility. Liposome or LESWs can deliver BoNT-A across the urothelial barrier and have therapeutic effects on decreasing frequency and urgency episodes without compromising voiding function; these treatment modalities might have potential in treating patients with sensory bladder disorders.

Author Contributions: Y.-H.J.: literature search and part of manuscript writing, W.-R.Y.: literature search and part of manuscript writing, H.-C.K.: critical comment and manuscript rearrangement. All authors have read and agreed to the published version of the manuscript.

References

1. Chen, L.C.; Kuo, H.C. Pathophysiology of refractory overactive bladder. *Low. Urin. Tract. Symptoms* **2019**, *11*, 177–181. [CrossRef]
2. Roehrborn, C.G.; Abrams, P.; Rovner, E.S.; Kaplan, S.A.; Herschorn, S.; Guan, Z. Efficacy and tolerability of tolterodine extended-release in men with overactive bladder and urgency urinary incontinence. *BJU Int.* **2006**, *97*, 1003–1006. [CrossRef]
3. Kuo, H.C.; Lee, K.S.; Na, Y.; Sood, R.; Nakaji, S.; Kubota, Y.; Kuroishi, K. Results of a randomized, double-blind, parallel-group, placebo- and active-controlled, multicenter study of mirabegron, a β3-adrenoceptor agonist, in patients with overactive bladder in Asia. *Neurourol. Urodyn.* **2015**, *34*, 685–692. [CrossRef]
4. Engstrom, G.; Henningsohn, L.; Steineck, G.; Leppert, J. Self-assessed health, sadness and happiness in relation to the total burden of symptoms from the lower urinary tract. *BJU Int.* **2005**, *95*, 810–815. [CrossRef]
5. Hu, T.W.; Wagner, T.H.; Bentkover, J.D.; LeBlanc, K.; Piancentini, A.; Stewart, W.F.; Corey, R.; Zhou, S.Z.; Hunt, T.L. Estimated economic costs of overactive bladder in the United States. *Urology* **2003**, *61*, 1123–1128. [CrossRef]
6. Rosen, R.; Altwein, J.; Boyle, P.; Kirby, R.S.; Lukacs, B.; Meuleman, E.; O'Leary, M.P.; Puppo, P.; Chris, R.; Giuliano, F. Lower urinary tract symptoms and male sexual dysfunction: The Multinational Survey of the Ageing Male (MSAM-7). *Eur. Urol.* **2003**, *44*, 637–649. [CrossRef]
7. Kuo, H.C. Pathophysiology of lower urinary tract symptoms in aged men without bladder outlet obstruction. *Urol. Int.* **2000**, *64*, 86–92. [CrossRef]
8. Milson, I.; Abrams, P.; Cardozo, L.; Roberts, R.G.; Thuroff, J.; Wein, A.J. How widespread are the symptoms of an overactive bladder and how are they managed? A population based prevalence study. *BJU Int.* **2001**, *87*, 760–766. [CrossRef]
9. Chuang, Y.C.; Liu, S.P.; Lee, K.S.; Liao, L.; Wang, J.; Yoo, T.K.; Chu, R.; Sumarsono, B. Prevalence of overactive bladder in China, Taiwan and South Korea: Results from a cross-sectional, population-based study. *Low. Urin. Tract. Symptoms* **2019**, *11*, 48–55. [CrossRef]
10. Temml, C.; Heidler, S.; Ponholzer, A.; Madersbacher, S. Prevalence of the overactive bladder syndrome by applying the International Continence Society definition. *Eur. Urol.* **2005**, *48*, 622–627. [CrossRef]
11. Birder, L. Role of the urothelium in bladder function. *Scand. J. Urol. Nephrol. Suppl.* **2004**, *215*, 48–53. [CrossRef]
12. Ong, H.L.; Kuo, H.C. Urothelial dysfunction and sensory protein expressions in patients with urological or systemic diseases and hypersensitive bladder. *Urol. Sci.* **2017**, *28*, 128–134. [CrossRef]
13. Brady, C.M.; Apostolidis, A.N.; Harper, M.; Yiangou, Y.; Beckett, A.; Jacques, T.S.; Freeman, A.; Scaravilli, F.; Fowler, C.J.; Anand, P. Parallel changes in bladder suburothelial vanilloid receptor TRPV1 and pan-neuronal marker PGP9.5 immunoreactivity in patients with neurogenic detrusor overactivity after intravesical resiniferatoxin treatment. *BJU Int.* **2004**, *93*, 770–776. [CrossRef]
14. Brady, C.; Apostolidis, A.; Yiangou, Y.; Baecker, P.A.; Ford, A.P.; Freeman, A.; Jacques, T.S.; Fowler, C.J.; Anand, P. P2X3-immunoreactive nerve fibers in neurogenic detrusor overactivity and the effect of intravesical resiniferatoxin (RTX). *Eur. Urol.* **2004**, *46*, 247–253. [CrossRef]
15. Smet, P.J.; Moore, K.H.; Jonavicius, J. Distribution and colocalization of calcitonin gene-related peptide, tachykinins, and vasoactive intestinal peptide in normal and indiopathic unstable human urinary bladder. *Lab. Invest.* **1997**, *77*, 37–49.
16. Cruz, F.; Avelino, A.; Cruz, C.; Nagy, I. Sensory fibers immunoreactive to the vanilloid receptor protein: Distribution in the urinary bladder. *Neurourol. Urodyn.* **2000**, *19*, 456.
17. De Groat, W.D. A neurological basis for the overactive bladder. *Urology* **1997**, *50*, 36. [CrossRef]
18. Fowler, C.J.; Beck, R.O.; Gerrard, S.; Betts, C.D.; Fowler, C.G. Intravesical capsaicin for treatment of detrusor hyperreflexia. *J. Neurol. Neurosurg. Psychiatry* **1994**, *57*, 169–173. [CrossRef]
19. Kuo, H.C. Effectiveness of intravesical resiniferatoxin for anticholinergic treatment refractory detrusor overactivity due to nonspinal cord lesions. *J. Urol.* **2003**, *170*, 835–839. [CrossRef]

20. Cruz, F.; Guimaräes, M.; Silva, C.; Reis, M. Suppression of bladder hyperreflexia by intravesical resiniferatoxin. *Lancet* **1997**, *350*, 640–641. [CrossRef]
21. Khera, M.; Somogyi, G.T.; Kiss, S.; Boone, T.B.; Smith, C.P. Botulinum toxin A inhibits ATP release from bladder urothelium after chronic spinal cord injury. *Neurochem. Int.* **2004**, *45*, 987–993. [CrossRef]
22. Avelino, A.; Cruz, C.; Nagy, I.; Cruz, F. Vanilloid receptor 1 expression in the rat urinary tract. *Neuroscience* **2002**, *109*, 787–798. [CrossRef]
23. Yiangou, Y.; Facer, P.; Ford, A.; Brady, C.; Wisteman, O.; Fowler, C.C.; Anand, P. Capsaicin receptor VR1 and ATP-gated ion channel P2X3 in human urinary bladder. *BJU Int.* **2001**, *87*, 774–779. [CrossRef] [PubMed]
24. Birder, L.A.; Kanai, A.J.; de Groat, W.C.; Kiss, S.; Nealen, M.L.; Burke, N.E.; Dineley, K.E.; Watkins, S.; Reynolds, I.J.; Caterina, M.J. Vanilloid receptor expression suggests a sensory role for urinary bladder epithelial cells. *Proc. Natl. Acad. Sci. USA* **2001**, *98*, 13396–13401. [CrossRef]
25. Birder, L.; Andersson, K.E. Urothelial signaling. *Physiol. Rev.* **2013**, *93*, 653–680. [CrossRef]
26. Smet, P.J.; Edyvane, K.A.; Jonavicius, J.; Marshall, V.R. Distribution of NADPH- diaphorase-positive nerves supplying the human urinary bladder. *J. Autonom. Nerv. Syst.* **1994**, *47*, 109–113. [CrossRef]
27. Morrison, J.; Wen, J.; Kibble, A. Activation of pelvic afferent nerves from the rat bladder during filling. *Scand. J. Urol. Nephrol.* **1999**, *201*, 73–75. [CrossRef]
28. Gabella, G. The structural relations between nerve fibers and muscle cells in the urinary bladder of the rat. *J. Neurocytol.* **1995**, *24*, 159–187. [CrossRef]
29. Abbasian, B.; Shair, A.; O'Gorman, D.B.; Pena-Diaz, A.M.; Brennan, L.; Engelbrecht, K.; Koenig, D.W.; Reid, G.; Burton, J.P. Potential Role of Extracellular ATP Released by Bacteria in Bladder Infection and Contractility. *mSphere* **2019**, *4*. [CrossRef]
30. Vannucchi, M.G.; Traini, C.; Guasti, D.; Del Popolo, G.; Faussone-Pellegrini, M.S. Telocytes subtypes in human urinary bladder. *J. Cell. Mol. Med.* **2014**, *18*, 2000–2008. [CrossRef]
31. Wiseman, O.J.; Fowler, C.J.; Landon, D.N. The role of the human bladder lamina propria myofibroblasts. *BJU Int.* **2003**, *91*, 89–93. [CrossRef] [PubMed]
32. Sui, G.P.; Rothery, S.; Dupont, E.; Fry, C.H.; Severs, N.J. Gap junctions and connexin expression in human suburothelial interstitial cells. *BJU Int.* **2002**, *90*, 119–129. [CrossRef] [PubMed]
33. Yoshida, M.; Miyamae, K.; Iwashida, H.; Otani, M.; Inadome, A. Management of detrusor dysfunction in the elderly: Changes in acetylcholine and adenosine triphosphaterelease during ageing. *Urology* **2004**, *63*, 17–23. [CrossRef] [PubMed]
34. Avelino, A.; Cruz, F. TRPVI (vanilloid receptor) in the urinary tract: Expression, function and clinical applications. Naunyn. Schmiedebergs. *Arch. Pharmacol.* **2006**, *373*, 287–299. [CrossRef]
35. Shie, J.H.; Kuo, H.C. Higher level of cell apoptosis and abnormal E-cadherin expression in the urothelium are associated with inflammation in patients with interstitial cystitis/painful bladder syndrome. *BJU Int.* **2011**, *108*, E136e41. [CrossRef]
36. Shie, J.H.; Kuo, H.C. Pathologic mechanism of the therapeutic effect of botulinum toxin A on interstitial cystitis and painful bladder syndrome. *Tzu. Chi. Med. J.* **2012**, *24*, 170–177. [CrossRef]
37. Shie, J.H.; Liu, H.T.; Kuo, H.C. Increased cell apoptosis of the urothelium is mediated by inflammation in interstitial cystitis/painful bladder syndrome. *Urology* **2012**, *79*, 484.e7–484.e13. [CrossRef]
38. Apostolidis, A.; Jacques, T.S.; Freeman, A.; Kalsi, V.; Popat, R.; Gonzales, G.; Datta, S.N.; Ghazi-Noori, S.; Elneil, S.; Dasgupta, P.; et al. Histological changes in the urothelium and suburothelium of human overactive bladder following intradetrusor injections of botulinum neurotoxin type A for the treatment of neurogenic or idiopathic detrusor overactivity. *Eur. Urol.* **2008**, *53*, 1245–1253. [CrossRef]
39. Kuo, H.; Liu, H.T.; Tyagi, P.; Chancellor, M.B. Urinary nerve growth factor levels in urinary tract diseases with or without frequency urgency symptoms. *Low. Urin. Tract. Symptoms* **2010**, *2*, 88–94. [CrossRef]
40. Liu, H.T.; Kuo, H.C. Urinary nerve growth factor levels are increased in patients with bladder outlet obstruction with overactive bladder symptoms and reduced after successful medical treatment. *Urology* **2008**, *72*, 104–108. [CrossRef]
41. Lowe, E.M.; Anand, P.; Terenghi, G.; Williams-Chestnut, R.E.; Sinicropi, D.V.; Osborne, J.L. Increased nerve growth factor levels in the urinary bladder of women with idiopathic sensory urgency and interstitial cystitis. *Br. J. Urol.* **1997**, *79*, 572–577. [CrossRef] [PubMed]

42. Shie, J.H.; Kuo, H.C. Pathophysiology of urothelial dysfunction in patients with interstitial cystitis/ bladder pain syndrome: Increased apoptosis and decreased junctional protein expression in the urothelium due to suburothelial inflammation. *Tzu. Chi. Med. J.* **2009**, *21*, 103–109. [CrossRef]
43. Kuo, H.C. Novel treatment of interstitial cystitis/bladder pain syndrome based on pathophysiology. *Clin. Investig.* **2012**, *2*, 1085–1100. [CrossRef]
44. Yamaguchi, O.; Honda, K.; Nomiya, M.; Shishido, K.; Kakizaki, H.; Tanaka, H.; Yamanishi, T.; Homma, Y.; Takeda, M.; Araki, I.; et al. Defining overactive bladder as hypersensitivity. *Neurourol. Urodyn.* **2007**, *26*, 904–907. [CrossRef] [PubMed]
45. Simpson, L.L. Kinetic studies on the interaction between botulinum toxin type A and the cholinergic neuromuscular junction. *J. Pharmaco.l Exp. Ther.* **1980**, *212*, 16–21.
46. Coelho, A.; Dinis, P.; Pinto, R.; Gorgal, T.; Silva, C.; Silva, A.; Silva, J.; Cruz, C.D.; Cruz, F.; Avelino, A. Distribution of the high-affinity binding site and intracellular target of botulinum toxin type A in the human bladder. *Eur Urol.* **2010**, *57*, 884–890. [CrossRef] [PubMed]
47. Aoki, K.R.; Guyer, B. Botulinum toxin type A and other botulinum toxin serotypes: A comparative review of biochemical and pharmacological actions. *Eur. J. Neurol.* **2001**, *8* (Suppl. 5), 21–29. [CrossRef]
48. Dong, M.; Yeh, F.; Tepp, W.H.; Dean, C.; Johnson, E.A.; Janz, R.; Chapman, E.R. SV2 is the protein receptor for botulinum neurotoxin A. *Science* **2006**, *312*, 592–596. [CrossRef]
49. Coelho, A.; Cruz, F.; Cruz, C.D.; Avelino, A. Spread of onabotulinumtoxinA after bladder injection. Experimental study using the distribution of cleaved SNAP-25 as the marker of the toxin action. *Eur. Urol.* **2012**, *61*, 1178–1184. [CrossRef]
50. Hanna-Mitchell, A.T.; Wolf-Johnston, A.S.; Barrick, S.R.; Kanai, A.J.; Chancellor, M.B.; de Groat, W.C.; Birder, L.A. Effect of botulinum toxin A on urothelial-release of ATP and expression of SNARE targets within the urothelium. *Neurourol. Urodyn.* **2015**, *34*, 79–84. [CrossRef]
51. Apostolidis, A.; Popat, R.; Yiangou, Y.; Cockayne, D.; Ford, A.P.; Davis, J.B.; Dasgupta, P.; Fowler, C.J.; Anand, P. Decreased sensory receptors P2X3 and TRPV1 in suburothelial nerve fibers following intradetrusor injections of Botulinum toxin for human detrusor overactivity. *J. Urol.* **2005**, *174*, 977–982. [CrossRef]
52. Kessler, T.M.; Danuser, H.; Schumacher, M.; Studer, U.E.; Burkhard, F.C. Botulinum A toxin injections into the detrusor: An effective treatment in idiopathic and neurogenic detrusor overactivity? *Neurourol. Urodyn.* **2005**, *24*, 231–236. [CrossRef] [PubMed]
53. Kuo, H.C. Clinical effects of suburothelial injection of botulinum A toxin in patients with non-neurogenic detrusor overactivity refractory to anticholinergics. *Urology* **2005**, *66*, 94–98. [CrossRef] [PubMed]
54. Kuo, H.C. Urodynamic evidence of effectiveness of botulinum A toxin injection in treatment of detrusor overactivity refractory to anticholinergic agents. *Urology* **2004**, *63*, 868–872. [CrossRef] [PubMed]
55. Sahai, A.; Khan, M.S.; Dasgupta, P. Efficacy of botulinum toxin-A for treating idiopathic detrusor overactivity: Results from a single center, randomized, double-blind, placebo controlled trial. *J. Urol.* **2007**, *177*, 2231–2236. [CrossRef]
56. Brubaker, L.; Richter, H.E.; Visco, A.; Mahajan, S.; Nygaard, I.; Braun, T.M.; Barber, M.D.; Menefee, S.; Schaffer, J.; Weber, A.M.; et al. Refractory idiopathic urge urinary incontinence and botulinum A injection. *J. Urol.* **2008**, *180*, 217–222. [CrossRef]
57. Popat, R.; Apostolidis, A.; Kalsi, V.; Gonzales, G.; Fowler, C.J.; Dasgupta, P. A comparison between the response of patients with idiopathic detrusor overactivity and neurogenic detrusor overactivity to the first intradetrusor injection of botulinum-A toxin. *J. Urol.* **2005**, *174*, 984989. [CrossRef]
58. Rajkumar, G.N.; Small, D.R.; Mustafa, A.W.; Conn, G. A prospective study to evaluate the safety, tolerability, efficacy and durability of response of intravesical injection of botulinum toxin type A into detrusor muscle in patients with refractory idiopathic detrusor overactivity. *BJU Int.* **2005**, *96*, 848–852. [CrossRef]
59. Werner, M.; Schmid, D.M.; Schussler, B. Efficacy of botulinum-A toxin in the treatment of detrusor overactivity incontinence: A prospective nonrandomized study. *Am. J. Obstet. Gynecol.* **2005**, *192*, 1735–1740. [CrossRef]
60. Kuo, H.C. Reduction of urgency severity is associated with long-term therapeutic effect after intravesical onabotulinumtoxinA injection for idiopathic detrusor overactivity. *Neurourol. Urodyn.* **2011**, *30*, 1497–1502. [CrossRef]
61. Liu, H.T.; Kuo, H.C. Intravesical botulinum toxin A injections plus hydrodistension can reduce nerve growth factor production and control bladder pain in interstitial cystitis. *Urology* **2007**, *70*, 463–468. [CrossRef] [PubMed]

62. Liu, H.T.; Chancellor, M.B.; Kuo, H.C. Urinary nerve growth factor levels are elevated in patients with detrusor overactivity and decreased in responders to detrusor botulinum toxin-A injection. *Eur. Urol.* **2009**, *56*, 700–706. [CrossRef] [PubMed]
63. Liu, H.T.; Kuo, H.C. Urinary nerve growth factor level could be a potential biomarker for diagnosis of overactive bladder. *J. Urol.* **2008**, *179*, 2270–2274. [CrossRef] [PubMed]
64. Liu, H.T.; Tyap, P.; Chancellor, M.B.; Kuo, H.C. Urinary nerve growth factor level is increased in patients with interstitial cystitis/painful bladder syndrome and decreased in responders to treatment. *BJU Int.* **2009**, *104*, 1476–1481. [CrossRef]
65. Chuang, Y.C.; Yoshimura, N.; Huang, C.C.; Wu, M.; Chiang, P.H.; Chancellor, M.B. Intravesical botulinum toxin A administration inhibits COX-2 and EP4 expression and suppresses bladder hyperactivity in cyclophosphamide-induced cystitis in rats. *Eur. Urol.* **2009**, *56*, 159–166. [CrossRef] [PubMed]
66. Wagg, A.; Cardozo, L.; Chapple, C.; De Ridder, D.; Kelleher, C.; Kirby, M.; Milsom, I.; Vierhout, M. Overactive bladder syndrome in older people. *BJU Int.* **2007**, *99*, 502–509. [CrossRef]
67. Chapple, C.R.; Cruz, F.; Cardozo, L.; Staskin, D.; Herschorn, S.; Choudhury, N.; Stoelzel, M.; Heesakkers, J.; Siddiqui, E. Safety and Efficacy of Mirabegron: Analysis of a Large Integrated Clinical Trial Database of Patients with Overactive Bladder Receiving Mirabegron, Antimuscarinics, or Placebo. *Eur. Urol.* **2020**, *77*, 119–128. [CrossRef]
68. Wennberg, A.L.; Molander, U.; Fall, M.; Edlund, C.; Peeker, R.; Milsom, I. A longitudinal population-based survey of urinary incontinence, overactive bladder, and other lower urinary tract symptoms in women. *Eur. Urol.* **2009**, *55*, 783–791. [CrossRef]
69. Geppetti, P.; Nassini, R.; Materazzi, S.; Benemei, S. The concept of neurogenic inflammation. *BJU Int.* **2008**, *101*, 2–6. [CrossRef]
70. Seki, S.; Sasaki, K.; Fraser, M.O.; Igawa, Y.; Nishizawa, O.; Chancellor, M.B.; de Groat, W.C.; Yoshimura, N. Immunoneutralization of nerve growth factor in lumbosacral spinal cord reduces bladder hyperreflexia in spinal cord injured rats. *J. Urol.* **2002**, *168*, 2269–2274. [CrossRef]
71. Chuang, Y.C.; Fraser, M.O.; Yu, Y.; Chancellor, M.B.; de Groat, W.C.; Yoshimura, N. The role of bladder afferent pathways in bladder hyperactivity induced by the intravesical administration of nerve growth factor. *J. Urol.* **2001**, *165*, 975–979. [CrossRef]
72. Kuo, H.C. Overactive bladder is a dynamic syndrome. *Eur. Urol.* **2009**, *55*, 792–793. [CrossRef] [PubMed]
73. Anger, J.T.; Weinberg, A.; Suttorp, M.J.; Litwin, M.S.; Shekelle, P.G. Outcomes of intravesical botulinum toxin for idiopathic overactive bladder syndromes: A systemic review of the literature. *J. Urol.* **2010**, *183*, 2258–2264. [CrossRef] [PubMed]
74. Nitti, V.W.; Dmochowski, R.; Herschorn, S.; Sand, P.; Thompson, C.; Nardo, C.; Yan, X.; Haag-Molkenteller, C.; EMBARK Study Group. OnabotulinumtoxinA for the treatment of patients with overactive bladder and urinary incontinence: Results of a phase 3, randomized, placebo-controlled trial. *J. Urol.* **2013**, *189*, 2186–2193.
75. Chapple, C.; Sievert, K.D.; MacDiarmid, S.; Khullar, V.; Radziszewski, P.; Nardo, C.; Thompson, C.; Zhou, J.; Haag-Molkenteller, C. OnabotulinumtoxinA 100U significantly improves all idiopathic overactive bladder symptoms and quality of life in patients with overactive bladder and urinary incontinence: A randomised, double-blind, placebo-controlled trial. *Eur. Urol.* **2013**, *64*, 249–256. [CrossRef] [PubMed]
76. Rovner, E.; Kennelly, M.; Schulte-Baukloh, H.; Zhou, J.; Haag-Molkenteller, C.; Dasgupta, P. Urodynamic results and clinical outcomes with intradetrusor injections of onabotulinumtoxinA in a randomized, placebo-controlled dose-finding study in idiopathic overactive bladder. *Neurourol. Urodyn.* **2011**, *30*, 556–562. [CrossRef] [PubMed]
77. Dmochowski, R.; Chapple, C.; Nitti, V.W.; Chancellor, M.; Everaert, K.; Thompson, C.; Daniell, G.; Zhou, J.; Haag-Molkenteller, C. Efficacy and safety of onabotulinumtoxinA for idiopathic overactive bladder: A double-blind, placebo-controlled, randomized, dose ranging trial. *J. Urol.* **2010**, *184*, 2416–2422. [CrossRef]
78. Lightner, D.J.; Gomelsky, A.; Souter, L.; Vasavada, S.P. Diagnosis and Treatment of Overactive Bladder (Non-Neurogenic) in Adults: AUA/SUFU Guideline Amendment 2019. *J. Urol.* **2019**, *202*, 558–563. [CrossRef]
79. Lucas, M.G.; Bosch, R.J.; Burkhard, F.C.; Cruz, F.; Madden, T.B.; Nambiar, A.K.; Neisius, A.; de Ridder, D.J.; Tubaro, A.; Turner, W.H.; et al. European Association of Urology. EAU guidelines on assessment and nonsurgical management of urinary incontinence. *Eur. Urol.* **2012**, *62*, 1130–1142. [CrossRef]
80. Kuo, H.C.; Liao, C.H.; Chung, S.D. Adverse events of intravesical botulinum toxin A injections for idiopathic detrusor overactivity: Risk factors and influence on treatment outcome. *Eur. Urol.* **2010**, *58*, 919–926. [CrossRef]

81. Kuo, H.C. Bladder base/trigone injection is safe and as effective as bladder body injection of onabotulinumtoxinA for idiopathic detrusor overactivity refractory to antimuscarinics. *Neurourol. Urodyn.* **2011**, *30*, 1242–1248.
82. Schulte-Baukloh, H.; Weiss, C.; Stolze, T.; Herholz, J.; Stürzebecher, B.; Miller, K.; Knispel, H.H. Botulinum-A toxin detrusor and sphincter injection in treatment of overactive bladder syndrome: Objective outcome and patient satisfaction. *Eur. Urol.* **2005**, *48*, 984–990. [CrossRef] [PubMed]
83. Smith, C.P.; Nishiguchi, J.; O'Leary, M.; Yoshimura, N.; Chancellor, M.B. Single-institution experience in 110 patients with botulinum toxin A injection into bladder or urethra. *Urology* **2005**, *65*, 37–41. [CrossRef] [PubMed]
84. Schmid, D.M.; Sauermann, P.; Werner, M.; Schuessler, B.; Blick, N.; Muentener, M.; Strebel, R.T.; Perucchini, D.; Scheiner, D.; Schaer, G.; et al. Experience with 100 cases treated with botulinum-A toxin injections in the detrusor muscle for idiopathic overactive bladder syndrome refractory to anticholinergics. *J. Urol.* **2006**, *176*, 177–185. [CrossRef]
85. Kuo, H.C. Will suburothelial injection of small dose of botulinum A toxin have similar therapeutic effects and less adverse events for refractory detrusor overactivity? *Urology* **2006**, *68*, 993–997. [CrossRef]
86. Karsenty, G.; Elzayat, E.; Delapparent, T.; St-Denis, B.; Lemieux, M.C.; Corcos, J. Botulinum toxin type a injections into the trigone to treat idiopathic overactive bladder do not induce vesicoureteral reflux. *J. Urol.* **2007**, *177*, 1011–1114. [CrossRef]
87. Kuo, H.C. Comparison of effectiveness of detrusor, suburothelial and bladder base injections of botulinum toxin a for idiopathic detrusor overactivity. *J. Urol.* **2007**, *178*, 1359–1363. [CrossRef]
88. Tincello, D.G.; Kenyon, S.; Abrams, K.R.; Mayne, C.; Toozs-Hobson, P.; Taylor, D.; Slack, M. Botulinum toxin a versus placebo for refractory detrusor overactivity in women: A randomised blinded placebo-controlled trial of 240 women (the RELAX study). *Eur. Urol.* **2012**, *62*, 507–514. [CrossRef]
89. Fowler, C.J.; Auerbach, S.; Ginsberg, D.; Hale, D.; Radziszewski, P.; Rechberger, T.; Patel, V.D.; Zhou, J.; Thompson, C.; Kowalski, J.W. OnabotulinumtoxinA improves health-related quality of life in patients with urinary incontinence due to idiopathic overactive bladder: A 36-week, double-blind, placebo-controlled, randomized, dose-ranging trial. *Eur. Urol.* **2012**, *62*, 148–157. [CrossRef]
90. Denys, P.; Le Normand, L.; Ghout, I.; Costa, P.; Chartier-Kastler, E.; Grise, P.; Hermieu, J.F.; Amarenco, G.; Karsenty, G.; Saussine, C.; et al. Efficacy and safety of low doses of onabotulinumtoxinA for the treatment of refractory idiopathic overactive bladder: A multicentre, double-blind, randomised, placebo-controlled dose-ranging study. *Eur. Urol.* **2012**, *61*, 520–529.
91. Liao, C.H.; Kuo, H.C. Increased risk of large post-void residual urine and decreased long-term success rate after intravesical onabotulinumtoxinA injection for refractory idiopathic detrusor overactivity. *J. Urol.* **2013**, *189*, 1804–1810. [CrossRef]
92. Mangera, A.; Apostolidis, A.; Andersson, K.E.; Dasgupta, P.; Giannantoni, A.; Roehrborn, C.; Novara, G.; Chapple, C. An updated systematic review and statistical comparison of standardised mean outcomes for the use of botulinum toxin in the management of lower urinary tract disorders. *Eur. Urol.* **2014**, *65*, 981–990. [CrossRef] [PubMed]
93. Wang, C.C.; Lee, C.L.; Kuo, H.C. Efficacy and Safety of Intravesical OnabotulinumtoxinA Injection in Patients with Detrusor Hyperactivity and Impaired Contractility. *Toxins* **2016**, *8*, E82. [CrossRef]
94. Onem, K.; Bayrak, O.; Demirtas, A.; Coskun, B.; Dincer, M.; Kocak, I.; Onur, R.; Turkish Urology Academy, Incontinence/Neurourology Study Group. Efficacy and safety of onabotulinumtoxinA injection in patients with refractory overactive bladder: First multicentric study in Turkish population. *Neurourol. Urodyn.* **2018**, *37*, 263–268. [CrossRef]
95. Chuang, Y.C.; Yoshimura, N.; Huang, C.C.; Chiang, P.H.; Chancellor, M.B. Intravesical botulinum toxin A administration produces analgesia against acetic acid induced bladder pain response in rats. *J. Urol.* **2004**, *172*, 1529–1532. [CrossRef] [PubMed]
96. Kuo, H.C. Preliminary results of suburothelial injection of botulinum a toxin in the treatment of chronic interstitial cystitis. *Urol. Int.* **2005**, *75*, 170–174. [CrossRef] [PubMed]
97. Cui, M.; Aoki, K.R. Botulinum toxin type A (BTX-A) reduces inflammatory pain in the rat formalin model. *Cephalalgia* **2000**, *20*, 414–418.
98. Smith, C.P.; Radziszewski, P.; Borkowski, A.; Somogyi, G.T.; Boone, T.B.; Chancellor, M.B. Botulinum toxin a has antinociceptive effects in treating interstitial cystitis. *Urology* **2004**, *64*, 871–875. [CrossRef] [PubMed]

99. Giannantoni, A.; Costantini, E.; Di Stasi, S.M.; Tascini, M.C.; Bini, V.; Porena, M. Botulinum A toxin intravesical injections in the treatment of painful bladder syndrome: A pilot study. *Eur. Urol.* **2006**, *49*, 704–709. [CrossRef]
100. Giannantoni, A.; Porena, M.; Costantini, E.; Zucchi, A.; Mearini, L.; Mearini, E. Botulinum A toxin intravesical injection in patients with painful bladder syndrome: 1-year followup. *J. Urol.* **2008**, *179*, 1031–1034. [CrossRef]
101. Hanno, P.M.; Erickson, D.; Moldwin, R.; Faraday, M.M.; American Urological Association. Diagnosis and treatment of interstitial cystitis/bladder pain syndrome: AUA guideline amendment. *J. Urol.* **2015**, *193*, 1545–1553. [CrossRef]
102. Kuo, H.C.; Chancellor, M.B. Comparison of intravesical botulinum toxin type A injections plus hydrodistention with hydrodistention alone for the treatment of refractory interstitial cystitis/painful bladder syndrome. *BJU Int.* **2009**, *104*, 657–661. [CrossRef] [PubMed]
103. Giannantoni, A.; Mearini, E.; Del Zingaro, M.; Proietti, S.; Porena, M. Two-year efficacy and safety of botulinum a toxin intravesical injections in patients affected by refractory painful bladder syndrom+e. *Curr. Drug Deliv.* **2010**, *7*, 1–4. [CrossRef] [PubMed]
104. Pinto, R.; Lopes, T.; Frias, B.; Silva, A.; Silva, J.A.; Silva, C.M.; Cruz, C.; Cruz, F.; Dinis, P. Trigonal injection of botulinum toxin A in patients with refractory bladder pain syndrome/interstitial cystitis. *Eur. Urol.* **2010**, *58*, 360–365. [CrossRef] [PubMed]
105. Chung, S.D.; Kuo, Y.C.; Kuo, H.C. Intravesical OnabotulinumtoxinA Injections for Refractory Painful Bladder Syndrome. *Pain Physician* **2012**, *15*, 197–202.
106. Shie, J.H.; Liu, H.T.; Wang, Y.S.; Kuo, H.C. Immunohistochemical evidence suggests repeated intravesical application of botulinum toxin A injections may improve treatment efficacy of interstitial cystitis/bladder pain syndrome. *BJU Int.* **2013**, *111*, 638–646. [CrossRef]
107. Kuo, H.C. Repeated onabotulinumtoxin-a injections provide better results than single injection in treatment of painful bladder syndrome. *Pain Physician* **2013**, *16*, E15–E23.
108. Lee, C.L.; Kuo, H.C. Intravesical botulinum toxin a injections do not benefit patients with ulcer type interstitial cystitis. *Pain Physician* **2013**, *16*, 109–116.
109. Pinto, R.; Lopes, T.; Costa, D.; Barros, S.; Silva, J.; Silva, C.; Cruz, C.; Dinis, P.; Cruz, F. Ulcerative and nonulcerative forms of bladder pain syndrome/interstitial cystitis do not differ in symptom intensity or response to onabotulinum toxin A. *Urology* **2014**, *83*, 1030–1034. [CrossRef]
110. Wang, J.; Wang, Q.; Wu, Q.; Chen, Y.; Wu, P. Intravesical Botulinum Toxin A Injections for Bladder Pain Syndrome/Interstitial Cystitis: A Systematic Review and Meta-Analysis of Controlled Studies. *Med. Sci. Monit.* **2016**, *22*, 3257–3267. [CrossRef]
111. Kuo, H.C.; Jiang, Y.H.; Tsai, Y.C.; Kuo, Y.C. Intravesical botulinum toxin-A injections reduce bladder pain of interstitial cystitis/bladder pain syndrome refractory to conventional treatment - A prospective, multicenter, randomized, double-blind, placebo-controlled clinical trial. *Neurourol. Urodyn.* **2016**, *35*, 609–614. [CrossRef]
112. Pinto, R.A.; Costa, D.; Morgado, A.; Pereira, P.; Charrua, A.; Silva, J.; Cruz, F. Intratrigonal OnabotulinumtoxinA Improves Bladder Symptoms and Quality of Life in Patients with Bladder Pain Syndrome/Interstitial Cystitis: A Pilot, Single Center, Randomized, Double-Blind, Placebo Controlled Trial. *J. Urol.* **2018**, *199*, 998–1003. [CrossRef] [PubMed]
113. Dowson, C.; Watkins, J.; Khan, M.S.; Dasgupta, P.; Sahai, A. Repeated botulinum toxin type A injections for refractory overactive bladder: Medium-term outcomes, safety profile, and discontinuation rates. *Eur. Urol.* **2012**, *61*, 834–839. [CrossRef] [PubMed]
114. Mohee, A.; Khan, A.; Harris, N.; Eardley, I. Long-term outcome of the use of intravesical botulinum toxin for the treatment of overactive bladder (OAB). *BJU Int.* **2013**, *111*, 106–113. [CrossRef] [PubMed]
115. Kuo, Y.C.; Kuo, H.C. Adverse Events of Intravesical OnabotulinumtoxinA Injection between Patients with Overactive Bladder and Interstitial Cystitis–Different Mechanisms of Action of Botox on Bladder Dysfunction? *Toxins* **2016**, *8*, 75. [CrossRef]
116. Dowson, C.; Sahai, A.; Watkins, J.; Dasgupta, P.; Khan, M.S. The safety and efficacy of botulinum toxin-A in the management of bladder oversensitivity: A randomised double-blind placebo-controlled trial. *Int. J. Clin. Pract.* **2011**, *65*, 698–704. [CrossRef]
117. Fraser, M.O.; Chuang, Y.C.; Tyagi, P.; Yokoyama, T.; Yoshimura, N.; Huang, L.; De Groat, W.C.; Chancellor, M.B. Intravesical liposomes administration: A novel treatment for hyperactive bladder in the rat. *Urology* **2003**, *61*, 656–663. [CrossRef]

118. Chuang, Y.C.; Tyagi, P.; Huang, C.C.; Yoshimura, N.; Wu, M.; Kaufman, J.; Chancellor, M.B. Urodynamic and immunohistochemical evaluation of intravesical botulinum toxin A delivery using liposomes. *J. Urol.* **2009**, *182*, 786–792. [CrossRef]
119. Kuo, H.C.; Liu, H.T.; Chuang, Y.C.; Birder, L.A.; Chancellor, M.B. Pilot study of liposome-encapsulated onabotulinumtoxinA for patients with overactive bladder: A single-center study. *Eur. Urol.* **2014**, *65*, 1117–1124. [CrossRef]
120. Chuang, Y.C.; Kaufmann, J.H.; Chancellor, D.; Chancellor, M.B.; Kuo, H.C. Bladder instillation of Liposome encapsulated onabotulinumtoxinA improves overactive bladder symptoms: A prospective, multicenter, double-blind randomized trial. *J. Urol.* **2014**, *192*, 1743–1749. [CrossRef]
121. Chuang, Y.C.; Kuo, H.C. A prospective, multicenter, double-blind, randomized trial of bladder instillation of liposome formulation onabotulinumtoxinA for interstitial cystitis/bladder pain syndrome. *J. Urol.* **2017**, *198*, 376–382. [CrossRef]
122. Li, H.; Zhang, Z.; Peng, J.; Xin, Z.; Li, M.; Yang, B.; Fang, D.; Tang, Y.; Guo, Y. Treatment with low-energy shock wave alleviates pain in an animal model of uroplakin 3A-induced autoimmune interstitial cystitis/painful bladder syndrome. *Investig. Clin. Urol.* **2019**, *60*, 359–366. [CrossRef] [PubMed]
123. Wang, H.J.; Lee, W.C.; Tyagi, P.; Huang, C.C.; Chuang, Y.C. Effects of low energy shock wave therapy on inflammatory moleculars, bladder pain, and bladder function in a rat cystitis model. *Neurourol. Urodyn.* **2017**, *36*, 1440–1447. [CrossRef] [PubMed]
124. Chuang, Y.C.; Huang, T.L.; Tyagi, P.; Huang, C.C. Urodynamic and Immunohistochemical Evaluation of Intravesical Botulinum Toxin A Delivery Using Low Energy Shock Waves. *J. Urol.* **2016**, *196*, 599–608. [CrossRef] [PubMed]
125. Nageib, M.; El-Hefnaw, A.S.; Zahran, M.H.; El-Tabey, N.A.; Sheir, K.Z.; Shokeir, A.A. Delivery of intravesical botulinum toxin A using low-energy shockwaves in the treatment of overactive bladder: A preliminary clinical study. *Arab. J. Urol.* **2019**, *17*, 216–220. [CrossRef]

18

The Pharmacological Mechanism of Diabetes Mellitus-Associated Overactive Bladder and Its Treatment with Botulinum Toxin A

Chung-Cheng Wang [1,2], Yung-Hong Jiang [3] and Hann-Chorng Kuo [3,*]

1 Department of Urology, En Chu Kong Hospital, New Taipei City 23702, Taiwan; ericwcc@ms27.hinet.net
2 Department of Biomedical Engineering, Chung Yuan Christian University, Taoyuan City 32023, Taiwan
3 Department of Urology, Hualien Tzu Chi Hospital, Buddhist Tzu Chi Medical Foundation and Tzu Chi University, Hualien 97002, Taiwan; redeemer1019@yahoo.com.tw
* Correspondence: hck@tzuchi.com.tw

Abstract: Diabetes mellitus (DM) is an independent risk factor for overactive bladder (OAB). The pathophysiology of DM-associated OAB is multifactorial and time-dependent. Diabetic bladder dysfunction is highly associated with diabetic complications, mainly including diabetic neuropathy and atherosclerosis. Chronic systemic inflammation and bladder urothelial inflammation may contribute to the onset of OAB. Intravesical botulinum toxin A (BoNT-A) injection has proved to be a successful treatment for idiopathic and neurogenic OAB. BoNT-A can inhibit the efferent pathways of the bladder as well as the chronic inflammation and hypersensitivity via the afferent pathways. We conducted a review of the published literature in Pubmed using a combination of two keywords, namely "botulinum toxin A" (BoNT-A) and "overactive bladder", with or without the additional keywords "detrusor overactivity", "diabetes mellitus", "inflammation", and "urodynamic study". We also reviewed the experience of our research teams, who have published several studies of the association between DM and OAB. Since limited data support the effectiveness and safety of BoNT-A for treating patients with DM-associated OAB, a comprehensive evaluation of diabetic complications and urodynamic study is needed before treatment. In the future, it is imperative to explore the clinical characteristics and inflammatory biomarkers of diabetes as determining predictors of the treatment efficacy.

Keywords: diabetes mellitus; overactive bladder; inflammation; botulinum toxin

Key Contribution: Through inhibiting chronic inflammation and hypersensitivity of urinary bladder, intravesical BoNT-A injection appears to be effective and safe in patients with DM-associated OAB. A comprehensive evaluation of DM complications and urodynamic studies is needed before treatment.

---

1. Introduction

Overactive bladder (OAB) and diabetes mellitus (DM) are common health threats and both increase in incidence and prevalence with advancing age. Several epidemiological studies have shown that OAB is more common in patients with type 2 DM than in the general population, and women with DM treated with insulin have higher odds (OR 3.5, 95% CI 1.6–7.9) of urge incontinence than those treated with non-insulin medication [1,2]. A study investigating the prevalence and correlation of urinary incontinence and OAB conducted in Taiwan showed that women who were elderly and menopausal and had a history of DM or hypertension and higher body mass index were significantly predisposed to an OAB [3]. Higher glycosylated hemoglobin levels represented an independent predictor of OAB symptoms among DM patients [4]. Even in early-stage DM, type 2 DM in male patients age <45 years had more OAB symptoms and erectile dysfunction than the controls [5]. Regarding OAB management, a study of 36,560 OAB patients in the US found that patients with DM are more persistent and adherent to OAB medications and have higher odds of filling a second medication prescription than patients without DM [6]. These factors may imply that DM is an important risk factor of OAB, but conventional oral medication is usually not as effective for OAB patients with DM.

We conducted a review of the published literature in Pubmed, using a combination of two keywords, namely "botulinum toxin A" (BoNT-A) and "overactive bladder" with or without the additional keywords "detrusor overactivity", "diabetes mellitus", "inflammation", and "urodynamic study". We reviewed the pathophysiology of DM-associated OAB, the anti-inflammatory effects of BoNT-A, and the clinical evidence for intravesical BoNT-A injection in patients with DM-associated OAB. We aimed to clarify the role of BoNT-A treatment in these patients.

2. Urodynamic Finding in Patients with DM-Associated OAB

Traditionally, diabetic cystopathy is considered as a triad of decreased bladder sensation, increased bladder capacity, and impaired emptying function [7]. Recent clinical and experimental evidence suggests that storage problems such as OAB and detrusor overactivity are common manifestations in early DM. Table 1 summarizes the urodynamic findings of patients with diabetic bladder dysfunction [8–12]. These studies showed that patients (both sexes) with DM had progressive, diverse bladder dysfunction depending on the stage of DM. In addition, diabetic bladder dysfunction is highly associated with other diabetic complications. Majima et al. analyzed the impact of DM on bladder function and found that the presence of both diabetic retinopathy and nephropathy was correlated with the presence of detrusor underactivity [9]. Patients with only diabetic retinopathy had the highest percentage of detrusor hyperactivity and impaired contractility (DHIC). Interestingly, a sub-population of patients reported in our literature search has normal detrusor contractility patterns, but develop detrusor overactivity, which was seen only in cases with neither retinopathy nor diabetic nephropathy. Furthermore, Lee et al. studied urodynamic characteristics and sensory bladder function in type 2 DM women at a mean age of 66.9 years [11]. The electrophysiological evidence indicated an association between impaired A-delta as well as C-fiber bladder afferent pathways and poor emptying function in the women with detrusor underactivity. However, patients with detrusor overactivity had similar current perception threshold values as those in the normal detrusor function group. Ho et al. compared the urodynamic finding in women with DM with and without OAB [13]. Compared to DM without OAB, the women with DM and OAB were more likely to have increased bladder sensation, detrusor overactivity, impaired voiding dysfunction, and a higher percentage of bladder outlet obstruction (BOO). Because of the very different presentations of diabetic bladder dysfunction, we suggest patients with DM-associated OAB undergo a comprehensive evaluation for possible diabetic complications and urodynamic studies before treatment of refractory DM-associated OAB.

Table 1. Summary of urodynamic findings in patients with diabetes.

Author [reference]	Patients (*n*)	Mean Age (years)	DM Duration (years)	DO	DHIC	DU	Normal	SUI
Majima [9]	57M	65.8	10	5 (9%)	18 (32%)	22 (39%)	12 (23%)	NA
Karoli [8]	44F	54.8	11.6	10 (23%)	NA	5 (11%)	9 (16%)	22 (48%)
Bansal [10]	52M	61.3	11	20 (39%)	NA	41 (79%)	NA	NA
Gali [12]	21M + 19F	64.5	10.9	7 (18%)	24 (60%)	4 (10%)	5 (13%)	NA
Lee [11]	86F	66.9	11.4	12 (14%)	NA	30 (35%)	33 (38%)	NA

DO: detrusor overactivity; DHIC: detrusor hyperactivity and impaired contractility; DU: detrusor underactivity; SUI: stress urinary incontinence; NA: not available.

3. Pathophysiology of DM-Associated OAB

The pathophysiology of DM-associated bladder dysfunction is multifactorial and time-dependent. From experimental and human studies, these changes can be a result of an alteration in the physiology of the detrusor smooth muscle cells, bladder innervation, extracellular matrix, or urothelial dysfunction [14]. In studies of streptozocin (STZ)-induced acute diabetic rats, the up-regulation of M2 and M3 muscarinic biosynthesis in the urinary bladder could lead to increased reactivity to acetylcholine, which results in detrusor overactivity [15,16]. In rats with type 2 DM on a high-fat diet, compared with controls, the diabetic bladders were hypertrophied and had increased volume per void and detrusor muscle contractility to the exogenous addition of carbachol in the compensated stage [17]. Progression from the compensated to decompensated state mainly involves decreased contractility to muscarinic stimulation. In addition, the alternation of the biomechanical behavior of the bladder wall induced by diuresis or diabetes is another important indicator of diabetic bladder dysfunction. In STZ-induced acute diabetic rats, the bladder wall could undergo rapid time-dependent structural and compositional remodeling, mainly including decreased collagen, increased elastin, and a nonlinear stress–strain relationship, and mechanical anisotropy, with greater tissue compliance in the circumferential direction than in the longitudinal direction [18,19].

In a prospective study of 120 type 2 DM patients using simple questionnaires, OAB severity and diabetic peripheral neuropathy were significantly correlated [20]. This finding was similar to that in another study in which the OAB group of women with type 2 DM had a significantly greater mean 5 Hz current perception threshold test value at the big toe compared to diabetic women without OAB [21]. This finding indicated that the hyposensitivity of unmyelinated C fiber afferents at the distal extremities heralded the early stages of diabetic bladder dysfunction. These studies suggest that multiple factors contribute to the occurrence and progression of diabetic bladder dysfunction.

The alternations of the urothelial and underlying lamina propria have been reported that are associated with OAB and diabetic cystopathy. In STZ diabetic rats 9 weeks after onset, scanning electron microscopy showed defective urothelial cells present in the bladders compared with controls, indicating a significant breach of the urothelial barrier [22]. In these diabetic rats, about 20% of the epithelium showed cellular disruption and death within the mucosal lining and umbrella cell loss. In addition, DM had significantly upregulated urothelial gene expression and receptors mainly for glucose metabolism (aldose reductase and sorbitol dehydrogenase), cell survival, cell-signaling receptors (acetylcholine receptors AChR-M2 and AChR-M3, purinergic receptors P2X2 and P2X3), and cell death. The compromised barrier function and alterations in urothelial mechanosensitivity and cell signaling contributed to bladder overactivity.

The findings of the animal studies have been further corroborated by a human study. Bladder mucosa was biopsied from 19 DM-associated OAB patients, 14 OAB patients without DM, and 10 healthy controls [23]. Decreased expression of urothelial junction protein (E-cadherin and ZO-1) and increased urothelial inflammation (mast cells) were noted in the non-diabetic OAB and diabetic OAB patients. The P2X3 protein expression in DM-associated OAB patients was significantly greater than that in OAB patients without DM and controls. However, E-cadherin, mast cells, ZO-1, apoptotic cells, and M2 and M3 muscarinic proteins were comparable between the OAB patients with and without DM. These findings suggest that urothelial dysfunction and chronic urothelial inflammation contribute to the pathogeneses of OAB. However, DM does not aggravate the severity of urothelial inflammation in OAB patients.

4. Diabetes and Bladder Inflammation

Chronic inflammation plays a potential role in the pathogenesis of type 2 DM [24]. The possible mechanisms to explain insulin resistance in type 2 DM include oxidative stress, endoplasmic reticulum stress, lipotoxicity, and glucotoxicity. These cellular stresses may induce an inflammatory response or they are exacerbated by inflammation. The vicious cycle of chronic inflammation and related stresses is associated with several diabetic complications, including atherosclerosis, neuropathy, retinopathy, nephropathy, and cystopathy.

Accumulating evidence suggests the roles of several inflammation biomarkers in obesity-induced insulin resistance. Acute-phase proteins such as C-reactive protein (CRP) and pro-inflammatory cytokines (interleukin (IL)-1β and IL-6, and tumor necrosis factor-α), and chemokines are increased in obese and type 2 DM patients, and these markers are reduced when patients are engaged in an intensive lifestyle intervention causing body weight loss [25]. In an 11-year cohort study, the inflammatory biomarkers C-reactive protein and pro-adrenomedullin were independently associated with cardiovascular events and all-cause mortality in type 2 DM patients [26]. Additionally, compared with controls, elevated serum levels of tumor necrotic factor-α and decreased neuregulin-4 (a novel adipokine) were found in diabetic patients and correlated with the severity of diabetic peripheral neuropathy [27,28]. Yeniel et al. assessed atherosclerosis indicators and blood perfusion in the bladder necks in women with OAB. They found that the OAB severity correlated with systemic atherosclerosis and impaired vascular perfusion of the urinary bladder [29]. In diabetic mice, Inouye et al. found that Evans blue extravasation in bladder vessels, an index of peripheral and neurogenic inflammation, correlated with bladder dysfunction [30]. Furthermore, Xiao et al. showed that compared with controls and diuretic groups, diabetic mice have bladders with higher levels of nitrotyrosine (a biomarker of NO-dependent, reactive nitrogen species-induced nitrative stress) and Mn superoxide dismutase (representing the activity of free radical scavengers) [31].

Recently, Hughes Jr. et al. showed that the NLRP3 inflammasome, an intracellular sensor that detects endogenous danger signals and environmental irritants, can sense diabetic metabolites and induce inflammation implicated in diabetic complications and neurodegeneration [32]. Compared to NLRP3 genes of knocked out non-diabetic mice, NLRP3 genes of knocked out diabetic mice had a higher serum glucose level but similar voiding volume, voiding frequency, voiding efficiency, severity of bladder inflammation, bladder Aδ-fibers, and C-fibers density. Interestingly, bladder inflammation and bladder decompression in BOO rats can be inhibited by NLRP3 inhibitor glyburide which might be effective to treat diabetic bladder dysfunction via the similar pathway [33]. In addition, Szasz et al. proposed another possible mechanism of diabetic bladder dysfunction via Toll-like receptor 4 (TLR4) activation. Innate immune system activation via TLR4 leads to inflammation and oxidative stress which causes bladder hypertrophy and hypercontractility [34]. Unlike wild type streptozotocin mice, TLR4 knock out diabetic mice were protected from diabetes-induced bladder dysfunction despite similar levels of hyperglycemia. These evidences, taken together, suggest that inflammatory pathways could be a component of a strategy to prevent or control diabetes and its associated complications.

5. Inhibition of Chronic Inflammation and Hypersensitivity by Intravesical Botulinum Toxin A Injection

Injection of botulinum toxin A (BoNT-A) into the detrusor muscle has emerged as a successful treatment for idiopathic and neurogenic detrusor overactivity [35,36]. Figure 1 summarizes some possible mechanisms that have been proposed to support its clinical efficacy for patients with DM-associated OAB [37]. Firstly, BoNT-A is well known for its ability to block the neuronal release of acetylcholine at the neuromuscular junction and therefore to inhibit abnormal smooth muscle contractions. Secondly, BoNT-A not only inhibits the efferent pathway of the bladder but also suppresses hypersensitivity via the afferent pathway. Thirdly, BoNT-A has anti-inflammatory effects and blocks noxious neurotransmitter release from the urothelium, including substance P, calcitonin gene-related peptide, and adenosine triphosphate (ATP). Finally, BoNT-A could be transported both anterogradely and retrogradely along either motor or sensory axons for bi-directional delivery between peripheral tissues or the central nerve system. Significant accumulation of the radio-labeled BoNT-A was noted in the lumbosacral dorsal root ganglia after bladder injection in normal rats [38,39]. Thus, BoNT-A might block not only acetylcholine release from motor nerve terminals but also central synaptic transmission, including glutamate, noradrenaline, dopamine, ATP, gamma-aminobutyric acid, and glycine. Since the pathophysiology of DM-associated OAB consists of afferent and efferent neuropathy, chronic inflammation and urothelial dysfunction, intravesical BoNT-A injection might be effective to treat DM-associated OAB.

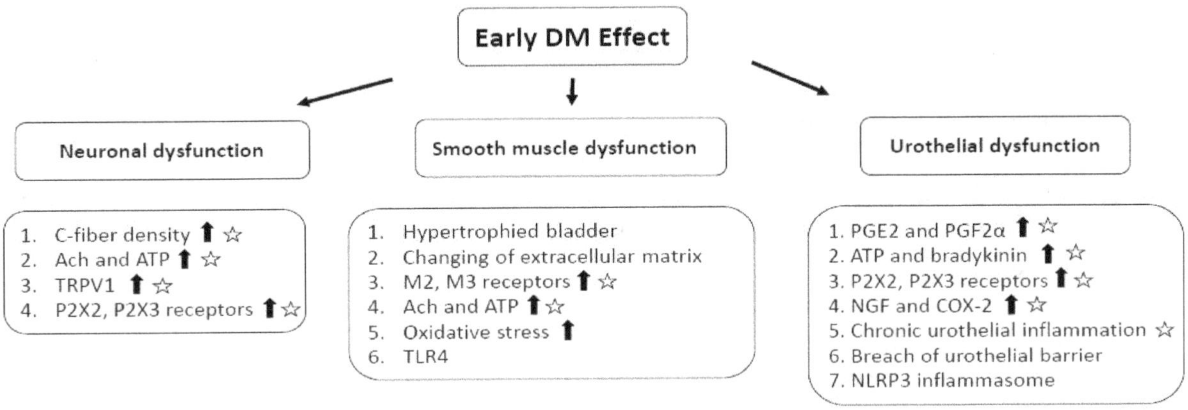

Figure 1. The early effect of diabetes mellitus on the innervation or function of the neuronal component, detrusor smooth muscle, and urothelium. Pentagram sign implies the possible mechanism of BoNT-A to support the clinical efficacy for DM-associated overactive bladder (OAB). The arrow means "increase".

Several experimental studies could support the clinical use of BoNT-A in treatment of DM-associated OAB. In acute and chronic inflammation in a rat model, BoNT-A significantly inhibited the release of substance P and calcitonin gene-related peptide after acute and chronic bladder injury [40]. In spinal-cord-injured rats, BoNT-A reversed the ratio of excitatory (ATP) and inhibitory (nitric oxide) urothelial transmitters and decreased non-voiding bladder contraction frequency [41]. In BOO-induced detrusor overactivity in rats, the expressions of nerve growth factor and transient receptor potential vanilloid 1 (TRPV1) proteins in the urothelium were significantly higher in the BOO group than in the control group and the expressions decreased significantly with BoNT-A detrusor injections [42]. In children with neurogenic detrusor overactivity, BoNT-A detrusor injections led to significant reductions in muscarinic M2, M3, P2X2, and purinergic P2X1, P2X2, and P2X3 receptors [43]. In another neurogenic bladder study in 15 children with myelodysplasia, urinary transforming growth factor beta-1 and nerve growth factor declined following intradetrusor BoNT-A injection [44]. These animal and clinical studies of BoNT-A strengthen the evidence of its therapeutic effects in diabetic patients with OAB. Since muscarinic M3 and P2X3 protein expressions in the bladders of DM-associated OAB patients were significantly higher than those in the controls, BoNT-A detrusor injection may provide an alternative treatment for these patients [23].

6. Clinical Outcomes of Intravesical Botulinum Toxin A Injection for Patients with DM-Associated OAB

Although numerous laboratory and clinical findings support that BoNT-A inhibits overactivity and chronic inflammation of OAB by different pathways, very few clinical studies have investigated intravesical BoNT-A treatment of patients with DM-associated OAB. Wang et al. reported the first retrospective study to compare the efficacy and safety of intravesical 100 U onabotulinumtoxinA injection in 48 patients with refractory type 2 DM-associated OAB [45]. During the 6-month follow-up period, similar success rates were noted between the diabetic and non-diabetic OAB groups (DM, 56% versus non-DM, 61%, $p = 0.128$). The disappearance rate of detrusor overactivity proved by videourodynamic studies was also similar in both groups (DM, 56.3%, versus non-DM, 47.8%, $p = 0.41$). However, the patients with DM more commonly had adverse events such as large postvoid residual urine volumes and general weakness than the non-DM group.

One hypothesis is that early phase DM causes compensated bladder function, and late-phase DM causes decompensated bladder function [46,47]. Thus, DHIC, a paradoxical condition involving both the storage and voiding phases of bladder function, could happen during the transition from OAB to underactive bladder in DM patients. An interesting study comparing the efficacy and safety of intravesical onabotulinumtoxinA injection in patients with DHIC or OAB showed that the OAB symptoms in both groups significantly improved during the 3-month follow-up period [48]. However, the mean duration of therapeutic efficacy in patients with DHIC was significantly shorter than that of patients with OAB (4.9 ± 4.8 months versus 7.2 ± 3.3 months, $p = 0.03$). Additionally, the incidences of adverse events including acute urinary retention, large postvoid residual urine volume, urinary tract infection, gross hematuria, and general weakness were comparable in both groups.

Furthermore, Kuo et al. analyzed the adverse events after intravesical BoNT-A injection in 217 patients with idiopathic detrusor overactivity [49]. The results showed that male sex, large baseline postvoid residual urine, comorbidities, and higher doses of BoNT-A (>100 U) were risk factors for adverse events after BoNT-A injection for OAB. However, the occurrence of adverse events did not affect treatment outcome. As a result, intravesical BoNT-A injection is still recommended in patients with DM-associated OAB who develop DHIC. Patients should be informed of the possibility of shorter therapeutic duration and adverse events before injection.

7. Conclusions

Based on recent basic and clinical studies, intravesical BoNT-A injection appears to be effective and safe in patients with DM-associated OAB. However, this hypothesis requires further validation through randomized controlled clinical studies. A comprehensive evaluation of DM complications and urodynamic studies is needed before BoNT-A treatment for DM-associated OAB to avoid the occurrence of adverse events. Finally, it is important to explore the status of the clinical characteristics and inflammatory biomarkers of DM as determining predictors of BoNT-A treatment efficacy in the future.

Author Contributions: Conceptualization, H.-C.K.; methodology, C.-C.W.; formal analysis, C.-C.W. and Y.-H.J.; writing manuscript-draft, C.-C.W. and Y.-H.J.; writing—review and editing, H.-C.K.; supervision, H.-C.K. All authors have read and agreed to the published version of the manuscript.

Acknowledgments: The authors thank the staff of Formosa Medical Editors for assistance with manuscript preparation.

References

1. Xu, D.; Zhao, M.; Huang, L.; Wang, K. Overactive bladder symptom severity, bother, help-seeking behavior, and quality of life in patients with type 2 diabetes: A path analysis. *Health Qual. Life Outcomes* **2018**, *16*, 1. [CrossRef] [PubMed]
2. Jackson, R.A.; Vittinghoff, E.; Kanaya, A.M.; Miles, T.P.; Resnick, H.E.; Kritchevsky, S.B.; Simonsick, E.M.; Brown, J.S. Urinary incontinence in elderly women: Findings from the Health, Aging, and Body Composition Study. *Obstet. Gynecol.* **2004**, *104*, 301–307. [CrossRef] [PubMed]
3. Chen, G.D.; Hu, S.W.; Chen, Y.C.; Lin, T.L.; Lin, L.Y. Prevalence and correlations of anal incontinence and constipation in Taiwanese women. *Neurourol. Urodyn.* **2003**, *22*, 664–669. [CrossRef] [PubMed]
4. Chiu, A.F.; Huang, M.H.; Wang, C.C.; Kuo, H.C. Higher glycosylated hemoglobin levels increase the risk of overactive bladder syndrome in patients with type 2 diabetes mellitus. *Int. J. Urol.* **2012**, *19*, 995–1001. [CrossRef] [PubMed]
5. Wang, C.C.; Chancellor, M.B.; Lin, J.M.; Hsieh, J.H.; Yu, H.J. Type 2 diabetes but not metabolic syndrome is associated with an increased risk of lower urinary tract symptoms and erectile dysfunction in men aged <45 years. *BJU Int.* **2010**, *105*, 1136–1140. [CrossRef] [PubMed]
6. Johnston, S.; Janning, S.W.; Haas, G.P.; Wilson, K.L.; Smith, D.M.; Reckard, G.; Quan, S.-P.; Bukofzer, S. Comparative persistence and adherence to overactive bladder medications in patients with and without diabetes. *Int. J. Clin. Pract.* **2012**, *66*, 1042–1051. [CrossRef] [PubMed]
7. Moller, C.F.; Olesen, K.P. Diabetic cystopathy. IV: Micturition cystourethrography compared with urodynamic investigation. *Dan. Med. Bull.* **1976**, *23*, 291–294.
8. Karoli, R.; Bhat, S.; Fatima, J.; Priya, S. A study of bladder dysfunction in women with type 2 diabetes mellitus. *Indian J. Endocrinol. Metab.* **2014**, *18*, 552–557. [CrossRef]

9. Majima, T.; Matsukawa, Y.; Funahashi, Y.; Takai, S.; Kato, M.; Yamamoto, T.; Gotoh, M. Urodynamic analysis of the impact of diabetes mellitus on bladder function. *Int. J. Urol.* **2019**, *26*, 618–622. [CrossRef]
10. Bansal, R.; Agarwal, M.M.; Modi, M.; Mandal, A.K.; Singh, S.K. Urodynamic profile of diabetic patients with lower urinary tract symptoms: Association of diabetic cystopathy with autonomic and peripheral neuropathy. *Urology* **2011**, *77*, 699–705. [CrossRef]
11. Lee, W.C.; Wu, H.P.; Tai, T.Y.; Yu, H.J.; Chiang, P.H. Investigation of urodynamic characteristics and bladder sensory function in the early stages of diabetic bladder dysfunction in women with type 2 diabetes. *J. Urol.* **2009**, *181*, 198–203. [CrossRef] [PubMed]
12. Gali, A.; Mucciardi, G.; Buttice, S.; Subba, E.; D'Amico, C.; Lembo, F.; Magno, C. Correlation between advanced glycation end-products, lower urinary tract symptoms and bladder dysfunctions in patients with type 2 diabetes mellitus. *Low. Urin. Tract. Symptoms* **2017**, *9*, 15–20. [CrossRef] [PubMed]
13. Ho, C.H.; Tai, H.C.; Yu, H.J. Urodynamic findings in female diabetic patients with and without overactive bladder symptoms. *Neurourol. Urodyn.* **2010**, *29*, 424–427. [CrossRef] [PubMed]
14. Yoshimura, N.; Chancellor, M.B.; Andersson, K.E.; Christ, G.J. Recent advances in understanding the biology of diabetes-associated bladder complications and novel therapy. *BJU Int.* **2005**, *95*, 733–738. [CrossRef]
15. Tong, Y.C.; Chin, W.T.; Cheng, J.T. Alterations in urinary bladder M2-muscarinic receptor protein and mRNA in 2-week streptozotocin-induced diabetic rats. *Neurosci. Lett.* **1999**, *277*, 173–176. [CrossRef]
16. Tong, Y.C.; Cheng, J.T. Alteration of M(3) subtype muscarinic receptors in the diabetic rat urinary bladder. *Pharmacology* **2002**, *64*, 148–151. [CrossRef]
17. Klee, N.S.; Moreland, R.S.; Kendig, D.M. Detrusor contractility to parasympathetic mediators is differentially altered in the compensated and decompensated states of diabetic bladder dysfunction. *Am. J. Physiol. Renal. Physiol.* **2019**, *317*, F388–F398. [CrossRef]
18. Gray, M.A.; Wang, C.C.; Sacks, M.S.; Yoshimura, N.; Chancellor, M.B.; Nagatomi, J. Time-dependent alterations of select genes in streptozotocin-induced diabetic rat bladder. *Urology* **2008**, *71*, 1214–1219. [CrossRef]
19. Wang, C.C.; Nagatomi, J.; Toosi, K.K.; Yoshimura, N.; Hsieh, J.H.; Chancellor, M.B.; Chancellor, M.B.; Sacks, M.S. Diabetes-induced alternations in biomechanical properties of urinary bladder wall in rats. *Urology* **2009**, *73*, 911–915. [CrossRef]
20. Tanik, N.; Tanik, S.; Albayrak, S.; Zengin, K.; Inan, L.E.; Caglayan, E.K.; Celikbilek, A.; Kirboga, K.; Gurdal, M. Association Between Overactive Bladder and Polyneuropathy in Diabetic Patients. *Int. Neurourol. J.* **2016**, *20*, 232–239. [CrossRef]
21. Lee, W.C.; Wu, H.C.; Huang, K.H.; Wu, H.P.; Yu, H.J.; Wu, C.C. Hyposensitivity of C-fiber afferents at the distal extremities as an indicator of early stages diabetic bladder dysfunction in type 2 diabetic women. *PLoS ONE* **2014**, *9*, e86463. [CrossRef] [PubMed]
22. Hanna-Mitchell, A.T.; Ruiz, G.W.; Daneshgari, F.; Liu, G.; Apodaca, G.; Birder, L.A. Impact of diabetes mellitus on bladder uroepithelial cells. *Am. J. Physiol. Regul. Integr. Comp. Physiol.* **2013**, *304*, R84–R93. [CrossRef] [PubMed]
23. Wang, C.C.; Kuo, H.C. Urothelial Dysfunction and Chronic Inflammation in Diabetic Patients with Overactive Bladder. *Low. Urin. Tract. Symptoms* **2017**, *9*, 151–156. [CrossRef] [PubMed]
24. Donath, M.Y.; Shoelson, S.E. Type 2 diabetes as an inflammatory disease. *Nat. Rev. Immunol.* **2011**, *11*, 98–107. [CrossRef] [PubMed]
25. Esser, N.; Legrand-Poels, S.; Piette, J.; Scheen, A.J.; Paquot, N. Inflammation as a link between obesity, metabolic syndrome and type 2 diabetes. *Diabetes Res. Clin. Pract.* **2014**, *105*, 141–150. [CrossRef]
26. Landman, G.W.; Kleefstra, N.; Groenier, K.H.; Bakker, S.J.; Groeneveld, G.H.; Bilo, H.J.; Van Hateren, K.J. Inflammation biomarkers and mortality prediction in patients with type 2 diabetes (ZODIAC-27). *Atherosclerosis* **2016**, *250*, 46–51. [CrossRef]
27. Ristikj-Stomnaroska, D.; Risteska-Nejashmikj, V.; Papazova, M. Role of Inflammation in the Pathogenesis of Diabetic Peripheral Neuropathy. *Open Access Maced. J. Med. Sci.* **2019**, *7*, 2267–2270. [CrossRef]
28. Yan, P.; Xu, Y.; Zhang, Z.; Gao, C.; Zhu, J.; Li, H.; Wan, Q. Decreased plasma neuregulin 4 levels are associated with peripheral neuropathy in Chinese patients with newly diagnosed type 2 diabetes: A cross-sectional study. *Cytokine* **2019**, *113*, 356–364. [CrossRef]

29. Yeniel, A.O.; Ergenoglu, A.M.; Meseri, R.; Kismali, E.; Ari, A.; Kavukcu, G.; Aydin, H.H.; Ak, H.; Atay, S.; Itil, I.M. Is overactive bladder microvasculature disease a component of systemic atheroscleorosis? *Neurourol. Urodyn.* **2018**, *37*, 1372–1379. [CrossRef]
30. Inouye, B.M.; Hughes, F.M., Jr.; Jin, H.; Lutolf, R.; Potnis, K.C.; Routh, J.C.; Rouse, D.C.; Foo, W.-C.; Purves, J.T. Diabetic bladder dysfunction is associated with bladder inflammation triggered through hyperglycemia, not polyuria. *Res. Rep. Urol.* **2018**, *10*, 219–225. [CrossRef]
31. Xiao, N.; Wang, Z.; Huang, Y.; Daneshgari, F.; Liu, G. Roles of polyuria and hyperglycemia in bladder dysfunction in diabetes. *J. Urol.* **2013**, *189*, 1130–1136. [CrossRef] [PubMed]
32. Hughes, F.M., Jr.; Hirshman, N.A.; Inouye, B.M.; Jin, H.; Stanton, E.W.; Yun, C.E.; Davis, L.G.; Routh, J.C.; Purves, J.T. NLRP3 promotes diabetic bladder dysfunction and changes in symptom-specific bladder innervation. *Diabetes* **2019**, *68*, 430–440. [CrossRef] [PubMed]
33. Hughes, F.M., Jr.; Sexton, S.J.; Ledig, P.D.; Yun, C.E.; Jin, H.; Purves, J.T. Bladder decompensation and reduction in nerve density in a rat model of chronic bladder outlet obstruction are attenuated with the NLRP3 inhibitor glyburide. *Am. J. Physiol. Renal. Physiol.* **2019**, *316*, F113–F120. [CrossRef] [PubMed]
34. Szasz, T.; Wenceslau, C.F.; Burgess, B.; Nunes, K.P.; Webb, R.C. Toll-like receptor 4 activation contributes to diabetic bladder dysfunction in a murine model of type 1 diabetes. *Diabetes* **2016**, *65*, 3754–3764. [CrossRef]
35. Kuo, Y.C.; Kuo, H.C. Botulinum toxin injection for lower urinary tract dysfunction. *Int. J. Urol.* **2013**, *20*, 40–55. [CrossRef]
36. Kuo, H.C. Urodynamic evidence of effectiveness of botulinum A toxin injection in treatment of detrusor overactivity refractory to anticholinergic agents. *Urology* **2004**, *63*, 868–872. [CrossRef]
37. Jhang, J.F.; Kuo, H.C. Botulinum toxin A and lower urinary tract dysfunction: Pathophysiology and mechanisms of action. *Toxins* **2016**, *8*, 120. [CrossRef]
38. Akaike, N.; Shin, M.-C.; Wakita, M.; Torii, Y.; Harakawa, T.; Ginnaga, A.; Kato, K.; Kaji, R.; Kozaki, S. Transsynaptic inhibition of spinal transmission by A2 botulinum toxin. *J. Physiol.* **2013**, *591*, 1031–1043. [CrossRef]
39. Papagiannopoulou, D.; Vardouli, L.; Dimitriadis, F.; Apostolidis, A. Retrograde transport of radiolabelled botulinum neurotoxin type A to the CNS after intradetrusor injection in rats. *BJU Int.* **2016**, *117*, 697–704. [CrossRef]
40. Lucioni, A.; Bales, G.T.; Lotan, T.L.; McGehee, D.S.; Cook, S.P.; Rapp, D.E. Botulinum toxin type A inhibits sensory neuropeptide release in rat bladder models of acute injury and chronic inflammation. *BJU Int.* **2008**, *101*, 366–370. [CrossRef]
41. Smith, C.P.; Gangitano, D.; Munoz, A.; Salas, N.A.; Boone, T.B.; Aoki, K.R.; Francis, J.; Somogyi, G.T. Botulinum toxin type A normalizes alterations in urothelial ATP and NO release induced by chronic spinal cord injury. *Neurochem. Int.* **2008**, *52*, 1068–1075. [CrossRef] [PubMed]
42. Ha, U.S.; Park, E.Y.; Kim, J.C. Effect of botulinum toxin on expression of nerve growth factor and transient receptor potential vanilloid 1 in urothelium and detrusor muscle of rats with bladder outlet obstruction-induced detrusor overactivity. *Urology* **2011**, *78*, 721. [CrossRef] [PubMed]
43. Schulte-Baukloh, H.; Priefert, J.; Knispel, H.H.; Lawrence, G.W.; Miller, K.; Neuhaus, J. Botulinum toxin A detrusor injections reduce postsynaptic muscular M2, M3, P2X2, and P2X3 receptors in children and adolescents who have neurogenic detrusor overactivity: A single-blind study. *Urology* **2013**, *81*, 1052–1057. [CrossRef] [PubMed]
44. Top, T.; Sekerci, C.A.; Isbilen-Basok, B.; Tanidir, Y.; Tinay, I.; Isman, F.K.; Akbal, C.; Şimşek, F.; Tarcan, T. The effect of intradetrusor botulinum neurotoxin type A on urinary NGF, TGF BETA-1, TIMP-2 levels in children with neurogenic detrusor overactivity due to myelodysplasia. *Neurourol. Urodyn.* **2017**, *36*, 1896–1902. [CrossRef] [PubMed]
45. Wang, C.C.; Liao, C.H.; Kuo, H.C. Diabetes mellitus does not affect the efficacy and safety of intravesical onabotulinumtoxina injection in patients with refractory detrusor overactivity. *Neurourol. Urodyn.* **2014**, *33*, 1235–1239. [CrossRef] [PubMed]
46. Daneshgari, F.; Liu, G.; Birder, L.; Hanna-Mitchell, A.T.; Chacko, S. Diabetic bladder dysfunction: Current translational knowledge. *J. Urol.* **2009**, *182* (Suppl. 6), S18–S26. [CrossRef]
47. Chancellor, M.B. The overactive bladder progression to underactive bladder hypothesis. *Int. Urol. Nephrol.* **2014**, *46* (Suppl. 1), S23–S27. [CrossRef]

48. Wang, C.C.; Lee, C.L.; Kuo, H.C. Efficacy and Safety of Intravesical OnabotulinumtoxinA Injection in Patients with Detrusor Hyperactivity and Impaired Contractility. *Toxins* **2016**, *8*, 82. [CrossRef]
49. Kuo, H.C.; Liao, C.H.; Chung, S.D. Adverse events of intravesical botulinum toxin a injections for idiopathic detrusor overactivity: Risk factors and influence on treatment outcome. *Eur. Urol.* **2010**, *58*, 919–926. [CrossRef]

19

Mechanism of Action of Botulinum Toxin A in Treatment of Functional Urological Disorders

Yu-Hua Lin [1,2,3], Bing-Juin Chiang [1,4,5] and Chun-Hou Liao [1,4,*]

1 Divisions of Urology, Department of Surgery, Cardinal Tien Hospital, New Taipei City 23148, Taiwan; jorgesuperowl@gmail.com (Y.-H.L.); bingjuinchiang@gmail.com (B.-J.C.)
2 Department of Chemistry, Fu Jen Catholic University, New Taipei City 24205, Taiwan
3 Graduate Institute of Biochemical and Pharmaceutical Science, Fu Jen Catholic University, New Taipei City 24205, Taiwan
4 College of Medicine, Fu-Jen Catholic University, New Taipei City 24205, Taiwan
5 School of Life Science, College of Science, National Taiwan Normal University, Taipei 11677, Taiwan
* Correspondence: liaoch22@gmail.com

Abstract: Intravesical botulinum toxin (BoNT) injection is effective in reducing urgency and urinary incontinence. It temporarily inhibits the detrusor muscle contraction by blocking the release of acetylcholine (Ach) from the preganglionic and postganglionic nerves in the efferent nerves. BoNT-A also blocks ATP release from purinergic efferent nerves in the detrusor muscle. In afferent nerves, BoNT-A injection markedly reduces the urothelial ATP release and increases nitric oxide (NO) release from the urothelium. BoNT-A injection in the urethra or bladder has been developed in the past few decades as the treatment method for detrusor sphincter dyssyndergia, incontinence due to neurogenic or idiopathic detrusor overactivity, sensory disorders, including bladder hypersensitivity, overactive bladder, and interstitial cystitis/chronic pelvic pain syndrome. Although the FDA only approved BoNT-A injection treatment for neurogenic detrusor overactivity and for refractory overactive bladder, emerging clinical trials have demonstrated the benefits of BoNT-A treatment in functional urological disorders. Cautious selection of patients and urodynamic evaluation for confirmation of diagnosis are crucial to maximize the successful outcomes of BoNT-A treatment.

Keywords: botulinum toxin; functional urology disorder; human

Key Contribution: This article reviewed the mechanism of action of botulinum toxin A in treatment of different urological disorders.

---

1. Introduction

Botulinum toxin (BoNT), one of the most potent natural neurotoxins known for centuries, has been found with emerging medical efficacy in the past few decades [1,2]. BoNT was initially documented with the symptoms of foodborne botulism in the 18th century [3]. A botulism outbreak after a funeral dinner with smoked ham in 1895 led to the discovery of the pathogen Clostridium botulinum by Emile Pierre van Ermengem, Professor of Bacteriology at the University of Ghent [3]. Acute BoNT poisoning was initially observed with vomiting, intestinal spasms, mydriasis, ptosis, dysphagia, and finally respiratory failure [4]. It may take 3–6 months to recover from botulinum intoxication [4]. Since BoNT was discovered as the produced toxin from the bacterium Clostridium botulinum, it has been widely used to treat neuropathic pain syndromes and dystonic disease [5–8].

Botulinum toxin A (BoNT-A) has been used for the treatment of lower urinary tract disease (LUTD) since the late 1980s. Dykstra et al. reported injection of BoNT-A to the external urethral sphincter in men with spinal cord injury (SCI) for the treatment of detrusor-sphincter dyssynergia (DSD) in

1988 [9]. The treatment of SCI patients with neurogenic detrusor overactivity (DO) using detrusor BoNT-A injections at multiple sites was also developed [10]. Idiopathic DO and overactive bladder (OAB) patients were also reported with successful treatment with intravesical BoNT-A injection [11,12]. Maria et al. first described the therapeutic effects of BoNT-A injection for patients with benign prostatic hyperplasia (BPH) with voiding dysfunction in 2003 [13]. However, the latest randomized controlled trial investigating the efficacy of BoNT-A injection for BPH-related lower urinary tract symptoms (LUTS) demonstrated no significant difference between the treatment group and the placebo [14]. Moreover, BoNT-A intravesical injection treatment has been developed for interstitial cystitis/bladder pain syndrome (IC/BPS) because of its anti-inflammatory effects [15,16]. As the uses of BoNT-A expand in the field of urology, understanding its mechanisms and clinical effects is essential.

2. Mechanism of Action of BoNT-A

BoNT is a neurotoxin protein, which comprises a 50-kDa light chain and a 100 kDa heavy chain linked by a disulfide bond [17]. Seven serotypes of BoNT has been identified, and the most commonly used type in medicine is BoNT-A [17]. BoNT enters the presynaptic neuron membrane through binding of the heavy-chain C-terminal to the synaptic vesicle protein (SV2) [18]. After toxin endocytosis, the disulfide bond of BoNT is cleaved. The light-chain protein, which is the true active moiety, is then linked to the synaptosomal nerve associated protein 25 (SNAP-25) [18]. SNAP-25 is a protein with essential function for the binding of vesicles to the cell membrane and signal transduction. By binding the light-chain protein of BoNT-A to SNAP-25 and other SNAP families, BoNT-A inhibits neurotransmitters' exocytosis from the vesicles; hence, the affected neuromuscular junctions become paralyzed [18].

A clinical study confirmed SV2 and SNAP-25 immunoreactive fibers are distributed over the suburothelial and muscular layers instead of the urothelium in human bladder [19]. SV2 or SNAP-25 protein is not expressed within the urothelial or muscular cells [19]. The SV2 are expressed more abundantly in the cholinergic and parasympathetic fibers, as compared to the less than half expression to the sensory and sympathetic nerves. These findings suggest that the parasympathetic nerves are the main target of BoNT-A action in the human urinary bladder [19]. Other clinical studies associated with animal models demonstrated the SV2 expression in the human and rat bladder mucosae, as well as synaptosomal nerve-associated protein 23 (SNAP-23) and SNAP-25 in the urothelial cells and mucosa (differed in intensity) from the rat and human bladder [20]. SNAP-23 is a homologous target membrane SNAP receptor (t-SNARE) and is structurally and functionally similar to SNAP-25. SNAP-23 may be cleaved by BoNT-A, but human SNAP-23 is more resistant to botulinum [21,22]. The distribution pattern of SNAP-23 is different from that of SNAP-25: SNAP-23 is expressed mainly within the superficial or apical layer of urothelial layer, while SNAP-25 is detected throughout the urothelial layer [20]. SNAP-23 also interacts to multiple vesicle-associated membrane protein and syntaxin [23]. Since the urothelium is considered both a barrier as well as a significant signal transduction gate, the release of other neurotransmitters such as glutamate, adenosine triphosphate (ATP), neurotrophins, or NO may be affected after BoNT-A injection [24,25].

In clinical studies, BoNT-A inhibits the release of acetylcholine (Ach) and other neurotransmitters at the neuromuscular junction in human striated muscle [26]. Further neural modulating effects are observed by influencing the α and γ motor neurons after BoNT-A treatment (the α and γ motor neurons innervate the extrafusal and the intrafusal muscle fibers, respectively) [26]. Intravesical BoNT-A administration results in SNAP-25 cleavage, which inhibits the vesicular noradrenaline release. This action may prevent the α- and β3-adrenoceptors activation, and the reaction additionally affects the bladder neck contracture and detrusor relaxation [27]. A clinical study with receptor analysis conducted after BoNT-A injection treatment to the human bladders with neurogenic detrusor overactivity (NDO) showed significant reduction of the M2 and M3 muscarinic receptors as well as the P2X purinoceptor 2 (P2X2) and P2X purinoceptor 3 (P2X3) in the muscle layer [28]. This indicates that BoNT-A hinders DO through both sensory and motor features.

In addition, the ATP receptor P2X3 is critical for peripheral pain responses and afferent pathways controlling the urinary bladder volume reflexes [29–31]. In an animal model study, P2X3-null mice presented a marked hyporeflexia of the urinary bladder [29]. This result indicates that ATP plays an important role in mediating bladder fullness sensation and is crucial in the pathophysiology of OAB. In clinical studies, the human bladder, P2X3, and the transient receptor potential vanilloid subfamily-1 (TRPV1) are observed in the suburothelial layer [30]. A clinical study on the receptor profiles in biopsies from NDO or idiopathic DO patients showed a decreased P2X3 and TRPV1 immunoreactivity in the sensory nerve fiber after BoNT-A intravesical injection treatment [31]. The degree of decrease in the TRPV1 and P2X3 immunoreactivity is found to be correlated to clinical improvement (reduction of frequency and urgency status) [31]. Clinical studies with intravesical BoNT-A injections demonstrated significant inhibition of ATP and neurotrophin release and an increase of nitric oxide (NO) release from the human urothelial cells [24,30].

Animal models have shown possible mechanisms of action of BoNT-A injection treatment in interstitial cystitis/bladder pain syndrome (IC/BPS). In the isolated rat bladder model of acute injury and chronic inflammation, a significant amount of reduced calcitonin gene-related peptide and substance P from the afferent nerve terminals is observed [32,33]. The results suggest that BoNT-A injection treatment is a solution method of neurogenic inflammation in patients with IC/BPS [32,33]. TRPV1 inflammatory sensitization is found to play a vital role in inflammatory pain mediation [34]. Some proinflammatory agents (e.g., nerve growth factor, ATP, and IGF-I) sensitize rat nociceptors by promoting the recruitment of TRPV1 channels to the neuronal surface [34]. In preclinical studies, BoNT-A injection into oocytes expressing TRPV1 was found to block the TRPV1 membrane translocation by affecting protein kinase C (PKC) signaling [35]. The inhibition of the inflammatory sensitization of TRPV1 receptors by BoNT-A may also describe the therapeutic effects of BoNT-A injection to medication refractory IC/BPS. In an animal model study, BoNT-A has been shown to inhibit the ATP release from the urothelium in chronic bladder inflammation [36]. In clinical studies, reduction of the nerve growth factor and brain-derived neurotrophic levels in patients with IC/BPS after intravesical BoNT-A injection has demonstrated an analgesic effect [37,38]. BoNT-A conducted direct analgesic effects through exocytosis suppression of sensory neurotransmitters over the peripheral nociceptive neurons. However, indirect analgesic effects seemed also present with decreased spinal cord neuronal activity and with prevention of central sensitization as verified in some other clinical studies [39,40].

In a preclinical study for LUTS that related to prostate enlargement, BoNT-A injection has been reported to induce prostate atrophy and activate the apoptotic pathway in rats, which may result in reduced sympathetic stimulation of the prostate [41]. BoNT-A injection in a rat model revealed prostate weight reduction and reduced level of tyrosine hydroxylase-positive sympathetic nerve fibers and synaptophysin-positive cells in the epithelium [42,43]. In clinical studies, human prostate injection of BoNT-A has demonstrated apoptotic activity at the epithelial and stromal components of the prostate [44]. The reaction subsequently reduced the anatomical obstruction [44]. A clinical study comparing intraprostatic BoNT-A and normal saline injections demonstrated a significant contractile function reduction while maintaining relaxation response by presenting reduced prostatic urethral pressure response to intravenous norepinephrine and electrostimulation [45].

3. BoNT-A Treatment in OAB and DO

OAB is a clinical syndrome characterized by urinary urgency, usually accompanied by frequency and nocturia, with or without urinary incontinence, in the absence of urinary tract infection or other pathology [46]. Treatment of OAB is typically initiated with behavioral therapy, followed by oral medications including antimuscarinics or beta-agonists [47]. A large-scale study showed 46.2% of OAB patients discontinued medical treatment due to poor response or less effective as expected after treatment [48]. DO was defined as a urodynamic observation characterized by involuntary detrusor contraction during the bladder-filling phase [49]. DO is usually associated with symptoms of urgency, which is defined as a complaint of sudden, compelling desire to pass urine that is difficult to defer [50].

DO has been noticed in those with disturbances in the nerve, detrusor muscular, or urothelial levels [50]. Ach plays a key role in mediating bladder contraction through muscarinic receptors and detrusor muscle, and mediating ATP through purinergic receptors (P2X) stimulation has also been associated with bladder contraction [30].

In the central nervous system (CNS), the prefrontal cerebral cortex, the L-region of the pontine micturition center, and the lumbar spinal cord play the essential role of detrusor contraction inhibition [50]. A spinal cord lesion above the lumbosacral cord level may cause inhibitory pathway dysfunction, which further disturbs the voluntary control of micturition and results in NDO [50]. The sacral spinal reflex is known to be mediated by the unmyelinated C-fibers and is active in patients with SCI and NDO [50]. For idiopathic detrusor overactivity (IDO), although there is no specific central or peripheral neurologic dysfunction, increased expression of P2X2, TRPV1, and muscarinic receptors over the urothelium have been found in a clinical study [51].

Several clinical studies have demonstrated BoNT-A's efficacy in urgency and urinary incontinence reduction [10]. In the efferent nerves, BoNT-A injection temporarily inhibits the detrusor muscle contraction by blocking the Ach release via cleaving SNAP-25 from both the preganglionic and postganglionic nerve [24]. BoNT-A also blocks ATP release from the purinergic efferent nerves in the detrusor muscle [52]. In the afferent nerves, BoNT-A injection markedly reduced urothelial ATP release [53,54]. NO inhibits the afferent nerve conduction in the bladder detrusor and BoNT-A injection facilitates increased NO release from the urothelium [54]. In summary, BoNT-A injection has effects involving the efferent and afferent nerve pathways.

4. BoNT-A Treatment for DSD in Patients with Spinal Cord Injury

DSD is characterized by involuntary contraction of the external urethral sphincter during a detrusor contraction and is caused by CNS injury between the sacral spinal cord and pontine micturition center [55]. High post-void urine amount, incomplete emptying, and increased intravesical pressure during voiding phase are noticed in the SCI patient with DSD. BoNT-A injection to the urethral sphincter has demonstrated sphincter relaxation by blocking Ach from the presynaptic vesicles at the neuromuscular junction [9,56,57]. Although DSD patient receiving BoNT-A injection over the urethral sphincter may experience incontinence, most of the patients were satisfied by the treatment effects of significant urethral pressure reduction, increased voiding volume, and decreased urinary incontinence episodes [56,57].

5. BoNT-A Injection for Dysfunctional Voiding (DV) or Bladder Neck Dysfunction (BND)

DV is characterized by voiding intermittency or urine flow rate fluctuation due to involuntary contraction of the periurethral striated muscle during voiding in non-neurological deficit individuals [49]. As BoNT-A injection treatment has been successfully used in SCI patients with DSD, it has been developed for adults with non-neurogenic voiding dysfunction. Fowler's syndrome consists of challenging symptoms of poor external urethral sphincter relaxation without neurological or anatomical abnormality, which may cause voiding difficulty and even urinary retention [58]. Patients with non-neurogenic voiding dysfunction classically present with open bladder neck but poorly relaxed urethral sphincter and normal-to-high voiding pressure during micturition by urodynamic study and are mostly refractory to medical treatment [59]. Several recent clinical studies have shown BoNT-A injection to the external urethral sphincter could be a safe and efficient treatment method for refractory DV patients [60–62]. Post-treatment, improvements were noticed in several clinical aspects in those studies, such as maximal flow rate, voided urine amount, decreased detrusor voiding pressure, international prostate symptom score (IPSS), and quality of life index. However, only the total IPSS and voided volume improvements were significantly greater than those in the placebo group in a randomized controlled double-blind study [62].

Some DV patients without strong electromyographic activity may have similar symptoms of DV due to poor relaxation of the pelvic floor muscle and the urethral sphincter [63]. Poor bladder neck relaxation in BND may lead to weak stream and increased residual urine amount after voiding [63]. Recent studies demonstrated that BoNT-A injections in the external urethral sphincter, pelvic floor muscle, or bladder neck may offer promising therapeutic effects for DV symptoms improvement [61,64,65]. Synchronous significant reduction of the bladder outlet resistance and the pelvic floor pressure were observed in a study after BoNT-A injection treatment to the pelvic floor muscle, which indicates a more complex mechanism in DV symptoms. Further evidence is necessary to explain the pathophysiology of BoNT-A action in DV or bladder neck dysfunction.

6. BoNT-A Injection for IC/BPS

IC/BPS is a clinical syndrome described as having "An unpleasant sensation (pain, pressure, discomfort) perceived to be related to urinary bladder, associated with lower urinary tract symptoms of more than 6 weeks duration, in the absence of infection or other identifiable causes" [62]. Though the real pathophysiology of IC/BPS has remained unclear for decades, recent studies have progressed in molecular biology, which have focused on urothelial dysfunction and neurogenic inflammation and could explain some part of the disease [61–66]. Urothelial defect with surface glycosaminoglycan and associated dysregulation of urothelial permeability has been established as one of the pathogenesis of IC/BPS [65]. IC/BPS also had upregulated P2X3 receptors and with increasing ATP release in the urothelium [66]. TRPV1 is a capsaicin receptor that detects bladder pain. A recent clinical study found that the increased inflammation severity correlated with a high TRPV1-immunoreactive nerve fibers and nerve growth factor (NGF) in IC/BPS expression and the correlation is directly positive to the clinical symptoms [67]. Substance P, a neurotransmitter secreted from the sensory nerve and a key cytokine in inflammatory process and pain, was also found with increased expression in the bladder nerve fibers of IC/BPS patients [68]. NGF, a neuropeptide involved in the regulation of growth released by the mast cell in the inflammatory process, was found with increased expression in the bladder mucosa, urine, and serum of IC/BPS patients [69,70]. NGF is also believed to play a pivotal role in the pathogenesis of IC/BPS.

BoNT-A injections improved urothelial function in IC/BPS patients by P2X3 and TRPV1 receptor expression reduction in the urothelium, which may be the chronic pain control mechanism [71]. BoNT-A injections inhibit the sensory neurotransmitters that further reduce pain sensation [71]. Various clinical studies have shown decreased NGF mRNA expression in the bladder for those who responded to intravesical BoNT-A injection treatment [72,73]. Recent clinical evidence suggests that BoNT-A stops the inflammation process in the bladder [74,75]. Declined tryptase expression was discovered over the urothelium after repeated BoNT-A injection, which indicated the reduction of mast cell activity in the treated IC/BPS patients' bladder [74]. Furthermore, BoNT-A injection treatment was found with decreased vascular endothelial growth factor (VEGF) and attenuated vasculogenesis in the bladder of IC/BPS patients [75]. Apoptotic signaling also decreased in evidence after BoNT-A injection treatment [75].

7. BoNT-A Injection for BPH

BPH is the most common cause of bladder outlet obstruction in men. The prostate growth's anatomical obstruction may be the main reason for lower urinary tract symptoms, but inflammation, infection, and metabolic disorders can also be possible etiologies [76]. The prostate is innervated with the parasympathetic and sympathetic nerves [77]. The cholinergic nerves and muscarinic receptors are present in the fibromuscular stroma of the prostate, which can explain the previous beneficial effects of BoNT-A intraprostatic injection treatments [78–81]. However, a recent randomized controlled trial stated that high placebo effects appeared persistent and may be associated with the symptom improvement [14]. Several studies have shown that BoNT-A injection into prostate can effectively reduce pain in men with chronic prostatitis [82]. The effect of BoNT-A on male LUTS might result from anti-inflammation effect but not reducing the prostate volume [82]. Currently, BoNT-A injection treatment remains the less-common indication for men with BPH and lower urinary tract symptoms.

8. Conclusions

BoNT-A injections are widely used in functional urology disorders, and therapeutic benefits have been noticed across a wide range of lower urinary tract diseases. However, approval for indication has been obtained only for management of idiopathic OAB and NDO owing to SCI or multiple sclerosis. The United States and some other countries also approved use for the detrusor hyperactivity with impaired contractile function. Moreover, for IC/BPS patients' refractory to medical treatment, BoNT-A injections are considered the standard of treatment according to different guidelines. The pathophysiology of BoNT-A injection to different functional disorders is increasingly revealed in various clinical trials, and with promising therapeutic results of novel BoNT-A applications, including DV, BPH, and chronic prostatitis. However, not all patients of functional urology disorders refractory to conventional therapy can benefit from BoNT-A treatment, possibly because the underlying pathophysiology of these diseases has not been entirely clarified.

List of Abbreviations

Ach	acetylcholine
ATP	adenosine triphosphate
BND	bladder neck dysfunction
BoNT	botulinum toxin
BoNT-A	Botulinum toxin A
BPH	benign prostatic hyperplasia
CNS	central nervous system
DO	detrusor overactivity
DSD	detrusor-sphincter dyssynergia
DV	dysfunctional voiding
IC/BPS	interstitial cystitis/bladder pain syndrome
IDO	idiopathic detrusor overactivity
IPSS	international prostate symptom score
LUTD	lower urinary tract disease
LUTS	lower urinary tract symptoms
NDO	neurogenic detrusor overactivity
NGF	nerve growth factor
NO	nitric oxide
OAB	overactive bladder
P2X	purinergic receptors
P2X2	P2X purinoceptor 2
P2X3	P2X purinoceptor 3
PKC	protein kinase C
SCI	spinal cord injury
SNAP	synaptosomal nerve associated protein
SNAP-25	synaptosomal nerve associated protein 25
SNAP-23	synaptosomal nerve associated protein 23
SNARE	SNAP receptor
SV2	synaptic vesicle protein
t-SNARE	target membrane SNAP receptor
TRPV1	transient receptor potential vanilloid subfamily-1
VEGF	vascular endothelial growth factor

References

1. Naumann, M.; Jankovic, J. Safety of botulinum toxin type a: A systematic review and meta-analysis. *Curr. Med Res. Opin.* **2004**, *20*, 981–990. [CrossRef] [PubMed]
2. Fonfria, E.; Maignel, J.; Lezmi, S.; Martin, V.; Splevins, A.; Shubber, S.; Kalinichev, M.; Foster, K.; Picaut, P.; Krupp, J. The expanding therapeutic utility of botulinum neurotoxins. *Toxins* **2018**, *10*, 208. [CrossRef] [PubMed]
3. Erbguth, F.J. Historical notes on botulism, clostridium botulinum, botulinum toxin, and the idea of the therapeutic use of the toxin. *Mov. Disord. Off. J. Mov. Disord. Soc.* **2004**, *19*, S2–S6. [CrossRef] [PubMed]
4. Arnon, S.S.; Schechter, R.; Inglesby, T.V.; Henderson, D.A.; Bartlett, J.G.; Ascher, M.S.; Eitzen, E.; Fine, A.D.; Hauer, J.; Layton, M.; et al. Botulinum toxin as a biological weapon: Medical and public health management. *JAMA* **2001**, *285*, 1059–1070. [CrossRef] [PubMed]
5. Scott, A.B. Botulinum toxin injection of eye muscles to correct strabismus. *Trans. Am. Ophthalmol. Soc.* **1981**, *79*, 734–770. [PubMed]
6. Charles, P.D. Botulinum neurotoxin serotype a: A clinical update on non-cosmetic uses. *Am. J. Health-Syst. Pharm. AJHP Off. J. Am. Soc. Health-Syst. Pharm.* **2004**, *61*, S11–S23. [CrossRef]
7. Brown, E.A.; Schutz, S.G.; Simpson, D.M. Botulinum toxin for neuropathic pain and spasticity: An overview. *Pain Manag.* **2014**, *4*, 129–151. [CrossRef]
8. Park, J.; Park, H.J. Botulinum toxin for the treatment of neuropathic pain. *Toxins* **2017**, *9*, 260. [CrossRef]
9. Dykstra, D.D.; Sidi, A.A.; Scott, A.B.; Pagel, J.M.; Goldish, G.D. Effects of botulinum a toxin on detrusor-sphincter dyssynergia in spinal cord injury patients. *J. Urol.* **1988**, *139*, 919–922. [CrossRef]
10. Schurch, B.; Stohrer, M.; Kramer, G.; Schmid, D.M.; Gaul, G.; Hauri, D. Botulinum-a toxin for treating detrusor hyperreflexia in spinal cord injured patients: A new alternative to anticholinergic drugs? Preliminary results. *J. Urol.* **2000**, *164*, 692–697. [CrossRef]
11. Schulte-Baukloh, H.; Weiss, C.; Stolze, T.; Sturzebecher, B.; Knispel, H.H. Botulinum-a toxin for treatment of overactive bladder without detrusor overactivity: Urodynamic outcome and patient satisfaction. *Urology* **2005**, *66*, 82–87. [CrossRef] [PubMed]
12. Kuo, H.C. Urodynamic evidence of effectiveness of botulinum A toxin injection in treatment of detrusor overactivity refractory to anticholinergic agents. *Urology* **2004**, *63*, 868–872. [CrossRef] [PubMed]
13. Maria, G.; Brisinda, G.; Civello, I.M.; Bentivoglio, A.R.; Sganga, G.; Albanese, A. Relief by botulinum toxin of voiding dysfunction due to benign prostatic hyperplasia: Results of a randomized, placebo-controlled study. *Urology* **2003**, *62*, 259–264. [CrossRef]
14. Marberger, M.; Chartier-Kastler, E.; Egerdie, B.; Lee, K.S.; Grosse, J.; Bugarin, D.; Zhou, J.; Patel, A.; Haag-Molkenteller, C. A randomized double-blind placebo-controlled phase 2 dose-ranging study of onabotulinumtoxina in men with benign prostatic hyperplasia. *Eur. Urol.* **2013**, *63*, 496–503. [CrossRef] [PubMed]
15. Smith, C.P.; Radziszewski, P.; Borkowski, A.; Somogyi, G.T.; Boone, T.B.; Chancellor, M.B. Botulinum toxin a has antinociceptive effects in treating interstitial cystitis. *Urology* **2004**, *64*, 871–875. [CrossRef] [PubMed]
16. Jhang, J.F.; Kuo, H.C. Novel treatment of chronic bladder pain syndrome and other pelvic pain disorders by onabotulinumtoxina injection. *Toxins* **2015**, *7*, 2232–2250. [CrossRef]
17. Rossetto, O.; Pirazzini, M.; Montecucco, C. Botulinum neurotoxins: Genetic, structural and mechanistic insights. *Nat. Rev. Microbiol.* **2014**, *12*, 535–549. [CrossRef]
18. Dong, M.; Yeh, F.; Tepp, W.H.; Dean, C.; Johnson, E.A.; Janz, R.; Chapman, E.R. Sv2 is the protein receptor for botulinum neurotoxin A. *Science* **2006**, *312*, 592–596. [CrossRef]
19. Coelho, A.; Dinis, P.; Pinto, R.; Gorgal, T.; Silva, C.; Silva, A.; Silva, J.; Cruz, C.D.; Cruz, F.; Avelino, A. Distribution of the high-affinity binding site and intracellular target of botulinum toxin type a in the human bladder. *Eur. Urol.* **2010**, *57*, 884–890. [CrossRef]
20. Hanna-Mitchell, A.T.; Wolf-Johnston, A.S.; Barrick, S.R.; Kanai, A.J.; Chancellor, M.B.; de Groat, W.C.; Birder, L.A. Effect of botulinum toxin a on urothelial-release of ATP and expression of snare targets within the urothelium. *Neurourol. Urodyn.* **2015**, *34*, 79–84. [CrossRef]

21. Vaidyanathan, V.V.; Yoshino, K.; Jahnz, M.; Dorries, C.; Bade, S.; Nauenburg, S.; Niemann, H.; Binz, T. Proteolysis of snap-25 isoforms by botulinum neurotoxin types A, C, and E: Domains and amino acid residues controlling the formation of enzyme-substrate complexes and cleavage. *J. Neurochem.* **1999**, *72*, 327–337. [CrossRef] [PubMed]
22. Banerjee, A.; Li, G.; Alexander, E.A.; Schwartz, J.H. Role of snap-23 in trafficking of H^+-ATPase in cultured inner medullary collecting duct cells. *Am. J. Physiol. Cell Physiol.* **2001**, *280*, C775–C781. [CrossRef] [PubMed]
23. Suh, Y.H.; Terashima, A.; Petralia, R.S.; Wenthold, R.J.; Isaac, J.T.R.; Roche, K.W.; Roche, P.A. A neuronal role for SNAP-23 in postsynaptic glutamate receptor trafficking. *Nat. Neurosci.* **2010**, *13*, 338–343. [CrossRef] [PubMed]
24. Cruz, F. Targets for botulinum toxin in the lower urinary tract. *Neurourol. Urodyn.* **2014**, *33*, 31–38. [CrossRef] [PubMed]
25. Smith, C.P.; Gangitano, D.A.; Munoz, A.; Salas, N.A.; Boone, T.B.; Aoki, K.R.; Francis, J.; Somogyi, G.T. Botulinum toxin type a normalizes alterations in urothelial atp and no release induced by chronic spinal cord injury. *Neurochem. Int.* **2008**, *52*, 1068–1075. [CrossRef]
26. Chancellor, M.B.; Fowler, C.J.; Apostolidis, A.; de Groat, W.C.; Smith, C.P.; Somogyi, G.T.; Aoki, K.R. Drug insight: Biological effects of botulinum toxin A in the lower urinary tract. *Nat. Clin. Pract. Urol.* **2008**, *5*, 319–328. [CrossRef]
27. Kanai, A.; Zabbarova, I.; Oefelein, M.; Radziszewski, P.; Ikeda, Y.; Andersson, K.E. Mechanisms of action of botulinum neurotoxins, beta3-adrenergic receptor agonists, and pde5 inhibitors in modulating detrusor function in overactive bladders: Ici-rs 2011. *Neurourol. Urodyn.* **2012**, *31*, 300–308. [CrossRef]
28. Schulte-Baukloh, H.; Priefert, J.; Knispel, H.H.; Lawrence, G.W.; Miller, K.; Neuhaus, J. Botulinum toxin a detrusor injections reduce postsynaptic muscular M_2, M_3, P_2X_2, and P_2X_3 receptors in children and adolescents who have neurogenic detrusor overactivity: A single-blind study. *Urology* **2013**, *81*, 1052–1057. [CrossRef]
29. Cockayne, D.A.; Hamilton, S.G.; Zhu, Q.M.; Dunn, P.M.; Zhong, Y.; Novakovic, S.; Malmberg, A.B.; Cain, G.; Berson, A.; Kassotakis, L.; et al. Urinary bladder hyporeflexia and reduced pain-related behaviour in p2x3-deficient mice. *Nature* **2000**, *407*, 1011–1015. [CrossRef]
30. Yiangou, Y.; Facer, P.; Ford, A.; Brady, C.; Wiseman, O.; Fowler, C.J.; Anand, P. Capsaicin receptor VR1 and atp-gated ion channel p2x3 in human urinary bladder. *BJU Int.* **2001**, *87*, 774–779. [CrossRef]
31. Apostolidis, A.; Popat, R.; Yiangou, Y.; Cockayne, D.; Ford, A.P.; Davis, J.B.; Dasgupta, P.; Fowler, C.J.; Anand, P. Decreased sensory receptors p2x3 and trpv1 in suburothelial nerve fibers following intradetrusor injections of botulinum toxin for human detrusor overactivity. *J. Urol.* **2005**, *174*, 977–982. [CrossRef]
32. Rapp, D.E.; Turk, K.W.; Bales, G.T.; Cook, S.P. Botulinum toxin type a inhibits calcitonin gene-related peptide release from isolated rat bladder. *J. Urol.* **2006**, *175*, 1138–1142. [CrossRef]
33. Lucioni, A.; Bales, G.T.; Lotan, T.L.; McGehee, D.S.; Cook, S.P.; Rapp, D.E. Botulinum toxin type a inhibits sensory neuropeptide release in rat bladder models of acute injury and chronic inflammation. *BJU Int.* **2008**, *101*, 366–370. [CrossRef] [PubMed]
34. Camprubi-Robles, M.; Planells-Cases, R.; Ferrer-Montiel, A. Differential contribution of snare-dependent exocytosis to inflammatory potentiation of trpv1 in nociceptors. *FASEB J. Off. Publ. Fed. Am. Soc. Exp. Biol.* **2009**, *23*, 3722–3733. [CrossRef]
35. Morenilla-Palao, C.; Planells-Cases, R.; Garcia-Sanz, N.; Ferrer-Montiel, A. Regulated exocytosis contributes to protein kinase c potentiation of vanilloid receptor activity. *J. Biol. Chem.* **2004**, *279*, 25665–25672. [CrossRef] [PubMed]
36. Smith, C.P.; Vemulakonda, V.M.; Kiss, S.; Boone, T.B.; Somogyi, G.T. Enhanced ATP release from rat bladder urothelium during chronic bladder inflammation: Effect of botulinum toxin a. *Neurochem. Int.* **2005**, *47*, 291–297. [CrossRef] [PubMed]
37. Pinto, R.; Lopes, T.; Silva, J.; Silva, C.; Dinis, P.; Cruz, F. Persistent therapeutic effect of repeated injections of onabotulinum toxin a in refractory bladder pain syndrome/interstitial cystitis. *J. Urol.* **2013**, *189*, 548–553. [CrossRef] [PubMed]
38. Kuo, H.C.; Chancellor, M.B. Comparison of intravesical botulinum toxin type A injections plus hydrodistention with hydrodistention alone for the treatment of refractory interstitial cystitis/painful bladder syndrome. *BJU Int.* **2009**, *104*, 657–661. [CrossRef]

39. Guo, B.L.; Zheng, C.X.; Sui, B.D.; Li, Y.Q.; Wang, Y.Y.; Yang, Y.L. A closer look to botulinum neurotoxin type a-induced analgesia. *Toxicon Off. J. Int. Soc. Toxinology* **2013**, *71*, 134–139. [CrossRef]
40. Vemulakonda, V.M.; Somogyi, G.T.; Kiss, S.; Salas, N.A.; Boone, T.B.; Smith, C.P. Inhibitory effect of intravesically applied botulinum toxin a in chronic bladder inflammation. *J. Urol.* **2005**, *173*, 621–624. [CrossRef]
41. Gorgal, T.; Charrua, A.; Silva, J.F.; Avelino, A.; Dinis, P.; Cruz, F. Expression of apoptosis-regulating genes in the rat prostate following botulinum toxin type A injection. *BMC Urol.* **2012**, *12*, 1. [CrossRef] [PubMed]
42. Nishiyama, Y.; Yokoyama, T.; Tomizawa, K.; Okamura, K.; Yamamoto, Y.; Matsui, H.; Oguma, K.; Nagai, A.; Kumon, H. Effects of purified newly developed botulinum neurotoxin type a in rat prostate. *Urology* **2009**, *74*, 436–439. [CrossRef] [PubMed]
43. Silva, J.; Pinto, R.; Carvallho, T.; Coelho, A.; Avelino, A.; Dinis, P.; Cruz, F. Mechanisms of prostate atrophy after glandular botulinum neurotoxin type a injection: An experimental study in the rat. *Eur. Urol.* **2009**, *56*, 134–140. [CrossRef] [PubMed]
44. Chuang, Y.C.; Chancellor, M.B. The application of botulinum toxin in the prostate. *J. Urol.* **2006**, *176*, 2375–2382. [CrossRef]
45. Lin, A.T.; Yang, A.H.; Chen, K.K. Effects of botulinum toxin a on the contractile function of dog prostate. *Eur. Urol.* **2007**, *52*, 582–589. [CrossRef]
46. Haylen, B.T.; de Ridder, D.; Freeman, R.M.; Swift, S.E.; Berghmans, B.; Lee, J.; Monga, A.; Petri, E.; Rizk, D.E.; Sand, P.K.; et al. An international urogynecological association (iuga)/international continence society (ics) joint report on the terminology for female pelvic floor dysfunction. *Int. Urogynecol. J.* **2010**, *21*, 5–26. [CrossRef]
47. Lightner, D.J.; Gomelsky, A.; Souter, L.; Vasavada, S.P. Diagnosis and treatment of overactive bladder (non-neurogenic) in adults: Aua/sufu guideline amendment 2019. *J. Urol.* **2019**, *202*, 558–563. [CrossRef]
48. Benner, J.S.; Nichol, M.B.; Rovner, E.S.; Jumadilova, Z.; Alvir, J.; Hussein, M.; Fanning, K.; Trocio, J.N.; Brubaker, L. Patient-reported reasons for discontinuing overactive bladder medication. *BJU Int.* **2010**, *105*, 1276–1282. [CrossRef]
49. Abrams, P.; Cardozo, L.; Fall, M.; Griffiths, D.; Rosier, P.; Ulmsten, U.; van Kerrebroeck, P.; Victor, A.; Wein, A. The standardisation of terminology of lower urinary tract function: Report from the standardisation sub-committee of the international continence society. *Neurourol. Urodyn.* **2002**, *21*, 167–178. [CrossRef]
50. Steers, W.D. Pathophysiology of overactive bladder and urge urinary incontinence. *Rev. Urol.* **2002**, *4*, S17–S18.
51. Birder, L.A.; de Groat, W.C. Mechanisms of disease: Involvement of the urothelium in bladder dysfunction. *Nat. Clin. Pract. Urol.* **2007**, *4*, 46–54. [CrossRef] [PubMed]
52. Lawrence, G.W.; Aoki, K.R.; Dolly, J.O. Excitatory cholinergic and purinergic signaling in bladder are equally susceptible to botulinum neurotoxin a consistent with co-release of transmitters from efferent fibers. *J. Pharmacol. Exp. Ther.* **2010**, *334*, 1080–1086. [CrossRef] [PubMed]
53. Khera, M.; Somogyi, G.T.; Kiss, S.; Boone, T.B.; Smith, C.P. Botulinum toxin a inhibits ATP release from bladder urothelium after chronic spinal cord injury. *Neurochem. Int.* **2004**, *45*, 987–993. [CrossRef] [PubMed]
54. Collins, V.M.; Daly, D.M.; Liaskos, M.; McKay, N.G.; Sellers, D.; Chapple, C.; Grundy, D. Onabotulinumtoxina significantly attenuates bladder afferent nerve firing and inhibits ATP release from the urothelium. *BJU Int.* **2013**, *112*, 1018–1026. [CrossRef]
55. Chancellor, M.B.; Kaplan, S.A.; Blaivas, J.G. Detrusor-external sphincter dyssynergia. *Ciba Found. Symp.* **1990**, *151*, 195–206.
56. Kuo, H.C. Satisfaction with urethral injection of botulinum toxin a for detrusor sphincter dyssynergia in patients with spinal cord lesion. *Neurourol. Urodyn.* **2008**, *27*, 793–796. [CrossRef]
57. Huang, M.; Chen, H.; Jiang, C.; Xie, K.; Tang, P.; Ou, R.; Zeng, J.; Liu, Q.; Li, Q.; Huang, J.; et al. Effects of botulinum toxin a injections in spinal cord injury patients with detrusor overactivity and detrusor sphincter dyssynergia. *J. Rehabil. Med.* **2016**, *48*, 683–687. [CrossRef]
58. Osman, N.I.; Chapple, C.R. Fowler's syndrome—a cause of unexplained urinary retention in young women? Nature reviews. *Urology* **2014**, *11*, 87–98.
59. Carlson, K.V.; Rome, S.; Nitti, V.W. Dysfunctional voiding in women. *J. Urol.* **2001**, *165*, 143–147. [CrossRef]

60. Panicker, J.N.; Seth, J.H.; Khan, S.; Gonzales, G.; Haslam, C.; Kessler, T.M.; Fowler, C.J. Open-label study evaluating outpatient urethral sphincter injections of onabotulinumtoxina to treat women with urinary retention due to a primary disorder of sphincter relaxation (fowler's syndrome). *BJU Int.* **2016**, *117*, 809–813. [CrossRef]
61. Jiang, Y.H.; Wang, C.C.; Kuo, H.C. Onabotulinumtoxina urethral sphincter injection as treatment for non-neurogenic voiding dysfunction—A randomized, double-blind, placebo-controlled study. *Sci. Rep.* **2016**, *6*, 38905. [CrossRef] [PubMed]
62. Jiang, Y.H.; Chen, S.F.; Jhang, J.F.; Kuo, H.C. Therapeutic effect of urethral sphincter onabotulinumtoxina injection for urethral sphincter hyperactivity. *Neurourol. Urodyn.* **2018**, *37*, 2651–2657. [CrossRef] [PubMed]
63. Kuo, H.C. Videourodynamic characteristics and lower urinary tract symptoms of female bladder outlet obstruction. *Urology* **2005**, *66*, 1005–1009. [CrossRef] [PubMed]
64. Abbott, J.A.; Jarvis, S.K.; Lyons, S.D.; Thomson, A.; Vancaille, T.G. Botulinum toxin type a for chronic pain and pelvic floor spasm in women: A randomized controlled trial. *Obstet. Gynecol.* **2006**, *108*, 915–923. [CrossRef] [PubMed]
65. Sacco, E.; Tienforti, D.; Bientinesi, R.; D'Addessi, A.; Racioppi, M.; Pinto, F.; Totaro, A.; Vittori, M.; D'Agostino, D.; Bassi, P. Onabotulinumtoxina injection therapy in men with luts due to primary bladder-neck dysfunction: Objective and patient-reported outcomes. *Neurourol. Urodyn.* **2014**, *33*, 142–146. [CrossRef] [PubMed]
66. Sun, Y.; Keay, S.; Lehrfeld, T.J.; Chai, T.C. Changes in adenosine triphosphate-stimulated ATP release suggest association between cytokine and purinergic signaling in bladder urothelial cells. *Urology* **2009**, *74*, 1163–1168. [CrossRef] [PubMed]
67. Liu, B.L.; Yang, F.; Zhan, H.L.; Feng, Z.Y.; Zhang, Z.G.; Li, W.B.; Zhou, X.F. Increased severity of inflammation correlates with elevated expression of TRPV1 nerve fibers and nerve growth factor on interstitial cystitis/bladder pain syndrome. *Urol. Int.* **2014**, *92*, 202–208. [CrossRef] [PubMed]
68. Pang, X.; Marchand, J.; Sant, G.R.; Kream, R.M.; Theoharides, T.C. Increased number of substance p positive nerve fibres in interstitial cystitis. *Br. J. Urol.* **1995**, *75*, 744–750. [CrossRef] [PubMed]
69. Mizumura, K.; Murase, S. Role of nerve growth factor in pain. *Handb. Exp. Pharmacol.* **2015**, *227*, 57–77. [PubMed]
70. Liu, H.T.; Kuo, H.C. Increased urine and serum nerve growth factor levels in interstitial cystitis suggest chronic inflammation is involved in the pathogenesis of disease. *PLoS ONE* **2012**, *7*, e44687. [CrossRef]
71. Apostolidis, A.; Dasgupta, P.; Fowler, C.J. Proposed mechanism for the efficacy of injected botulinum toxin in the treatment of human detrusor overactivity. *Eur. Urol.* **2006**, *49*, 644–650. [CrossRef] [PubMed]
72. Liu, H.T.; Kuo, H.C. Intravesical botulinum toxin a injections plus hydrodistension can reduce nerve growth factor production and control bladder pain in interstitial cystitis. *Urology* **2007**, *70*, 463–468. [CrossRef] [PubMed]
73. Liu, H.T.; Tyagi, P.; Chancellor, M.B.; Kuo, H.C. Urinary nerve growth factor level is increased in patients with interstitial cystitis/bladder pain syndrome and decreased in responders to treatment. *BJU Int.* **2009**, *104*, 1476–1481. [CrossRef] [PubMed]
74. Shie, J.H.; Liu, H.T.; Wang, Y.S.; Kuo, H.C. Immunohistochemical evidence suggests repeated intravesical application of botulinum toxin a injections may improve treatment efficacy of interstitial cystitis/bladder pain syndrome. *BJU Int.* **2013**, *111*, 638–646. [CrossRef]
75. Peng, C.H.; Jhang, J.F.; Shie, J.H.; Kuo, H.C. Down regulation of vascular endothelial growth factor is associated with decreased inflammation after intravesical onabotulinumtoxina injections combined with hydrodistention for patients with interstitial cystitis–clinical results and immunohistochemistry analysis. *Urology* **2013**, *82*, e1451–e1456.
76. Lloyd, G.L.; Marks, J.M.; Ricke, W.A. Benign prostatic hyperplasia and lower urinary tract symptoms: What is the role and significance of inflammation? *Curr. Urol. Rep.* **2019**, *20*, 54. [CrossRef]
77. White, C.W.; Xie, J.H.; Ventura, S. Age-related changes in the innervation of the prostate gland: Implications for prostate cancer initiation and progression. *Organogenesis* **2013**, *9*, 206–215. [CrossRef]
78. Antunes, A.A.; Srougi, M.; Coelho, R.F.; de Campos Freire, G. Botulinum toxin for the treatment of lower urinary tract symptoms due to benign prostatic hyperplasia. *Nat. Clin. Pract. Urol.* **2007**, *4*, 155–160. [CrossRef]

79. Rusnack, S.R.; Kaplan, S.A. The use of botulinum toxin in men with benign prostatic hyperplasia. *Rev. Urol.* **2005**, *7*, 234–236.
80. Sacco, E.; Bientinesi, R.; Marangi, F.; Totaro, A.; D'Addessi, A.; Racioppi, M.; Pinto, F.; Vittori, M.; Bassi, P. Patient-reported outcomes in men with lower urinary tract symptoms (luts) due to benign prostatic hyperplasia (bph) treated with intraprostatic onabotulinumtoxina: 3-month results of a prospective single-armed cohort study. *BJU Int.* **2012**, *110*, E837–E844. [CrossRef]
81. Hamidi Madani, A.; Enshaei, A.; Heidarzadeh, A.; Mokhtari, G.; Farzan, A.; Mohiti Asli, M.; Esmaeili, S. Transurethral intraprostatic botulinum toxin-A injection: A novel treatment for bph refractory to current medical therapy in poor surgical candidates. *World J. Urol.* **2013**, *31*, 235–239. [CrossRef] [PubMed]
82. Chen, C.H.; Tyagi, P.; Chuang, Y.C. Promise and the pharmacological mechanism of botulinum toxin A in chronic prostatitis syndrome. *Toxins* **2019**, *11*, 586. [CrossRef] [PubMed]

20

Effect of Botulinum Toxin A on Bladder Pain—Molecular Evidence and Animal Studies

Ting-Chun Yeh [1], Po-Cheng Chen [2], Yann-Rong Su [3] and Hann-Chorng Kuo [4,*]

1 Division of Urology, Department of Surgery, Taiwan Adventist Hospital, Taipei City 105, Taiwan; breadtree100@gmail.com
2 Department of Urology, En Chu Kong Hospital, New Taipei City 237, Taiwan; b90401049@ntu.edu.tw
3 Department of Urology, National Taiwan University Hospital Hsin-Chu Branch, Hsinchu City 300, Taiwan; yrsu@hch.gov.tw
4 Department of Urology, Hualien Tzu Chi Hospital, Buddhist Tzu Chi Medical Foundation and Tzu Chi University, Hualien City 970, Taiwan
* Correspondence: hck@tzuchi.com.tw

Abstract: Botulinum toxin A (BTX-A) is a powerful neurotoxin with long-lasting activity that blocks muscle contractions. In addition to effects on neuromuscular junctions, BTX-A also plays a role in sensory feedback loops, suggesting the potentiality for pain relief. Although the only approved indications for BTX-A in the bladder are neurogenic detrusor overactivity and refractory overactive bladder, BTX-A injections to treat bladder pain refractory to conventional therapies are also recommended. The mechanism of BTX-A activity in bladder pain is complex, with several hypotheses proposed in recent studies. Here we comprehensively reviewed properties of BTX-A in peripheral afferent and efferent nerves, the inhibition of nociceptive neurotransmitter release, the reduction of stretch-related visceral pain, and its anti-inflammatory effects on the bladder urothelium. Studies have also revealed possible effects of BTX-A in the human brain. However, further basic and clinical studies are warranted to provide solid evidence-based support in using BTX-A to treat bladder pain.

Keywords: botulinum toxin A; bladder pain; interstitial cystitis; molecular mechanism

Key Contribution: This article comprehensively reviewed molecular mechanisms of the analgesic effects of BTX-A and summarized the properties of BTX-A used to treat bladder pain in both peripheral and central nervous pathways.

---

1. Introduction

Botulinum toxin, one of the most powerful neurotoxins in nature, is produced by the anaerobic, Gram-positive organism, *Clostridium botulinum*. Exposure to the botulinum toxin can be fatal, since this can lead to flaccid paralysis of the muscles, dysautonomia, and subsequent respiratory failure [1]. Of the seven distinct serotypes (A through G), botulinum toxin A (BTX-A) shows the longest duration of activity in blocking transmission at the neuromuscular junctions, making it the most popular form for clinical use. In 1988, Dykstra et al. were the first to use BTX-A in a urological application by injecting it into the urethral sphincter to treat detrusor sphincter dyssynergia in spinal cord injury patients [2].

Nowadays, BTX-A injection has been widely used in lower urinary tract diseases and is approved for patients with both overactive bladder (OAB) and neurogenic detrusor overactivity (NDO). In addition to OAB and NDO, using a BTX-A injection to treat the pain of interstitial cystitis/bladder pain syndrome (IC/BPS) is recommended in patients refractory to conventional therapies [3]. IC/BPS is a long-time challenge for urologists who treat its multifactorial conditions and accompanying pain.

Recently, it was recognized that the disease not only has organ-specific syndromes, but also urogenital manifestations of regional or systemic abnormalities characterized by neuropathic pain [4].

The mechanism of BTX-A activity on bladder pain has been investigated: it possibly affects both afferent and efferent nerves, along with having an antinociceptive mode of action [5]. Here we reviewed current molecular and cellular evidence and related animal studies for a better general understanding of the mechanism of action of BTX-A in bladder pain.

2. Results

2.1. Basic Mechanism of Action of BTX-A

Inactive BTX-A is a single-chain polypeptide of 150 kDa. When BTX-A is pharmacologically activated, it is cleaved to a 100-kDa heavy chain and a 50-kDa light chain that are connected by a single disulfide bond as well as noncovalent bonds [1,6]. BTX-A inhibits or reduces muscle contractions by blocking vesicular neurotransmitter release at neuroglandular and neuromuscular junctions. Two types of presynaptic cell membrane surface receptors for BTX-A have been identified—gangliosides and the synaptic vesicle-associated protein-2 (SV2) family. BTX-A binds to nerve terminals because of the high affinity of its heavy chain for SV2 allowing the toxin to be endocytosed into synaptic vesicles [7]. The light chain of BTX-A is translocated across the vesicle membrane in an acidic environment, and is then released into the cytosol by reduction of the interchain disulfide bond. Following its release from vesicles, the light chain is able to cleave synaptosomal-associated protein 25 (SNAP25) proteins, a part of a heterotrimeric soluble N-ethylmaleimide-sensitive factor attachment protein receptor (SNARE) complex, thereby inhibiting the fusion of vesicles with the nerve terminal membrane, and ensuring the blockade of neurotransmitter release and consequent smooth muscle contractions [8].

When using BTX-A to treat lower urinary tract diseases, the net effect results in: (1) the paralysis of low-grade contractions of the unstable detrusor to increase bladder capacity and reduce detrusor pressure during filling and resting phases, and (2) the preservation of high-grade contractions of the detrusor to initiate micturition [9–11]. In addition to this effect, a significant reduction in the sensation of urinary urgency has been reported by patients with OAB, suggesting a sensory effect on the bladder [12]. The effects on sensory feedback loops explain the mechanism of BTX-A activity in relieving symptoms of detrusor overactivity as well as suggest a potential role for BTX-A in the relief of hyperalgesia-associated lower urinary tract disorders, such as IC/BPS and chronic pelvic pain syndrome [9].

2.2. BTX Effects on Peripheral Sensory Nerves

Chronic pain persisting from months to years can reduce people's quality of life and become a major health-care burden. The pathophysiology of chronic pain can be classified as inflammation, neuropathic pain, or dysfunction [13]. Jankovic et al. described the first clinical application of BTX on cervical focal dystonia and hemifacial spasms. They observed an improvement in the pain of these patients, supporting an antinociceptive or afferent-mediated activity by BTX-A [14]. This finding initiated an era of research on the analgesic effects of BTX-A. Figure 1 shows the proposed mechanism of BTX-A effects on peripheral sensory system.

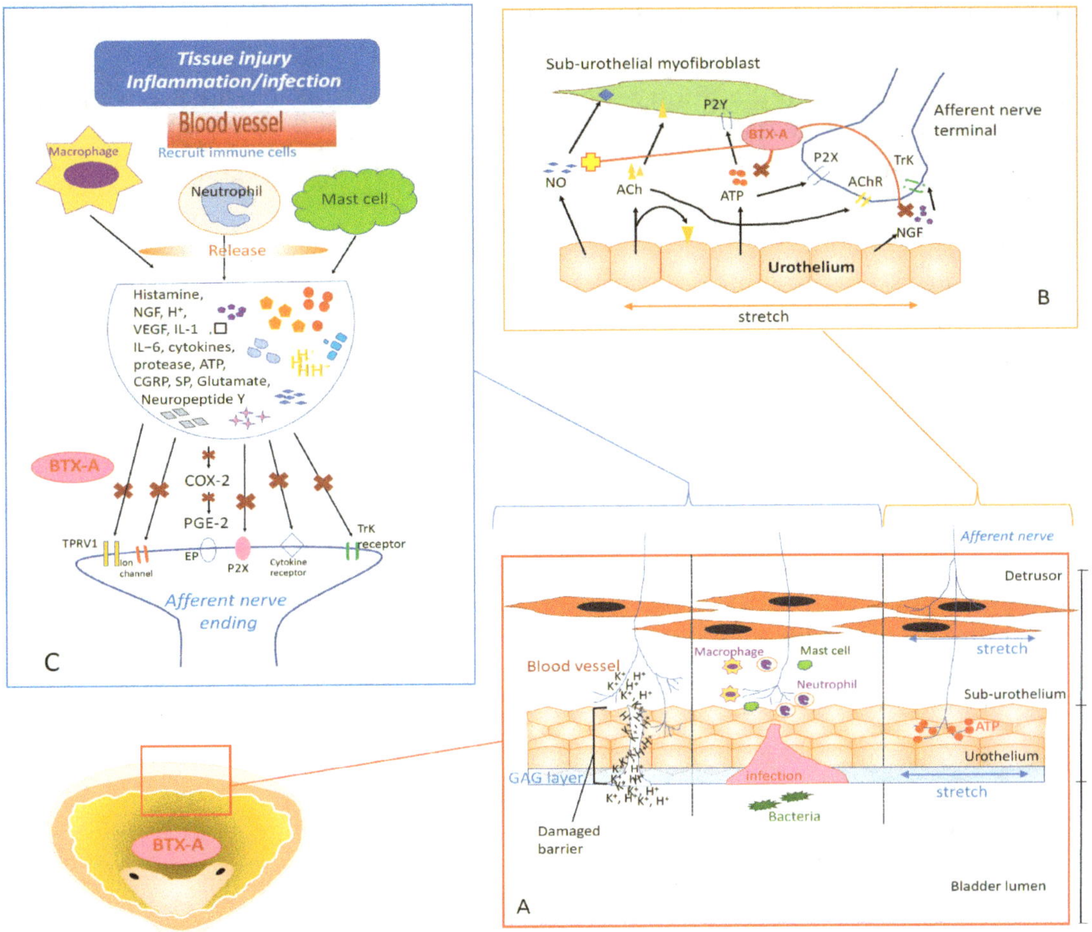

Figure 1. Mechanism of Intravesical BTX-A Effects on Peripheral Nervous System. (**A**) Afferent nerves innervate bladder sensation and carry information toward the central nervous system (CNS). Bladder-stretching is detected by the afferent nerve endings that extend into detrusor smooth muscles. The afferent nerve terminals extend into urothelium and sub-urothelial interstitium. These nerve terminals are sensitized when bacteria invade urothelium or high potassium ion penetrate after the urothelial barrier breaks down. (**B**) When bladder distention, the stretching urothelium releases neurotransmitters, including ATP, NGF, acetylcholine, and NO to activate afferent nerves. BTX-A blocks the afferent input by normalizing the balance of NO and ATP (blocks ATP and enhances NO). Besides, BTX-A dampens NGF, leads to attenuation of afferent excitability. (**C**) Immune cells including mast cells, macrophages and neutrophils were recruited by the cytokines released during bacterial infection or tissue damage. Histamine, interleukins, neuropeptides and more cytokines are subsequently released, which activates the bladder afferents.

2.2.1. Bladder Stretch (Spasm)-Related Visceral Pain

One possible pathomechanism of visceral pain has been proposed recently: tension-sensitive nerve terminals in the smooth muscle of hollow organs may respond to luminal distension or stretching [15,16]. In the bladder, BTX-A acts in detrusor muscle relaxation by inhibiting acetylcholine (Ach) release from parasympathetic nerve endings [17] (Figure 1, part B).

The transient receptor potential (TRP) superfamily of cationic ion channels is involved in many cellular functions and such channels are highly expressed in afferent neurons of the urinary bladder [18]. Members of the TRP channel superfamily include TRP vanilloid 1 (TRPV1), TRPV4, and TRP Ankyrin 1 (TRPA1), involved in the mechanosensory pathway of urothelial cells. Activation of such ion channels releases adenosine triphosphate (ATP), prostaglandin E2 (PGE2), and substance P, and causes visceral pain [18–20]. Therefore, it is inferred that the function of muscle paralysis by BTX-A is to help decrease bladder tension, reduce bladder spasms, downregulate such TRP channels, and consequently relieve bladder pain.

Chuang et al. had observed that intravesical BTX-A administration could significantly prolong the inter-contraction interval (ICI) of the bladder and produce analgesia against acetic acid-induced bladder pain in rats by inhibiting calcitonin gene-related peptide (CGRP) release from afferent nerve terminals [21].

When the bladder is distended, ligand-gated ion channel P2X purinoceptors 3 (P2X3) receptors on nerve endings in the bladder urothelium are activated by released ATP and evoke a neural discharge [22]. In an in vitro study, P2X3 subunits expressed by cultured IC bladder urothelial cells were upregulated during stretching; augmented ATP signaling in the bladder may explain IC symptoms [23]. Hanna-Mitchell et al. [24] and Collins et al. [25] demonstrated that the intravesical administration of BTX-A is effective in reducing stretch-induced ATP release in rats and mice models.

2.2.2. Inhibition of Nociceptive Neurotransmitter Release in Peripheral Endings

The antinociceptive effects of BTX-A were initially considered in simple muscle relaxation. Recent studies found muscle relaxation effects may not directly overlap with pain relief, which implies that the mechanism of action of BTX-A in pain relief is more complex than first thought and may have possible effects on sensory neurons [26,27]. Of note, the analgesic effects of BTX-A often persist longer than the neuroparalytic effects, which indicates that BTX-A affects pain fibers or sensory nerves.

Unmyelinated C-fibers and lightly myelinated Aδ-fibers are two types of nerve fibers that transmit sensory information from the bladder [28,29]. C-fibers are the primary nociceptive fibers that innervate the suburothelium of the bladder. Under normal conditions, C-fibers are silent but become activated in several pathological conditions, such as the alteration of potassium channels. Activated C-fibers result in increased excitability, the transmission of painful stimuli, and increased afferent drive that consequently contributes to detrusor hyperreflexia [29].

Nerve growth factor (NGF) influences C-fiber hyperexcitability in studies done by Vizzard et al. [30] and Seki et al. [31]. They observed increased NGF levels in the bladder, spinal cord, and lumbosacral dorsal root ganglia (DRG) in animals with spinal cord injury or chronic cystitis that exhibited bladder overactivity. Yoshimura et al. [32] set up a study to mimic this mechanism by intrathecally injecting NGF into female rats. Cystometrograms showed a reduction in ICI and voided volume, indicating bladder overactivity. Liu and Kuo [33] confirmed that intravesical BTX-A treatment can reduce NGF production to a normal level and control pain in IC/BPS patients.

C-fibers also release neuropeptides such as CGRP and substance P (SP), which are upregulated in patients with IC/BPS [34]. Numerous studies have shown that BTX-A blocks the release of nociceptive neurotransmitters from peripheral sensory nerves [35]. Durham et al. provided the first evidence that BTX-A directly decreases the release of CGRP from trigeminal neurons [36]. Welch et al. reported that BTX-A inhibits the release of CGRP, glutamate, and SP from cultured embryonic rat DRG [37]. BTX-A inhibition of the stimulated release of CGRP and SP from afferent nerve terminals has also been confirmed ex vivo by Lucioni et al. in rats with cyclophosphamide (CYP)-induced cystitis [38] and Rapp et al. in a capsaicin-evoked rat bladder model [39]. The antinociceptive effects of BTX-A in peripheral endings are depicted in Figure 2.

TRPV1 is a vanilloid receptor expressed in C-fibers that are involved in pain transmission after activation by heat, capsaicin, or resiniferatoxin [40]. A previous study showed that increased severity of inflammation correlated with a higher expression of TRPV1-immunoreactive nerve fibers and NGF levels in bladder biopsies from IC/BPS patients [41].

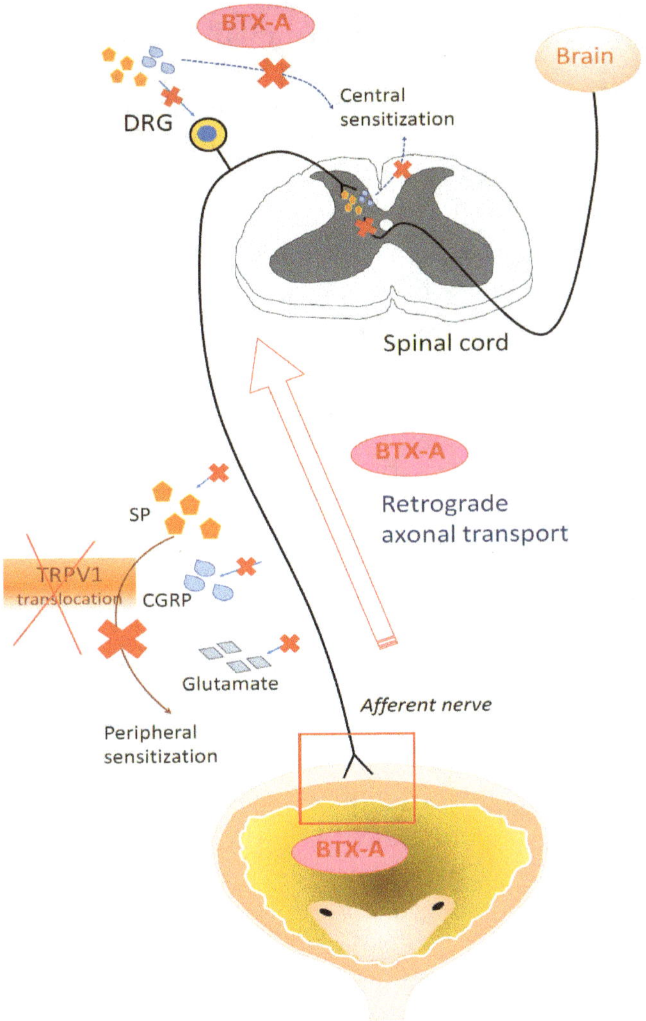

Figure 2. Illustration of Actions of BTX-A along the pain pathway. (1) BTX-A blocks the release of nociceptive neurotransmitters (SP, glutamate and CGRP) from afferent nerve endings and the translocation of TRPV receptor, leading to peripheral desensitization and results in attenuation of inflammation and pain. (2) Intravesical-injected BTX-A gains access to dorsal root ganglia (DRG) and spinal cord via retrograde axonal transport pathway. By blocking SP and CGRP there, BTX-A inhibits further central sensitization.

In addition to C-fibers, BTX-A may also affect Aδ-fibers. In an in vitro mouse preparation, BTX-A weakened both low- and high-threshold afferent units firing during bladder distension, suggesting that it acts on both Aδ- and C-fibers [25]. This same study revealed a five-fold increase in nitric oxide (NO) in urothelium after BTX-A administration. The increase in NO may have diminished afferent activity by acting as an inhibitory transmitter on myofibroblasts or the urothelium [42]. A balance in urothelial neurotransmitters between excitatory ATP and inhibitory NO has been proposed to modulate afferent activity and it would seem that BTX-A contributed to normalizing this balance [43].

2.2.3. Anti-inflammatory Effects of BTX-A in Bladder Urothelium

Inflammation-induced afferent sensitization to recruit immune cells is an important protective mechanism to resist infection in the urinary tract [44,45] (Figure 1, part C). However, prolonged inflammation may result in the long-lasting sensitization of afferents and lead to chronic pain [45]. Most experts believe that bladder pain can be attributed to chronic inflammation although the pathogenesis is still inconclusive due to contradictory histopathology results. However, an increase in proinflammatory mediators (histamine, NGF, and those released from mast cells) within the bladder and urine of IC/BPS patients has been widely reported, which is consistent with the hypothesis of inflammation causing bladder pain [46–48]. Cui et al. [49] were the first to describe the direct involvement of BTX-A in pain modulation after inhibiting inflammation. Formalin-induced edema and accompanying peripheral glutamate release were reduced by intraplantar BTX-A injection in rats.

To investigate the inflammatory-mediated pathophysiology of bladder pain, a range of irritants or immune stimulants, including CYP, lipopolysaccharide, acetic acid, acrolein, and protamine sulfate, have been administered in animal models [50]. Altered cystometry and an enhanced visceromotor response during bladder distension were shown in experimental animals, which mimicked a reduced bladder capacity and the hyperalgesia and allodynia observed in response to bladder distension in humans [45,51].

Chuang et al. [52] also reported that BTX-A intravesical injection reduced cyclooxygenase 2 (COX2) and PGE2 receptor expression in the bladders of rats with CYP-induced cystitis. In humans, Shie et al. [53] disclosed that repeated BTX-A injections significantly reduced the number of activated mast cells in the bladder. In another study, vascular endothelial growth factor (VEGF) expression and the apoptotic cell count were decreased in patients with IC/BPS after repeated BTX-A injections [54].

Increased Urothelial Permeability after Inflammation/Infection

Increased bladder permeability is believed to be a part of the underlying pathology of bladder hypersensitivity and hyperalgesia in IC/BPS patients or occur secondary to localized inflammation [45]. Many studies have pointed out that patients with IC/BPS, but not OAB, have a damaged or ulcerative, thin urothelium [55]. Liu et al. [56] confirmed results that identified mast cell infiltration in both the OAB and IC/BPS bladder wall, but showed reduced expression of the tight junction protein, zona occludens-1; E-cadherin was only detected in IC/BPS tissues. Glycosaminoglycan (GAG) replacement therapy with pentosane polysulfate (PPS) has been shown to improve bladder pain for some IC/BPS patients [57]. This may be due to the repair and recovery of a tight urothelial barrier maintained by GAG, the anti-inflammatory actions of PPS, and the inhibition of mast cell histamine release [58]. Although effects of BTX-A on urothelial barrier proteins have not been reported, it is reasonable to suggest that BTX-A injection may be beneficial for relieving bladder pain by inhibiting the localized inflammation of urothelium, reducing the numbers of activated mast cells [53], and blocking the subsequent release of inflammatory mediators, such as histamine, cytokines, and proteases, therefore desensitizing peripheral afferent nerve endings [59].

Amplified Sensory Symptoms after Inflammation

It has been observed that women with a history of recurrent urinary tract infection in childhood are more prone to be diagnosed with IC/BPS later in life [60]. This phenomenon may be due to a protective hypersensitive response during the remission process after a preceding bladder infection or inflammation. Basic studies have demonstrated that bladder insults in neonatal rats lead to a hypersensitive response to inflammation stimuli when tested in adults [61], and strengthens the spontaneous bladder distension-evoked activity of spinal visceral nociceptive neurons [62]. Altered spinal cord circuits regulate this situation because neonatal inflammation can prompt a downregulation of GABA (Aα-1) receptor microRNA and altered opioid peptide content in the dorsal horn [63,64].

2.3. BTX Effects in Bladder Urothelium and Lamina Propria

The bladder sensory system is complex and encompasses not only local afferent nerves, but also the bladder urothelium and lamina propria (LP), thus including the entire bladder mucosa. The urothelium was previously viewed as merely a passive blood-urine permeability barrier; however, it now apparently plays an active role in the bladder's sensory system by having certain "neuronal-like properties" [65]. In vitro studies have shown that some neurotransmitters, including NO, ATP, Ach, and prostaglandins, are released from the urothelium after the application of chemical or physical stressors [66]. BTX-A is able to bind to the toxin's receptor, SV2, within bladder urothelium and suppress hypotonic-evoked ATP release from rat urothelial cultures [24]. The LP lies between the urothelium and detrusor muscle, and contains mainly connective tissue, lymphatics, and abundant vasculatures [67]. The LP consists of afferent and efferent nerve endings, and acts as a "communication center" to integrate signals of the urothelium and local afferent nerve terminals [68]. Two specific kinds of cells, telocytes (Tc) and myofibroblasts (Myo), constitute a three-dimensional (3D) network structure in the LP that acts as a mass of stretch-receptors capable of perceiving physical and chemical stimuli and consequently behaving as a "functional syncytium" [69]. The Myo/Tc 3D network contributes to bladder compliance, avoids organ deformity and expresses muscarinic, vanilloid, and purinergic receptors that recognize signals from the urothelium and afferent nerve terminals to propagate information through this network to the bladder detrusor [69]. BTX-A was proposed to induce phenotypic changes in the Myo/Tc network, including the inhibition of expression of purinergic and SP receptors, and a reduction in the expression of contractile and gap junction proteins [70].

Nerve Sprouting and Exhaustion of BTX efficacy

The progressive loss of BTX-A efficacy can be seen during the treatment. When BTX-A was injected into a striated muscle, the efficacy persisted till antibodies against BTX-A were formed [71]. In the bladder, however, the phenomenon of losing BTX-A effectiveness may not work the same [68].

While BTX-A injection blocks nerve terminals, new nerve endings sprout to restore synaptic activity. Haferkamp et al. [72] biopsied the urothelium and LP of NDO patients, before and after the first BTX-A injection, and found axonal degeneration, nerve sprouting, and Schwann cell activation. In order to transduce signals correctly within the bladder sensory system, an appropriate distance between cells is necessary. Since sprouting is likely to be disorganized, the integration of signaling inside the LP system may be disturbed [71]. The excitation of new sprouting afferent nerve endings contributes to chronic neurogenic inflammation. Inflammation also activates the sensory nerve endings of the LP and causes the release of neuropeptides (SP, ATP, CGRP, neuropeptide Y) that mediate multidirectional interactions in Myo/Tc multicellular networks, and acts on endothelial, smooth muscle, and immune cells, and even back on nerve endings. These effects cause a positive feedback loop and turn into a vicious cycle [73]. The exhaustion of BTX efficacy is observed in NDO patients and may be due to the growth of afferent sprouts after repeated injections, which produce a chain reaction over time by maintaining and amplifying neurogenic inflammation [68].

2.4. BTX Effects in Central Nervous System

So far, the analgesic properties of BTX-A have been widely investigated in a variety of pain models. During investigations the following interesting observations were noted: (1) the effects induced by BTX-A administration are observed distantly from the site of injection; and (2) BTX-A affects not only the peripheral but also the central nervous system (CNS) [74]. In the experiments with radiolabeled BTX-A, the retrograde transport of BTX-A to the CNS has been recognized for decades [75]. However, the neurotoxin was thought to be possibly inactivated when reaching the CNS due to the slow rate of retrograde axonal transport [76]. Restani et al. observed that BTX-A was internalized by spinal cord motor neurons and underwent fast axonal retrograde transport by directly monitoring endocytosis and axonal transport of the neurotoxin [77].

The long-distance retrograde effects of BTX-A were thoroughly reported by Antonicci et al. [78]. They were the first to show that BTX-A applied in the peripheral nerves affected central circuits via retrograde transport and transcytosis [78]. The hypothesis of retrograde action of BTX-A in pain pathway is illustrated in Figure 2. In a rat bladder model, the concentrations of radiolabeled BTX-A increased over time in both L6-S1 dorsal root ganglia and L6-S1 spinal cord segments after injections it into the bladders of rats [79]. Because of its retrograde axonal transport to the CNS, the BTX-A neurotoxin may gain access to second-order neurons to affect these.

Interestingly, recent studies described how the unilateral injection of BTX-A can bilaterally reduce pain. These analgesic effects were shown in rat models of paclitaxel-induced peripheral neuropathy, carrageenan-induced hyperalgesia, and acidic saline-induced mirror pain [80–82]. Favre-Guilmard et al. [82] designed a carrageenan-induced pain model by subplantarly injecting BTX-A into experimental rats. Dramatic anti-hyperalgesia effects in uninjected contralateral hind paws of the rats were found in this study, which cannot be explained by the peripheral mechanism of BTX-A. These results suggested that BTX-A might have a central effect via the retrograde axonal transport system, which is also presumed to be the mechanism by which BTX-A acts to induce central neuropathic pain [83].

Intrathecal BTX-A administration by Coelho et al. [84] unlocks a brand new field of investigation into a deeper understanding of the actions of BTX-A [85]. This brilliant study, using animal models of severe bladder pain, described the administration of BTX-A via an alternative intrathecal route, which effectively functioned while undesirable side effects were avoided, including decreased detrusor pressure and increased post-void residual in bladder injections. This intrathecal route of administration was further investigated for intractable or refractory patterns of pain [6].

A recent breakthrough study using concurrent functional magnetic resonance imaging (fMRI) and urodynamic studies in female patients with multiple sclerosis and neurogenic overactive bladders reported that an intradetrusor injection of BTX-A increased the activity of most brain regions (cingulate body, prefrontal cortex, insula, and pontine micturition center) involved in the sensation and process of urinary urgency [86]. This was a pilot study to evaluate the possible effects of BTX-A at the level of the brain where sensory awareness is located. However, to date and to the best of our knowledge, no available evidence exists which directly demonstrates the effects of BTX-A on ascending bladder pain via a CNS system.

3. Conclusions

BTX-A is a promising option for treating bladder pain. Although the mechanisms involved are complicated, recent research efforts using a growing body of diverse expertise have been fruitful, especially in understanding the molecular architecture of the neurotoxin, as well as in the use of bioengineered animal models and in gaining electrophysiological-based insights. The analgesics effects of BTX-A are thought to be mainly mediated by muscle relaxation as well as the blockage of neurotransmitters and inflammatory substances. Recently, a hypothesis of BTX-A affecting the CNS via retrograde transportation to target neurotransmission in pain sensory circuits has been developed but is still very controversial when applied to humans [87]. Further research on the central action of BTX-A is important and will provide crucial information to better understand the pathophysiology of bladder pain. To date, BTX-A has only been approved by the U.S. Food and Drug Administration for NDO and OAB refractory to first-line therapy. This review comprehensively includes current molecular evidence of the effects of BTX-A on bladder pain. Further basic studies and clinical trials with a large number of patients are required in order to provide much more robust evidence-based support in using BTX-A to treat bladder pain.

4. Materials and Methods

This study is a literature review on the efficacy of BTX-A in bladder pain, focusing on molecular evidence and animal studies. A search for original and review articles was performed on PubMed, MEDLINE, Crossref, Embase, and Google Scholar databases using "botulinum toxin", "molecular model", "animal model", and "bladder pain" as search terms. To expand the scope of the search, we included the following terms: "interstitial cystitis", "hypersensitive bladder", "neuropathic pain", "pain management", "neurotoxin", "neurogenic bladder", and "botulinum toxin injections". This is a non-systemic review that was based on previously published articles. The search results were used to summarize current evidence for the possible molecular mechanism of action of BTX-A on bladder pain.

All papers identified were English-language, full-text papers. We also checked the reference lists of selected articles to identify any papers with potentially missed data.

Author Contributions: Conceptualization, H.-C.K.; methodology, T.-C.Y.; writing—original draft preparation, T.-C.Y.; writing—review and editing, T.-C.Y., P.-C.C. and Y.-R.S.; supervision, H.-C.K. All authors have read and agreed to the published version of the manuscript.

Acknowledgments: This work was greatly enhanced by Han-Chorng Kuo.

References

1. Arnon, S.S.; Schechter, R.; Inglesby, T.V.; Henderson, D.A.; Bartlett, J.G.; Ascher, M.S.; Eitzen, E.; Fine, A.D.; Hauer, J.; Layton, M.; et al. Botulinum toxin as a biological weapon: Medical and public health management. *JAMA* **2001**, *285*, 1059–1070. [CrossRef] [PubMed]
2. Dykstra, D.D.; Sidi, A.A.; Scott, A.B.; Pagel, J.M.; Goldish, G.D. Effects of botulinum A toxin on detrusor-sphincter dyssynergia in spinal cord injury patients. *J. Urol.* **1988**, *139*, 919–922. [CrossRef]
3. Giannantoni, A.; Bini, V.; Dmochowski, R.; Hanno, P.; Nickel, J.C.; Proietti, S.; Wyndaele, J.J. Contemporary management of the painful bladder: A systematic review. *Eur. Urol.* **2012**, *61*, 29–53. [CrossRef] [PubMed]
4. Pontari, M.A. Chronic prostatitis/chronic pelvic pain syndrome and interstitial cystitis: Are they related? *Curr. Urol. Rep.* **2006**, *7*, 329–334. [CrossRef] [PubMed]
5. Russell, A.; Kavia, R.; Dasgupta, P.; Sahai, A. The use of botulinum toxin for the treatment of urologic pain. *Curr. Opin. Urol.* **2013**, *23*, 570–578. [CrossRef] [PubMed]
6. Pirazzini, M.; Rossetto, O.; Eleopra, R.; Montecucco, C. Botulinum Neurotoxins: Biology, Pharmacology, and Toxicology. *Pharmacol. Rev.* **2017**, *69*, 200–235. [CrossRef]
7. Jiang, Y.H.; Liao, C.H.; Kuo, H.C. Current and potential urological applications of botulinum toxin A. *Nat. Rev. Urol.* **2015**, *12*, 519–533. [CrossRef]
8. Rummel, A. The long journey of botulinum neurotoxins into the synapse. *Toxicon* **2015**, *107*, 9–24. [CrossRef]
9. Chancellor, M.B.; Fowler, C.J.; Apostolidis, A.; de Groat, W.C.; Smith, C.P.; Somogyi, G.T.; Aoki, K.R. Drug Insight: Biological effects of botulinum toxin A in the lower urinary tract. *Nat. Clin. Pract. Urol.* **2008**, *5*, 319–328. [CrossRef]
10. Cruz, F.; Herschorn, S.; Aliotta, P.; Brin, M.; Thompson, C.; Lam, W.; Daniell, G.; Heesakkers, J.; Haag-Molkenteller, C. Efficacy and safety of onabotulinumtoxinA in patients with urinary incontinence due to neurogenic detrusor overactivity: A randomised, double-blind, placebo-controlled trial. *Eur. Urol.* **2011**, *60*, 742–750. [CrossRef]
11. Rovner, E.; Kennelly, M.; Schulte-Baukloh, H.; Zhou, J.; Haag-Molkenteller, C.; Dasgupta, P. Urodynamic results and clinical outcomes with intradetrusor injections of onabotulinumtoxinA in a randomized, placebo-controlled dose-finding study in idiopathic overactive bladder. *Neurourol. Urodyn.* **2011**, *30*, 556–562. [CrossRef]
12. Mangera, A.; Andersson, K.E.; Apostolidis, A.; Chapple, C.; Dasgupta, P.; Giannantoni, A.; Gravas, S.; Madersbacher, S. Contemporary management of lower urinary tract disease with botulinum toxin A: A systematic review of botox (onabotulinumtoxinA) and dysport (abobotulinumtoxinA). *Eur. Urol.* **2011**, *60*, 784–795. [CrossRef] [PubMed]
13. Fonfria, E.; Maignel, J.; Lezmi, S.; Martin, V.; Splevins, A.; Shubber, S.; Kalinichev, M.; Foster, K.; Picaut, P.; Krupp, J. The Expanding Therapeutic Utility of Botulinum Neurotoxins. *Toxins (Basel)* **2018**, *10*, 208. [CrossRef] [PubMed]
14. Jankovic, J.; Schwartz, K.; Donovan, D.T. Botulinum toxin treatment of cranial-cervical dystonia, spasmodic dysphonia, other focal dystonias and hemifacial spasm. *J. Neurol. Neurosurg. Psychiatry* **1990**, *53*, 633–639. [CrossRef] [PubMed]
15. Sengupta, J.N. Visceral pain: The neurophysiological mechanism. *Handb. Exp. Pharmacol.* **2009**. [CrossRef]
16. Jhang, J.F. Using Botulinum Toxin A for Treatment of Interstitial Cystitis/Bladder Pain Syndrome-Possible Pathomechanisms and Practical Issues. *Toxins (Basel)* **2019**, *11*, 641. [CrossRef]

17. Schurch, B.; Stohrer, M.; Kramer, G.; Schmid, D.M.; Gaul, G.; Hauri, D. Botulinum-A toxin for treating detrusor hyperreflexia in spinal cord injured patients: A new alternative to anticholinergic drugs? Preliminary results. *J. Urol.* **2000**, *164*, 692–697. [CrossRef]
18. Avelino, A.; Charrua, A.; Frias, B.; Cruz, C.; Boudes, M.; de Ridder, D.; Cruz, F. Transient receptor potential channels in bladder function. *Acta Physiol. (Oxf)* **2013**, *207*, 110–122. [CrossRef]
19. Andrade, E.L.; Ferreira, J.; Andre, E.; Calixto, J.B. Contractile mechanisms coupled to TRPA1 receptor activation in rat urinary bladder. *Biochem. Pharmacol.* **2006**, *72*, 104–114. [CrossRef]
20. Gevaert, T.; Vandepitte, J.; Hutchings, G.; Vriens, J.; Nilius, B.; De Ridder, D. TRPV1 is involved in stretch-evoked contractile changes in the rat autonomous bladder model: A study with piperine, a new TRPV1 agonist. *Neurourol. Urodyn.* **2007**, *26*, 440–450; discussion 451–453. [CrossRef]
21. Chuang, Y.C.; Yoshimura, N.; Huang, C.C.; Chiang, P.H.; Chancellor, M.B. Intravesical botulinum toxin a administration produces analgesia against acetic acid induced bladder pain responses in rats. *J. Urol.* **2004**, *172*, 1529–1532. [CrossRef] [PubMed]
22. Rong, W.; Spyer, K.M.; Burnstock, G. Activation and sensitisation of low and high threshold afferent fibres mediated by P2X receptors in the mouse urinary bladder. *J. Physiol.* **2002**, *541*, 591–600. [CrossRef] [PubMed]
23. Sun, Y.; Chai, T.C. Up-regulation of P2X3 receptor during stretch of bladder urothelial cells from patients with interstitial cystitis. *J. Urol.* **2004**, *171*, 448–452. [CrossRef] [PubMed]
24. Hanna-Mitchell, A.T.; Wolf-Johnston, A.S.; Barrick, S.R.; Kanai, A.J.; Chancellor, M.B.; de Groat, W.C.; Birder, L.A. Effect of botulinum toxin A on urothelial-release of ATP and expression of SNARE targets within the urothelium. *Neurourol. Urodyn.* **2015**, *34*, 79–84. [CrossRef]
25. Collins, V.M.; Daly, D.M.; Liaskos, M.; McKay, N.G.; Sellers, D.; Chapple, C.; Grundy, D. OnabotulinumtoxinA significantly attenuates bladder afferent nerve firing and inhibits ATP release from the urothelium. *BJU Int.* **2013**, *112*, 1018–1026. [CrossRef]
26. Giannantoni, A.; Gubbiotti, M.; Bini, V. Botulinum Neurotoxin A Intravesical Injections in Interstitial Cystitis/Bladder Painful Syndrome: A Systematic Review with Meta-Analysis. *Toxins (Basel)* **2019**, *11*, 510. [CrossRef]
27. Wheeler, A.; Smith, H.S. Botulinum toxins: Mechanisms of action, antinociception and clinical applications. *Toxicology* **2013**, *306*, 124–146. [CrossRef]
28. Takeda, M.; Mochizuki, T.; Yoshiyama, M.; Nakagomi, H.; Kobayashi, H.; Sawada, N.; Zakohji, H.; Du, S.; Araki, I. Sensor Mechanism and Afferent Signal Transduction of the Urinary Bladder: Special Focus on transient receptor potential Ion Channels. *Low Urin. Tract. Symptoms* **2010**, *2*, 51–60. [CrossRef]
29. Fowler, C.J.; Griffiths, D.; de Groat, W.C. The neural control of micturition. *Nat. Rev. Neurosci.* **2008**, *9*, 453–466. [CrossRef]
30. Vizzard, M.A. Changes in urinary bladder neurotrophic factor mRNA and NGF protein following urinary bladder dysfunction. *Exp. Neurol.* **2000**, *161*, 273–284. [CrossRef]
31. Seki, S.; Sasaki, K.; Fraser, M.O.; Igawa, Y.; Nishizawa, O.; Chancellor, M.B.; de Groat, W.C.; Yoshimura, N. Immunoneutralization of nerve growth factor in lumbosacral spinal cord reduces bladder hyperreflexia in spinal cord injured rats. *J. Urol.* **2002**, *168*, 2269–2274. [CrossRef]
32. Yoshimura, N.; Bennett, N.E.; Hayashi, Y.; Ogawa, T.; Nishizawa, O.; Chancellor, M.B.; de Groat, W.C.; Seki, S. Bladder overactivity and hyperexcitability of bladder afferent neurons after intrathecal delivery of nerve growth factor in rats. *J. Neurosci.* **2006**, *26*, 10847–10855. [CrossRef]
33. Liu, H.T.; Kuo, H.C. Intravesical botulinum toxin A injections plus hydrodistension can reduce nerve growth factor production and control bladder pain in interstitial cystitis. *Urology* **2007**, *70*, 463–468. [CrossRef]
34. Yu, S.J.; Xia, C.M.; Kay, J.C.; Qiao, L.Y. Activation of extracellular signal-regulated protein kinase 5 is essential for cystitis- and nerve growth factor-induced calcitonin gene-related peptide expression in sensory neurons. *Mol. Pain* **2012**, *8*, 48. [CrossRef] [PubMed]
35. Freund, B.; Schwartz, M. Temporal relationship of muscle weakness and pain reduction in subjects treated with botulinum toxin A. *J. Pain* **2003**, *4*, 159–165. [CrossRef]
36. Durham, P.L.; Cady, R.; Cady, R. Regulation of calcitonin gene-related peptide secretion from trigeminal nerve cells by botulinum toxin type A: Implications for migraine therapy. *Headache* **2004**, *44*, 35–42; discussion 42–43. [CrossRef]
37. Welch, M.J.; Purkiss, J.R.; Foster, K.A. Sensitivity of embryonic rat dorsal root ganglia neurons to Clostridium botulinum neurotoxins. *Toxicon* **2000**, *38*, 245–258. [CrossRef]

38. Lucioni, A.; Bales, G.T.; Lotan, T.L.; McGehee, D.S.; Cook, S.P.; Rapp, D.E. Botulinum toxin type A inhibits sensory neuropeptide release in rat bladder models of acute injury and chronic inflammation. *BJU Int.* **2008**, *101*, 366–370. [CrossRef]
39. Rapp, D.E.; Turk, K.W.; Bales, G.T.; Cook, S.P. Botulinum toxin type a inhibits calcitonin gene-related peptide release from isolated rat bladder. *J. Urol.* **2006**, *175*, 1138–1142. [CrossRef]
40. Andersson, K.E. TRP Channels as Lower Urinary Tract Sensory Targets. *Med. Sci. (Basel)* **2019**, *7*, 67. [CrossRef]
41. Liu, B.L.; Yang, F.; Zhan, H.L.; Feng, Z.Y.; Zhang, Z.G.; Li, W.B.; Zhou, X.F. Increased severity of inflammation correlates with elevated expression of TRPV1 nerve fibers and nerve growth factor on interstitial cystitis/bladder pain syndrome. *Urol. Int.* **2014**, *92*, 202–208. [CrossRef] [PubMed]
42. Smet, P.J.; Jonavicius, J.; Marshall, V.R.; de Vente, J. Distribution of nitric oxide synthase-immunoreactive nerves and identification of the cellular targets of nitric oxide in guinea-pig and human urinary bladder by cGMP immunohistochemistry. *Neuroscience* **1996**, *71*, 337–348. [CrossRef]
43. Smith, C.P.; Gangitano, D.A.; Munoz, A.; Salas, N.A.; Boone, T.B.; Aoki, K.R.; Francis, J.; Somogyi, G.T. Botulinum toxin type A normalizes alterations in urothelial ATP and NO release induced by chronic spinal cord injury. *Neurochem Int* **2008**, *52*, 1068–1075. [CrossRef] [PubMed]
44. Abraham, S.N.; Miao, Y. The nature of immune responses to urinary tract infections. *Nat. Rev. Immunol.* **2015**, *15*, 655–663. [CrossRef] [PubMed]
45. Grundy, L.; Caldwell, A.; Brierley, S.M. Mechanisms Underlying Overactive Bladder and Interstitial Cystitis/Painful Bladder Syndrome. *Front. Neurosci.* **2018**, *12*, 931. [CrossRef] [PubMed]
46. Jacobs, B.L.; Smaldone, M.C.; Tyagi, V.; Philips, B.J.; Jackman, S.V.; Leng, W.W.; Tyagi, P. Increased nerve growth factor in neurogenic overactive bladder and interstitial cystitis patients. *Can. J. Urol.* **2010**, *17*, 4989–4994. [PubMed]
47. Jhang, J.F.; Kuo, H.C. Pathomechanism of Interstitial Cystitis/Bladder Pain Syndrome and Mapping the Heterogeneity of Disease. *Int. Neurourol. J.* **2016**, *20*, S95-104. [CrossRef]
48. Kastrup, J.; Hald, T.; Larsen, S.; Nielsen, V.G. Histamine content and mast cell count of detrusor muscle in patients with interstitial cystitis and other types of chronic cystitis. *Br. J. Urol.* **1983**, *55*, 495–500. [CrossRef]
49. Cui, M.; Khanijou, S.; Rubino, J.; Aoki, K.R. Subcutaneous administration of botulinum toxin A reduces formalin-induced pain. *Pain* **2004**, *107*, 125–133. [CrossRef]
50. Fry, C.H.; Daneshgari, F.; Thor, K.; Drake, M.; Eccles, R.; Kanai, A.J.; Birder, L.A. Animal models and their use in understanding lower urinary tract dysfunction. *Neurourol. Urodyn.* **2010**, *29*, 603–608. [CrossRef]
51. DeBerry, J.J.; Schwartz, E.S.; Davis, B.M. TRPA1 mediates bladder hyperalgesia in a mouse model of cystitis. *Pain* **2014**, *155*, 1280–1287. [CrossRef] [PubMed]
52. Chuang, Y.C.; Yoshimura, N.; Huang, C.C.; Wu, M.; Chiang, P.H.; Chancellor, M.B. Intravesical botulinum toxin A administration inhibits COX-2 and EP4 expression and suppresses bladder hyperactivity in cyclophosphamide-induced cystitis in rats. *Eur. Urol.* **2009**, *56*, 159–166. [CrossRef] [PubMed]
53. Shie, J.H.; Liu, H.T.; Wang, Y.S.; Kuo, H.C. Immunohistochemical evidence suggests repeated intravesical application of botulinum toxin A injections may improve treatment efficacy of interstitial cystitis/bladder pain syndrome. *BJU Int.* **2013**, *111*, 638–646. [CrossRef] [PubMed]
54. Peng, C.H.; Jhang, J.F.; Shie, J.H.; Kuo, H.C. Down regulation of vascular endothelial growth factor is associated with decreased inflammation after intravesical OnabotulinumtoxinA injections combined with hydrodistention for patients with interstitial cystitis–clinical results and immunohistochemistry analysis. *Urology* **2013**, *82*, 1452.e1451-1456. [CrossRef]
55. Hurst, R.E.; Greenwood-Van Meerveld, B.; Wisniewski, A.B.; VanGordon, S.; Lin, H.; Kropp, B.P.; Towner, R.A. Increased bladder permeability in interstitial cystitis/painful bladder syndrome. *Transl. Androl. Urol.* **2015**, *4*, 563–571. [CrossRef]
56. Liu, H.T.; Shie, J.H.; Chen, S.H.; Wang, Y.S.; Kuo, H.C. Differences in mast cell infiltration, E-cadherin, and zonula occludens-1 expression between patients with overactive bladder and interstitial cystitis/bladder pain syndrome. *Urology* **2012**, *80*, 225.e213-228. [CrossRef]
57. Wyndaele, J.J.J.; Riedl, C.; Taneja, R.; Lovasz, S.; Ueda, T.; Cervigni, M. GAG replenishment therapy for bladder pain syndrome/interstitial cystitis. *Neurourol. Urodyn.* **2019**, *38*, 535–544. [CrossRef]

58. Chiang, G.; Patra, P.; Letourneau, R.; Jeudy, S.; Boucher, W.; Green, M.; Sant, G.R.; Theoharides, T.C. Pentosanpolysulfate inhibits mast cell histamine secretion and intracellular calcium ion levels: An alternative explanation of its beneficial effect in interstitial cystitis. *J. Urol.* **2000**, *164*, 2119–2125. [CrossRef]
59. Grundy, L.; Erickson, A.; Brierley, S.M. Visceral Pain. *Annu. Rev. Physiol.* **2019**, *81*, 261–284. [CrossRef]
60. Peters, K.M.; Killinger, K.A.; Ibrahim, I.A. Childhood symptoms and events in women with interstitial cystitis/painful bladder syndrome. *Urology* **2009**, *73*, 258–262. [CrossRef]
61. Randich, A.; Uzzell, T.; DeBerry, J.J.; Ness, T.J. Neonatal urinary bladder inflammation produces adult bladder hypersensitivity. *J. Pain* **2006**, *7*, 469–479. [CrossRef] [PubMed]
62. Ness, T.J.; Randich, A. Neonatal bladder inflammation alters activity of adult rat spinal visceral nociceptive neurons. *Neurosci. Lett.* **2010**, *472*, 210–214. [CrossRef] [PubMed]
63. Shaffer, A.D.; Ness, T.J.; Robbins, M.T.; Randich, A. Early in life bladder inflammation alters opioid peptide content in the spinal cord and bladder of adult female rats. *J. Urol.* **2013**, *189*, 352–358. [CrossRef] [PubMed]
64. Sengupta, J.N.; Pochiraju, S.; Kannampalli, P.; Bruckert, M.; Addya, S.; Yadav, P.; Miranda, A.; Shaker, R.; Banerjee, B. MicroRNA-mediated GABA Aalpha-1 receptor subunit down-regulation in adult spinal cord following neonatal cystitis-induced chronic visceral pain in rats. *Pain* **2013**, *154*, 59–70. [CrossRef]
65. Daly, D.M.; Collins, V.M.; Chapple, C.R.; Grundy, D. The afferent system and its role in lower urinary tract dysfunction. *Curr. Opin. Urol.* **2011**, *21*, 268–274. [CrossRef]
66. Kanai, A.; Fry, C.; Ikeda, Y.; Kullmann, F.A.; Parsons, B.; Birder, L. Implications for bidirectional signaling between afferent nerves and urothelial cells-ICI-RS 2014. *Neurourol. Urodyn.* **2016**, *35*, 273–277. [CrossRef]
67. Andersson, K.E.; McCloskey, K.D. Lamina propria: The functional center of the bladder? *Neurourol. Urodyn.* **2014**, *33*, 9–16. [CrossRef]
68. Traini, C.; Vannucchi, M.G. The Botulinum Treatment of Neurogenic Detrusor Overactivity: The Double-Face of the Neurotoxin. *Toxins (Basel)* **2019**, *11*, 614. [CrossRef]
69. Fry, C.H.; Vahabi, B. The Role of the Mucosa in Normal and Abnormal Bladder Function. *Basic Clin. Pharmacol. Toxicol.* **2016**, *119* (Suppl. 3), 57–62. [CrossRef]
70. Apostolidis, A.; Dasgupta, P.; Fowler, C.J. Proposed mechanism for the efficacy of injected botulinum toxin in the treatment of human detrusor overactivity. *Eur. Urol.* **2006**, *49*, 644–650. [CrossRef]
71. Dressler, D.; Adib Saberi, F. Botulinum Toxin: Mechanisms of Action. *Eur. Neurol.* **2005**, *53*, 3–9. [CrossRef] [PubMed]
72. Haferkamp, A.; Schurch, B.; Reitz, A.; Krengel, U.; Grosse, J.; Kramer, G.; Schumacher, S.; Bastian, P.J.; Buttner, R.; Muller, S.C.; et al. Lack of ultrastructural detrusor changes following endoscopic injection of botulinum toxin type a in overactive neurogenic bladder. *Eur. Urol.* **2004**, *46*, 784–791. [CrossRef] [PubMed]
73. Gouin, O.; Lebonvallet, N.; L'Herondelle, K.; Le Gall-Ianotto, C.; Buhe, V.; Plee-Gautier, E.; Carre, J.L.; Lefeuvre, L.; Misery, L. Self-maintenance of neurogenic inflammation contributes to a vicious cycle in skin. *Exp. Dermatol.* **2015**, *24*, 723–726. [CrossRef]
74. Pavone, F.; Luvisetto, S. Botulinum neurotoxin for pain management: Insights from animal models. *Toxins (Basel)* **2010**, *2*, 2890–2913. [CrossRef] [PubMed]
75. Wiegand, H.; Erdmann, G.; Wellhoner, H.H. 125I-labelled botulinum A neurotoxin: Pharmacokinetics in cats after intramuscular injection. *Naunyn Schmiedebergs Arch Pharmacol.* **1976**, *292*, 161–165. [CrossRef] [PubMed]
76. Black, J.D.; Dolly, J.O. Interaction of 125I-labeled botulinum neurotoxins with nerve terminals. I. Ultrastructural autoradiographic localization and quantitation of distinct membrane acceptors for types A and B on motor nerves. *J. Cell Biol.* **1986**, *103*, 521–534. [CrossRef]
77. Restani, L.; Giribaldi, F.; Manich, M.; Bercsenyi, K.; Menendez, G.; Rossetto, O.; Caleo, M.; Schiavo, G. Botulinum neurotoxins A and E undergo retrograde axonal transport in primary motor neurons. *PLoS Pathog.* **2012**, *8*, e1003087. [CrossRef]
78. Antonucci, F.; Rossi, C.; Gianfranceschi, L.; Rossetto, O.; Caleo, M. Long-distance retrograde effects of botulinum neurotoxin A. *J. Neurosci.* **2008**, *28*, 3689–3696. [CrossRef]
79. Papagiannopoulou, D.; Vardouli, L.; Dimitriadis, F.; Apostolidis, A. Retrograde transport of radiolabelled botulinum neurotoxin type A to the CNS after intradetrusor injection in rats. *BJU Int.* **2016**, *117*, 697–704. [CrossRef]
80. Bach-Rojecky, L.; Lackovic, Z. Central origin of the antinociceptive action of botulinum toxin type A. *Pharmacol. Biochem. Behav.* **2009**, *94*, 234–238. [CrossRef]

81. Bach-Rojecky, L.; Salkovic-Petrisic, M.; Lackovic, Z. Botulinum toxin type A reduces pain supersensitivity in experimental diabetic neuropathy: Bilateral effect after unilateral injection. *Eur. J. Pharmacol.* **2010**, *633*, 10–14. [CrossRef]
82. Favre-Guilmard, C.; Auguet, M.; Chabrier, P.E. Different antinociceptive effects of botulinum toxin type A in inflammatory and peripheral polyneuropathic rat models. *Eur. J. Pharmacol.* **2009**, *617*, 48–53. [CrossRef] [PubMed]
83. Park, J.; Chung, M.E. Botulinum Toxin for Central Neuropathic Pain. *Toxins (Basel)* **2018**, *10*, 224. [CrossRef] [PubMed]
84. Coelho, A.; Oliveira, R.; Rossetto, O.; Cruz, C.D.; Cruz, F.; Avelino, A. Intrathecal administration of botulinum toxin type A improves urinary bladder function and reduces pain in rats with cystitis. *Eur. J. Pain* **2014**, *18*, 1480–1489. [CrossRef] [PubMed]
85. Apostolidis, A. Words of wisdom. Re: Intrathecal administration of botulinum toxin type a improves urinary bladder function and reduces pain in rats with cystitis. *Eur. Urol.* **2015**, *67*, 816. [CrossRef]
86. Khavari, R.; Elias, S.N.; Pande, R.; Wu, K.M.; Boone, T.B.; Karmonik, C. Higher Neural Correlates in Patients with Multiple Sclerosis and Neurogenic Overactive Bladder Following Treatment with Intradetrusor Injection of OnabotulinumtoxinA. *J. Urol.* **2019**, *201*, 135–140. [CrossRef]
87. Kim, D.W.; Lee, S.K.; Ahnn, J. Botulinum Toxin as a Pain Killer: Players and Actions in Antinociception. *Toxins (Basel)* **2015**, *7*, 2435–2453. [CrossRef]

Permissions

All chapters in this book were first published by MDPI; hereby published with permission under the Creative Commons Attribution License or equivalent. Every chapter published in this book has been scrutinized by our experts. Their significance has been extensively debated. The topics covered herein carry significant findings which will fuel the growth of the discipline. They may even be implemented as practical applications or may be referred to as a beginning point for another development.

The contributors of this book come from diverse backgrounds, making this book a truly international effort. This book will bring forth new frontiers with its revolutionizing research information and detailed analysis of the nascent developments around the world.

We would like to thank all the contributing authors for lending their expertise to make the book truly unique. They have played a crucial role in the development of this book. Without their invaluable contributions this book wouldn't have been possible. They have made vital efforts to compile up to date information on the varied aspects of this subject to make this book a valuable addition to the collection of many professionals and students.

This book was conceptualized with the vision of imparting up-to-date information and advanced data in this field. To ensure the same, a matchless editorial board was set up. Every individual on the board went through rigorous rounds of assessment to prove their worth. After which they invested a large part of their time researching and compiling the most relevant data for our readers.

The editorial board has been involved in producing this book since its inception. They have spent rigorous hours researching and exploring the diverse topics which have resulted in the successful publishing of this book. They have passed on their knowledge of decades through this book. To expedite this challenging task, the publisher supported the team at every step. A small team of assistant editors was also appointed to further simplify the editing procedure and attain best results for the readers.

Apart from the editorial board, the designing team has also invested a significant amount of their time in understanding the subject and creating the most relevant covers. They scrutinized every image to scout for the most suitable representation of the subject and create an appropriate cover for the book.

The publishing team has been an ardent support to the editorial, designing and production team. Their endless efforts to recruit the best for this project, has resulted in the accomplishment of this book. They are a veteran in the field of academics and their pool of knowledge is as vast as their experience in printing. Their expertise and guidance has proved useful at every step. Their uncompromising quality standards have made this book an exceptional effort. Their encouragement from time to time has been an inspiration for everyone.

The publisher and the editorial board hope that this book will prove to be a valuable piece of knowledge for researchers, students, practitioners and scholars across the globe.

List of Contributors

Hung-Chieh Chiu
Department of Urology, China Medical University Hospital, Taichung 40447, Taiwan

Kuan-Chieh Chen
Department of Surgery, China Medical University Hospital, Taichung 40447, Taiwan

Chao-Hsiang Chang
Department of Urology, China Medical University Hospital, Taichung 40447, Taiwan
School of Medicine, China Medical University, Taichung 40402, Taiwan

Chung-Cheng Wang
Department of Urology, En Chu Kong Hospital, College of Medicine, National Taiwan University, Taipei 23702, Taiwan
Department of Biomedical Engineering, Chung Yuan Christian University, Chung-Li 32023, Taiwan

Cheng-Ling Lee
Department of Urology, Buddhist Tzu Chi General Hospital, and Tzu Chi University, Hualien 97002, Taiwan

David C. Moore, Joshua A. Cohn and Roger R. Dmochowski
Department of Urologic Surgery, Vanderbilt University Medical Center, Nashville, TN 37232-2765, USA

Jia-Fong Jhang
Department of Urology, Buddhist Tzu Chi General Hospital, Tzu Chi University, 707 Chung-Yang Road, Section 3, Hualien 970, Taiwan

Sheng-Fu Chen and Chia-Hwei Chang
Department of Urology, Buddhist Tzu Chi General Hospital and Tzu Chi University, 707, Section 3, Chung Yang Road, Hualian 970, Taiwan

Bin Chiu
Division of Urology, Department of Surgery, Far Eastern Memorial Hospital, Ban Ciao, New Taipei City 220, Taiwan

Shiu-Dong Chung
Division of Urology, Department of Surgery, Far Eastern Memorial Hospital, Ban Ciao, New Taipei City 220, Taiwan
Department of Urology, National Taiwan University Hospital, Taipei 100, Taiwan

Huai-Ching Tai
Department of Urology, National Taiwan University Hospital, Taipei 100, Taiwan

Lori A. Birder
Department of Medicine-Renal Electrolyte Division, University of Pittsburgh School of Medicine, Pittsburgh, PA 15261, USA
Pharmacology & Chemical Biology, University of Pittsburgh School of Medicine, Pittsburgh, PA 15261, USA

Fu-Shan Jaw
Institute of Biomedical Engineering, National Taiwan University, Taipei 10617, Taiwan

Stephen Shei-Dei Yang and Shang-Jen Chang
Division of Urology, Department of Surgery, Taipei Tzu Chi Hospital, The Buddhist Tzu Chi Medical Foundation, New Taipei 23142, Taiwan
School of Medicine, Buddhist Tzu Chi University, Hualien 97071, Taiwan

Chi-Wen Lo
Institute of Biomedical Engineering, National Taiwan University, Taipei 10617, Taiwan
Division of Urology, Department of Surgery, Taipei Tzu Chi Hospital, The Buddhist Tzu Chi Medical Foundation, New Taipei 23142, Taiwan
School of Medicine, Buddhist Tzu Chi University, Hualien 97071, Taiwan

Mei-Yi Wu
Department of Nephrology, Taipei Medical University-Shuang Ho Hospital, Taipei 23561, Taiwan

Chun-Hou Liao
College of Medicine, Fu-Jen Catholic University, New Taipei City 24205, Taiwan
Department of Urology, Cardinal Tien Hospital, New Taipei City 23148, Taiwan

Bing-Juin Chiang
College of Medicine, Fu-Jen Catholic University, New Taipei City 24205, Taiwan
Department of Urology, Cardinal Tien Hospital, New Taipei City 23148, Taiwan
Department of Life Science, College of Science, National Taiwan Normal University, Taipei 11677, Taiwan

Hann-Chorng Kuo
Department of Urology, Buddhist Tzu Chi General Hospital, and Tzu Chi University, Hualien 97002, Taiwan
School of Medicine, Tzu Chi University, Hualien 97004, Taiwan

Yu-Khun Lee
Department of Urology, Hualien Tzu Chi Hospital, Buddhist Tzu Chi Medical Foundation and Tzu Chi University, Hualien 970, Taiwan

Yao-Lin Kao
Department of Urology, National Cheng Kung University Hospital, College of Medicine, National Cheng Kung University, Tainan 704, Taiwan

Kuan-Hsun Huang
Department of Urology, Dalin Tzu Chi Hospital, Buddhist Tzu Chi Medical Foundation, Chiayi County 622, Taiwan

Yin-Chien Ou
Department of Urology, National Cheng Kung University Hospital, College of Medicine, National Cheng Kung University, Tainan 704, Taiwan
College of Medicine, Institute of Clinical Medicine, National Cheng Kung University, Tainan 704, Taiwan

Chien-Hsu Chen
Department of Urology 1, Kaohsiung Chang Gung Memorial Hospital, Chang Gung University College of Medicine, Kaohsiung 83301, Taiwan

Pradeep Tyagi
Department of Urology, University of Pittsburgh School of Medicine2, Pittsburgh, PA 15213, USA

Chin-Li Chen and En Meng
Division of Urology, Department of Surgery, Tri-Service General Hospital, National Defense Medical Center, 325, Section 2, Cheng-Gung Road, Taipei 114, Taiwan

Hsiu-Jen Wang
Department of Urology, Hualien Tzu Chi Hospital, Buddhist Tzu Chi Medical Foundation and Tzu Chi University, Hualien 970, Taiwan

Wan-Ru Yu
Department of Nursing, Hualien Tzu Chi Hospital, Buddhist Tzu Chi Medical Foundation and Tzu Chi University, Hualien 970, Taiwan

Hueih-Ling Ong
Department of Urology, Dalin Tzu Chi Hospital, Buddhist Tzu Chi Medical Foundation, Chiayi 622, Taiwan

Yi-Huei Chang and Huang Chi-Ping
Department of Urology, China Medical University Hospital, Taichung 40447, Taiwan
School of Medicine, China Medical University, Taichung 40402, Taiwan

Po-Jen Hsiao
Department of Urology, China Medical University Hospital, Taichung 40447, Taiwan
School of Medicine, China Medical University, Taichung 40402, Taiwan
Department of Urology, China Medical University Hsinchu Hospital, Hsinchu 302056, Taiwan

Hsi-Chin Wu and Eric Chieh-Lung Chou
Department of Urology, China Medical University Hospital, Taichung 40447, Taiwan
School of Medicine, China Medical University, Taichung 40402, Taiwan
Department of Urology, China Medical University Beigang Hospital, Beigang, Yunlin 651012, Taiwan

Po-Fan Hsieh
Department of Urology, China Medical University Hospital, Taichung 40447, Taiwan
School of Medicine, China Medical University, Taichung 40402, Taiwan
Graduate Institute of Biomedical Sciences, School of Medicine, China Medical University, Taichung 40402, Taiwan

Yuan-Hong Jiang
Department of Urology, Hualien Tzu Chi Hospital, Buddhist Tzu Chi Medical Foundation, Hualien 970, Taiwan
Department of Urology, Buddhist Tzu Chi University, Hualien 970, Taiwan

Yu-Hua Lin
Divisions of Urology, Department of Surgery, Cardinal Tien Hospital, New Taipei City 23148, Taiwan
Department of Chemistry, Fu Jen Catholic University, New Taipei City 24205, Taiwan
Graduate Institute of Biochemical and Pharmaceutical Science, Fu Jen Catholic University, New Taipei City 24205, Taiwan

Ting-Chun Yeh
Division of Urology, Department of Surgery, Taiwan Adventist Hospital, Taipei City 105, Taiwan

Po-Cheng Chen
Department of Urology, En Chu Kong Hospital, New Taipei City 237, Taiwan

Yann-Rong Su
Department of Urology, National Taiwan University Hospital Hsin-Chu Branch, Hsinchu City 300, Taiwan

Index

www.ingramcontent.com/pod-product-compliance
Lightning Source LLC
LaVergne TN
LVHW081032210926
848485LV00004B/1005
* 9 7 8 1 6 3 9 2 7 8 4 8 0 *